THE WHOLE HEALTH CATALOGUE

Shirley Linde

THE WHOLE HEALTH CATALOGUE

HOW TO STAY
WELL — CHEAPER

Rawson Associates Publishers, Inc.

NEW YORK

Library of Congress Cataloging in Publication Data
Linde, Shirley Motter.
  The whole health catalogue.
   1. Health. 2. Medicine, Popular. 3. Medical
care. I. Title. [DNLM: 1. Medicine—Popular works.
WB120 L743w]
RA776.L737 1977   613   77-77890
ISBN 0-89256-012-6
ISBN 0-89256-035-5 pbk.

Published simultaneously in Canada by
McClelland and Stewart, Ltd.
Manufactured in the United States of America
by Fairfield Graphics, Fairfield, Pennsylvania
Designed by Helen Barrow
Third Printing October 1978

CONTENTS

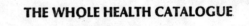

THE WHOLE HEALTH CATALOGUE

CHAPTER 1

Patient Power: How to Take Charge of Your Health

It is time for the patient to take the primary responsibility for his own health.

It is time for the patient to stop feeling ignorant of his body and of his health; to stop blindly accepting whatever he is told.

It is time for him to ask questions, to read, to understand. It is time for him to learn to recognize symptoms in his own body and to report them to his physician, and to give his ideas on what might be causing the problem. It is time for the patient to make the final decisions concerning his own body.

In essence, it is time for the patient to become an active part of the medical team in charge of his health . . . to stop being a Passive Patient, and to become an Active Patient.

There is a vast consumer movement underway in medicine in this country to do just this, to get patients more active in their own medical care. Perhaps we should call it Patient Power. We consider it a healthy part of the health care system because the more you can do for yourself, the better it is for you; and when you do need your doctor, the more you know about medicine, the better the two of you can work together to produce the best results.

None of this means ignoring your doctor. None of this means putting him down. He has vast skill and detailed knowledge vital to your health. You must work with him. But work with him as an Active Patient, knowledgeable in your own right. Your doctor is skilled, but he is also human so he makes mistakes; he is rushed; he is overworked; he is sometimes prejudiced for or against a particular medical approach.

And in the final analysis, to no one else is your body more important than to yourself. It is the most precious gift and vital possession you have.

Taking responsibility for your body is not simple. It means you have to assume the responsibility for taking the medicine your doctor prescribes, for dieting, taking vitamins, giving up cigarettes, whatever—and you can't blame someone else for any failures. But doing it will give you an exhilarating and satisfying sense of command and freedom of choice that you may never have had before.

The Whole Health Catalogue is designed for this in-command person who has decided to take charge of his own body and his own health. It's a maintenance manual for the Active Patient. It is to your health what a cookbook is to cooking, giving you facts on what to do before, during, and after you see your doctor. It may even give you an extra 20 years of life.

HOW TO SCORE A DOCTOR YOU ARE GOING TO

Ask yourself these questions about your doctor. Give him 4 points for every "Yes" answer.

SCORE

1. Did he do a complete medical history on your first visit, asking many specific questions about your past health and your family's? _____

2. Did he do a careful, complete physical examination at the first visit, and when he gives you a periodic physical exam now does he check all parts of your body including the inside of your mouth? _____

3. If you are a woman does he do a breast examination, pelvic examination, and a Pap smear? For men and women, a rectal examination? _____

4. Does he keep records and consult them at each visit? _____

5. Does he do routine laboratory exams of blood and urine at least once a year and report the findings to you? _____

6. Does he periodically take an electrocardiogram and measure your blood pressure and tell you what he finds? _____

7. Does he ask you about your eating habits and whether you exercise and whether you smoke or drink, and does he give you advice about these things when he should? _____

8. Does he refer you to other specialists or call in a consultant when advisable? _____

9. If he is a specialist, is he board certified? _____

10. Does he go to meetings, read journals, participate in continuing education programs? _____

11. Does he belong to several medical societies? _____

12. Does he do any patient education such as giving literature or recommending books? _____

13. Does he have someone to cover for him on days or evenings off and on vacations? _____

14. Is he willing to take phone call questions to save you making an office visit? _____

15. Does he make house calls if they are really necessary? (Most of them are *not* necessary.) _____

16. Does he spend enough time with you, giving you a chance to explain completely any problems that you might have? _____

17. Does he have a helpful attitude, so you feel you can discuss anything with him? _____

18. Does he treat you as a participant in your own health care rather than patronizingly putting you down for any opinions you might have? _____

19. Does he encourage you in things you want to try such as improving your diet, breast feeding, yoga, biofeedback? _____

20. Does he give you a complete diagnosis and explanation of any condition you might have so that you understand it? _____

21. If he wants you to have special tests or treatments, does he explain what they will be and why you need them and what any side effects might be that you should report to him? _____

22. Is he willing to label prescriptions as to contents if you ask him to? _____

23. Does he generally get good results with his treatments? (12 points) _____

If your doctor got 100, he could replace Marcus Welby. Anything over 80 is satisfactory. If you scored him less than that, look over the questions you answered "no" to; perhaps you can discuss them at your next visit. If he scored less than 70 and does not change on key areas you discuss with him and consider important, you may be happier with another doctor.

GETTING THE MOST FROM YOUR VISIT TO THE DOCTOR

Here's how to be an Active Patient and make your doctor-patient visits count.

When the nurse or doctor takes your medical history, answer all questions completely, including those about your family's medical background.

Tell your doctor everything, even if it is embarrassing or seems trivial. This is no time to give in to false modesty or pretend that you are a superman with no problems.

Don't make him play guessing games. Tell him as many details and clues as you can. If you have a hunch as to what it might be, or a fear about something, discuss it.

Make a list before you go of all symptoms and problems you want to mention and questions you want to ask, so you don't forget anything.

Write down the answers or instructions the doctor tells you, so you don't forget them.

At the end of his examination or when lab results are in, make sure your doctor tells you the diagnosis (or a discussion of several possible diagnoses if he hasn't yet zeroed in on one), that he explains his plan of treatment, and explains how effective you can expect that treatment to be.

And most important, when he gives you advice, follow it. If he gives you medicine, take it. It's absolutely astounding how many people pay money to a physician for advice and then ignore it.

If the treatment does not seem to be working or is causing a side effect, call him so that he can alter instructions. Do not stop taking medicines on your own.

Always call back or go back for a checkup when you are supposed to.

IF YOU WANT A WOMAN DOCTOR

Check your library for a nationwide *Directory of Women Physicians;* or you can buy one ($5) from the American Medical Women's Association, 1740 Broadway, New York, N.Y. 10019.

MAKING SHOTS HURT LESS

Three Australian researchers investigated and found punctures through dry skin hurt least; pain is substantially greater when the puncture is made through skin still damp with alcohol. So make sure the alcohol on your skin has dried before the nurse or doctor sticks the needle in. An intramuscular injection should be made in the arm or the outer surface of the thigh to be safer and less painful, *not* in the buttocks.

In Scotland blood for a blood count is taken from the back of the thumb instead of the fingertip. It hurts much less.

EMERGENCIES

Where is the nearest hospital to you that has an outpatient department or emergency ward? Determine this now. Then if you are faced with an emergency and cannot reach your doctor or have no regular doctor you can go to the emergency ward.

HOW TO FIND OUT WHAT YOUR DOCTOR REALLY MEANS

If you're like most people, listening to your doctor is like listening to a foreign language. You can't tell a coxalgia from a craniotomy.

But actually it's not as difficult as it sounds, no more difficult than CB jargon. Most medical words are based on Greek and Latin roots; learn the roots most usually used and you can figure out just about any words you hear or read.

The following list will give the basic parts of common medical words. By breaking it down to its component parts you can usually figure out the meaning of any medical word.

Meanwhile if he uses a bunch of big words and you don't know what he means, simply *tell* him you don't know what he means.

It is essential you know about your condition and understand exactly what to do.

WHEN YOUR DOCTOR SAYS:	THIS IS WHAT HE REALLY MEANS:
Arthro . . .	joint
. . . itis	inflammation
Arthritis	inflammation of a joint
Cardi . . .	heart
Carditis	inflammation of the heart
Colo . . .	colon
. . . ostomy	making an opening
Colostomy	making a new opening into the colon
Costa	rib
Intercostal	between the ribs
Coxa . . .	hip
. . . algia	pain
Coxalgia	pain in the hip
Cranio . . .	skull
. . . otomy	making an opening
Craniotomy	making a hole in the skull
Derma . . .	skin
. . . itis	inflammation
Dermatitis	inflammation of the skin
Encephal . . .	brain
Encephalitis	inflammation of the brain
Erythro . . .	red
. . . cyte	cell
Erythrocyte	red blood cell
Hepato . . .	liver
Hepatitis	inflammation of liver
Hyper . . .	much
Hyperthyroid	too much thyroid hormone
Hypo . . .	little
Hypothyroid	too little thyroid hormone
Hyster . . .	uterus
. . . ectomy	removal of
Hysterectomy	removal of the uterus
Leuko . . .	white
. . . cyte	cell
Leukocyte	white blood cell
Masto . . .	breast
Mastitis	inflammation of breast

WHEN YOUR DOCTOR SAYS:	THIS IS WHAT HE REALLY MEANS:	WHEN YOUR DOCTOR SAYS:	THIS IS WHAT HE REALLY MEANS:
Myo . . .	muscle	Phlebotomy	cutting into a vein
Myositis	inflammation of muscle	Pneumon . . .	lung
Orchi . . .	testicle	Pneumonitis	inflammation of lungs
. . . ectomy	removal of	Rhin . . .	nose
Orchidectomy	removal of the testicle	Rhinitis	inflammation of the nose
Phleb . . .	vein	Tracheo . . .	windpipe
. . . otomy	to cut into	Tracheotomy	cutting into windpipe

ABBREVIATIONS AND WHAT THEY MEAN

ACTH	adrenocorticotropic hormone	GI	gastrointestinal
BMR	basal metabolic rate	GP	general practitioner
BP	blood pressure	GU	genitourinary
C	centigrade	GYN	gynecology
Ca	calcium	Hb	hemoglobin
CA	carcinoma (cancer)	IM	intramuscular
CNS	central nervous system	IV	intravenous
DDS	doctor of dental surgery, dentist	mm	millimeter
D & C	dilatation and curettage (of uterus)	NYD	not yet diagnosed
doa	dead on arrival	OB	obstetrics
EEG	electroencephalogram	r	roentgen (measure of radiation)
EENT	eye, ear, nose, and throat	RBC	red blood count
EKG	electrocardiogram	TLC	tender loving care
F	Fahrenheit	WBC	white blood count

HOW TO READ THE PRESCRIPTION YOUR DOCTOR GIVES YOU

Rx	prescription
Sig	label
ac	before meals
ad lib	whenever you want
b i d	twice a day
cc	cubic centimeter
dr	dram
extr	extract
gm	gram
gr	grains
gt	drop
mg	milligrams
min	minim, a drop
od	right eye
os	left eye
pc	after meals
gd	every day
gh	every hour
q i d	four times a day
q s	as much as is sufficient
t i d	three times a day

WHAT YOUR LAB REPORT REALLY MEANS

The laboratory values shown at top of page 7 are considered normal or average. If your test results are higher or lower it doesn't necessarily mean you have a certain disease, but it does mean it is something to be checked into.

HOW TO REDUCE YOUR DOCTOR BILLS

Have a family physician. He can answer questions by phone; he knows what works best for you without experimenting. His office charges are almost always cheaper than going to a hospital emergency room.

Talk with your doctor about the cost of medical care. If your ability to pay is limited, be frank. Your doctor may refer you to free services or lower his fee.

Learn to tell your problems directly and completely. Your bill is often in direct proportion to how much time you spend with your doctor. Keep time short by being direct, brief, but give all details of your problem. Write symptoms down ahead of

LABORATORY VALUES

TEST:	NORMAL RANGE:	AN ABNORMAL VALUE COULD MEAN:
Albumin	3.7–5.5	Liver disease or poor nutrition.
Bilirubin	0.1–1.2	Liver disease or breakdown of the red blood cells.
Calcium	8.5–11.0	High value could mean loss of bone tissue. Low value could be caused by deficient diet, kidney disease, or vitamin D deficiency.
Cholesterol	125–235	High value could mean increased risk of heart attack, and hardening of the arteries.
Glucose	60–110	High values seen in diabetes; may be altered by other hormone upsets, diet, some medicines.
Hematocrit	40–52	Low value could mean anemia.
Hemoglobin	13–18	Low value could mean anemia. High values may mean chronic disease of the lung.
Phosphatase	2–4	Bone disease; obstruction of the bile duct.
Potassium	3.5–5	High value can mean breakdown of blood cells or kidney damage. Diuretics frequently lower the value.
Red blood cells	4.2–6 million	Low value could mean anemia from blood loss, poor blood formation, or blood cell destruction.
Sedimentation rate	0–10	High value can mean infection or other disease.
Sodium	136–145	Kidney disease; diseases of the adrenal gland; dehydration.
Transaminase	5–40	Liver disease; heart attack; cell injury.
Triglycerides	15–175	High levels could mean hardening of the arteries; alcoholism; increased risk of heart attack.
Urea nitrogen	6–26	Liver disease; kidney disease.
Uric acid	2–6	Gout; kidney disease; danger of kidney stones; leukemia; certain types of heart disease.
White blood cells	5,000–10,000	Low values could mean defective blood cell formation, certain forms of anemia, malaria, tuberculosis. High values could mean infections, leukemia, certain anemias, burns.

time so you do not forget anything. Never keep a secret, no matter how trivial or how embarrassing. Always tell your doctor the truth about everything, including a drinking problem, drugs, sexual problems. The quicker you get better the more money saved.

Be a detective. Play Doctor Watson to his Sherlock Holmes. If you have a hunch what might be causing something, tell him. Tell him if you have been to any foreign countries lately or have been exposed to someone with a disease.

Be your own early warning system. Often you can tell when something is going wrong inside your body by being alert to changes and checking them with your doctor. If bowel movements become very light in color, almost gray, it may mean something is wrong with your liver or gallbladder. Bright red or blackish tar-color may mean bleeding in the bowel. Green color usually means food poisoning, yellow may mean an upset in fat metabolism. (Sometimes of course, such color changes occur from food such as spinach, beets, carrots, or iron tablets).

Changes in the urine are also diagnostic of certain diseases. A brown to blackish urine usually means bleeding in the urinary tract; a lighter than normal yellow is usually seen with diabetes and with some anemias; liver and gallbladder disease cause a greenish tint; excess niacin can cause bright yellow urine; hepatitis a brownish urine.

Your sputum can also give you signals. A yellow-to-green color is evidence of lung infection. Reddish or brown color means there may be congestion in the lungs (usually from heart trouble).

HOW TO USE THE I.R.S. TO UNDERWRITE SOME MEDICAL BILLS

Don't forget your medical, dental, and medicine deductions on your federal (and sometimes state and city) income taxes.

HERE ARE SOME OF THE COSTS YOU CAN DEDUCT FROM YOUR INCOME TAX

- Some medical insurance premiums
- Supplementary medical insurance under Medicare

- Payments to physicians, surgeons, dentists, optometrists, chiropractors, osteopaths, chiropodists, podiatrists, psychiatrists, psychologists, and Christian Science practitioners
- Payments for hospital services, therapy, laboratory, surgical, obstetrical, diagnostic, dental and x-ray fees, nursing services (including nurse's board paid by you), and ambulances
- Charges for medical care included in the tuition fee of a college, private school, or retirement home
- Payments for psychiatric care
- A parent's transportation expenses for regular visits recommended as part of a child's therapy
- Payments for medicines, drugs, and prescribed vitamins that exceed 1 percent of your adjusted gross income

- A special food or beverage prescribed by a physician for the treatment of an illness
- Payment for transportation essential to medical care, including bus, taxi, train or plane fares, parking fees (or 6¢ per mile if you use your car)
- Meals and lodging that are a necessary part of medical care
- Payments for sending a mentally or physically handicapped child to a special school
- Payments for special equipment installed in a home or car for medical purposes
- Payments for artificial teeth and limbs, eyeglasses, hearing aids, crutches, guide dogs and their maintenance
- Cost of special telephone equipment for a deaf person

CHAPTER 2

How to Increase Your Life Expectancy

THE AVERAGE LIFE SPAN

Prehistoric man probably had an average life span of 20 years; Romans of the Roman Empire about 30 years; in 1850 it was about 40 years. A child born today in the United States can expect to live to age 72 as an average; new statistics indicate it may be to age 74.

In the U.S. almost 90 percent of the people who live to be 100 have at least one parent who lived to be at least 70, and sometimes grandparents who lived long also.

WHY WOMEN LIVE LONGER THAN MEN

A baby girl born today can expect to live to be 76; a boy to be only 69.

The major differences are that men have more heart disease, have a higher suicide rate, a higher rate of fatal car and other accidents, have more cirrhosis of the liver, respiratory cancers, and emphysema. Figures are changing as more women go out to work.

WHERE CAN YOU LIVE LONGEST?

Life expectancy of residents of Hawaii now leads those of the other 50 states, according to the National Center for Health Statistics. Other states with high life expectancy are Minnesota, Utah, North Dakota, and Nebraska.

Here is the run-down of the average life expectancy, state by state:

AREA	MALE	FEMALE
Hawaii	71.02	76.79
Utah	69.49	76.55
Minnesota	69.38	76.80
North Dakota	69.23	77.01
Wisconsin	69.15	76.04
Connecticut	69.04	75.94
Nebraska	68.85	76.61
Kansas	68.83	76.54
Iowa	68.83	76.50
South Dakota	68.49	76.19
Oregon	68.43	76.20
Colorado	68.40	75.43
Rhode Island	68.31	75.48
Idaho	68.20	76.10
California	68.19	75.37
Massachusetts	68.12	75.45
Washington	68.07	75.78
Vermont	67.76	75.77
New Jersey	67.52	74.38
New Hampshire	67.48	75.19
Oklahoma	67.40	75.70
Ohio	67.25	74.55
Maine	67.24	74.85
Indiana	67.23	74.72
Michigan	67.09	74.48
Texas	67.05	74.99
New York	66.95	74.15

AREA	MALE	FEMALE
Pennsylvania	66.90	74.06
Missouri	66.88	74.66
Montana	66.73	75.08
Arkansas	66.68	74.97
Florida	66.61	74.96
Arizona	66.57	75.04
New Mexico	66.51	74.51
Illinois	66.48	73.96
Maryland	66.47	74.17
Delaware	66.29	74.07
Virginia	66.26	74.17
Kentucky	66.22	74.31
Wyoming	66.19	75.19
Tennessee	66.15	74.26
Alaska	66.05	74.03
Nevada	65.60	73.32
West Virginia	65.56	73.74
North Carolina	64.94	73.78
Alabama	64.90	73.41
Louisiana	64.85	72.88
Georgia	64.27	73.01
Mississippi	64.06	72.40
South Carolina	63.85	72.29
District of Columbia	60.92	70.52

AND THE 10 BEST CITIES

Science Digest determined what they considered the 10 healthiest cities by investigating air pollution, quality of medical care, incidence of fatal auto accidents and killer diseases, and the average life span of residents. Their results were as follows:

1. Any city in Hawaii
2. Eugene, Ore.
3. San Francisco
4. St. Cloud, Minn.
5. Austin, Tex.
6. La Junta, Colo.
7. Utica, N.Y.
8. Kanab, Utah
9. Ketchikan, Alaska
10. Middletown, Conn.

THE WORST CITIES AND STATES, HEALTHWISE, WERE:

1. Washington, D.C., whose people have shorter lives than any other Americans.
2. New Jersey, No. 1 in cancer incidence.
3. Rhode Island, No. 1 in heart disease and No. 3 in cancer.
4. The entire industrialized Ohio River Valley from Wheeling, W.Va., to Pittsburgh with unhealthy air.

HOW TO CALCULATE YOUR LIFE EXPECTANCY

If you are age 20 to 65 and reasonably healthy, this test provides a life-insurance company's statistical view of your life expectancy.

Start with the number 72.

Sex: If you are male, subtract 3; female, add 4.

Life style: If you live in an urban area with population over 2 million, subtract 2. If you live in a town under 10,000 or on a farm, add 2. If you work behind a desk, subtract 3. If your work requires regular, heavy physical labor, add 3. If you exercise strenuously (tennis, running, swimming, etc.) five times a week for at least a half-hour, add 4. Two or three times a week, add 2. If you live with a spouse or friend, add 5. If not, subtract 1 for every ten years alone since age 25.

Psyche: Sleep more than 10 hours each night? Subtract 4. Are you intense, aggressive, easily angered? Subtract 3. Are you easygoing, relaxed, a follower? Add 3. Are you happy? Add 1. Unhappy? Subtract 2. Have you had a speeding ticket in the last year? Subtract 1.

Success: Earn over $50,000 a year? Subtract 2. If you finished college, add 1. If you have a graduate or professional degree, add 2 more. If you are 65 or over and still working, add 3.

Heredity: If any grandparent lived to 85, add 2. If all four grandparents lived to 80, add 6. If either parent died of a stroke or heart attack before the age of 50, subtract 4. If any parent, brother, or sister under 50 has (or had) cancer or a heart condition, or has had diabetes since childhood, subtract 3.

Health: Smoke more than two packs a day? Subtract 8. One to two packs? Subtract 6. One-half to one? Subtract 3. Drink the equivalent of a quarter bottle of liquor a day? Subtract 1. Overweight by fifty pounds or more? Subtract 8. Thirty to fifty pounds? Subtract 4. Ten to thirty pounds? Subtract 2. Men over 40, if you have annual checkups, add 2. Women, if you see a gynecologist once a year, add 2.

Age Adjustment: Between 30 and 40? Add 2. Between 40 and 50? Add 3. Between 50 and 70? Add 4. Over 70? Add 5.

Add up your score to get your life expectancy at this time. Now compare it to the national averages for various ages:

AGE NOW	MALE	FEMALE
0–10	69.4–69.8	76.9–77.2
11–19	69.8–70.3	77.3–77.5
20–29	70.3–71.2	77.5–77.8
30–39	71.3–72.1	77.9–78.4
40–49	72.2–73.5	78.4–79.4
50–59	73.7–76.1	79.5–81
60–69	76.4–80.2	81.2–83.6
70–79	80.7–85.9	83.9–87.7
80–85	86.6–90.0	88.2–91.1

HOW CAN THE AVERAGE PERSON MAKE HIS LIFE LONGER?

He can add an easy 8 years to his life, say insurance companies, by simply keeping blood pressure and cholesterol levels down, drinking moderately or not at all, not smoking, exercising, and maintaining normal weight.

Dr. Linus Pauling, two-time Nobel Prize winner, says the average person can extend his life expectancy by 24 years if he doesn't smoke cigarettes, drastically decreases the amount of sugar he eats, and takes the proper amount of vitamins.

Dr. Paul Dudley White, former White House cardiologist: "We can control our destiny by changing our ways of life. . . . Keep moving, keep thinking. Don't let your brain atrophy. Too many people die from disuse of their bodies."

National Center for Health Services Research and Development: "Individuals who follow seven basic health practices may add 11 years to their life span. These practices are usually sleeping 7 or 8 hours a day, eating breakfast almost every day, only occasionally eating between meals, maintaining a body weight close to ideal for your height, exercising frequently, drinking in moderation or not at all, and never smoking cigarettes."

American Medical Association: "Between the ages of 45 and 50, men who weigh 60 pounds more than they should have a death rate that is 67 per cent higher than that of men whose weight is normal. Each extra pound increases their chances of dying by a bit more than one percent."

A LOOK AT WHAT THE SCIENTIFIC EVIDENCE SHOWS

The big four leading causes of death in the United States are heart disease and stroke, cancer, diabetes, and accidents.

So the first order of business is to eliminate the major risk factors that increase your chances of getting these giant killers. Because these risk factors—such as high blood pressure, overweight, smoking, lack of exercise, high sugar consumption, high cholesterol and triglycerides in the blood— don't just add on to each other in their effect. *They multiply!* For example, if you are between the ages of 30 and 59 and have high blood pressure, your risk of dying of one of these major diseases in the next 10 years is more than twice that of a person who doesn't have high blood pressure. If you also smoke, your chances are three times normal. If you have high blood pressure *and* smoke *and* have high cholesterol, your risk of death is *five* times higher.

So if you correct one factor in your life that is increasing your risk of death, that's good. But if you correct two or three or four, it can have an even greater effect . . . by several hundred percent.

HOW TO CUSTOMIZE A LIVE-LONG PROGRAM TO YOUR OWN LIFE

There is a new branch of medicine called *predictive* medicine—not just preventive medicine, but *predictive* medicine—that takes many clues from your hereditary background, living style, diet, and laboratory studies and determines specifically what you are most in danger of dying from. From your personal health profile, a computer finds out what you should be alert for *before you ever have any signs or symptoms*. And the computer tells you what you can do to best prevent your premature death by preventing your particular danger diseases from happening. Two medical groups that will evaluate your particular risk profile, working through your physician, are: Periodic Individualized Evaluation, Inc., of Santa Monica, Calif., and InterHealth in San Diego and Los Angeles. The University of Wisconsin Center for Health Sciences, Madison, Wisconsin, has a simplified 20-minute version that is available to anyone for $5.

A computer consultation service called Cardio-Dial, free to physicians through Ciba Pharmaceutical Company, will figure up your risk of having a coronary, but not other diseases.

Medical groups that provide screening for detection of existing hidden disease as well as determining your risk factors for future problems are: Life Extension Institute clinics (in New York, Baltimore, Philadelphia, Chicago, Denver, Los Angeles, San Diego, and San Francisco), Executive Health Examiners (New York), Mayo Clinic (Rochester), Lahey Clinic (Boston), Scripps Clinic (La Jolla).

WHAT ABOUT SPECIAL VITAMINS AND MINERALS?

Animal research indicates that vitamins C and E will fight some of the chemical changes that seem to accompany aging, and so will the mineral selenium and the sulfur-containing amino acids, and two food additives you shouldn't object to called BHT and BHA. Look for the latter on processed food labels. All of these have definitely increased the life span of mice and rats and of cells in test tubes.

So far there has been no long-term research in humans to prove these things occur in humans. But every specialist in nutrition medicine that we talked to is taking at least some of these substances himself. Most of the nutritionists take 500 to 2000 mg of vitamin C per day, 400 to 800 units of vitamin E, and 25 to 100 mcg of selenium, plus high amounts of vitamin Bs, an all-round vitamin-mineral supplement, wheat germ, and brewer's yeast.

The foods in which these nutrients are high are: eggs, onions, brewer's yeast, wheat germ, bran, broccoli, cabbage, tomato, muscle meats, leafy vegetables, fish, whole wheat, vegetable oils (like corn, safflower, soybean, and cottonseed oils), liver, sprouts, citrus fruits, berries, sprouted seeds.

PUTTING IT ALL TOGETHER: 13 WAYS TO HAVE A LONGER LIFE

After talking to the experts, reading the research reports, and sifting through the recommendations of gerontologists and nutritionists and specialists in preventive medicine, we make these recommendations to you for adding years to your life span.

Read each of the items in the first column. If your answer is *no* to the items in the first column, then good for you . . . keep it up. If your answer is *yes,* read the suggestions for change in the right-hand column. Underline those that you are not currently doing. Look them over when you have completed the questions and you will see your own individually designed program, which if you seriously put into practice will reduce your risk of the killer diseases and add years to your life.

IS THIS YOU?	THEN TO LIVE LONGER DO THIS:
Is your blood pressure high?	Get it down to 120/80.
Do you smoke cigarettes?	Become a non-smoker.
Are you 10 pounds or more overweight?	Get your weight down to normal.
Is your cholesterol high?	If it is over 180, get it down.
Are you inactive, always sitting?	Set up a regular exercise program appropriate to your physical condition.
Do you tend to overreact to stress and tension?	Explore ways to relax more. Try meditation or some of the new therapies.
Do you constantly race against time, trying to pack more into every hour than you can handle?	Try to simplify your life. Enjoy life more.
Are you reckless?	Study safety measures and curb your need to show off.
Do you eat large amounts of sugar and drink sugared drinks?	Eliminate sugar from your diet as much as you can.
Do you drink a great deal of alcohol?	Keep alcohol to only moderate amounts.
Do you eat large amounts of refined starches?	Switch to whole-grain carbohydrates.
Do you eat junk food?	Switch to fresh foods with high nutrient content.
Do you ignore vitamin supplements?	Take supplementary vitamins, especially C and E.

CHAPTER 3

Threats to Survival—
The Killer Diseases
and How to
Cope with Them

Heart Disease and Strokes

HIDDEN HEART ATTACKS

The greatest danger of a heart attack is not knowing you've suffered it. Many people have minor heart attacks, without recognizing them, before they have a sudden severe one that possibly kills them. If you ever have had acute chest pain, blackouts after exertion, noticeable shortness of breath, or what seems to be severe indigestion and gas, see your doctor.

HOW TO DETERMINE IF YOUR CHEST PAIN IS HEART PAIN

Pain is usually in the center of the chest, not on the side; may be in one spot behind the breastbone or throughout the chest. Pain may extend into the shoulder, arms, neck, or jaw.

It is a heavy, crushing pain with a squeezing or pressing sensation, or like a band pulled tight around the chest; it usually is *not* a burning, sharp, or a stitchlike pain. Pain may be mild or severe, may last a few minutes or several hours.

The pain is usually brought on by exertion or emotion and is accompanied by a sense of impending doom.

The hands become cold and sweaty, the forehead covered with sweat. There may be shortness of breath; it is difficult to take a deep breath. There may be nausea or vomiting. There may be dizzi-

ness, light-headedness, or blacking out. There may be double vision. There may be paleness, or the face may be gray.

Pain from the heart is usually relieved by rest and nitroglycerine. Other chest pain can be caused by arthritis, an injured rib, respiratory infection, a pinched nerve, a stitch in the side from overexertion, hiatal hernia, an ulcer, gallbladder trouble, or even from magnesium or potassium deficiencies.

Tests: Cough and breathe deeply. If the pain is made worse, it is probably not heart attack pain.

Raise your arms above your head. Pain due to arthritis or bursitis will be aggravated by this maneuver; heart pain will not.

Turn your head and bend your neck. Pain originating in the neck will be aggravated; heart pain will not.

WHAT TO DO IF YOU HAVE EARLY WARNING SIGNS OF HEART ATTACK

Call a doctor immediately. Describe your symptoms carefully.

While waiting for the doctor to arrive, stay where you are. Lie down or sit, whichever is more comfortable. (If you are short of breath, sitting up will help most.)

If you are chilled, get warm; if you are overheated, have someone open a window or turn on air conditioning.

If your doctor is not available leave a message

with his service, then get to the closest hospital immediately. Use the fastest transportation available. Sometimes a car is faster than calling an ambulance; otherwise call an ambulance.

If nitroglycerine tablets are handy, place one under your tongue; it will help ease pain and stress.

If you are transporting a heart attack victim to the hospital, watch him carefully. If he loses consciousness, hold your ear to his chest. If you cannot hear a heartbeat, stop the car immediately, place the patient on a hard surface outside the car, and apply mouth-to-mouth breathing and chest resuscitation. Keep applying and have someone else call an ambulance.

WHAT ARE YOUR ODDS FOR A HEART ATTACK OR STROKE?

To determine your risk, answer the following questions and determine your score.

1. Are you overweight more than 30 pounds? 1 point.

2. What is your diastolic (the bottom number) blood pressure? 1 point if it is 90 to 100, and 2 points if it is over 100.

3. Do you smoke? If so, 1 point. For two packs a day, 2 points.

4. Do you regularly exercise or are you more sedentary? If sedentary, 1 point.

5. Do you or your parents or your family have diabetes? If someone in your family, 1 point; if you have it, 2 points.

6. Have your parents or any brothers or sisters had a heart attack or stroke before age 60? If yes, 1 point.

7. Do you have a high cholesterol level? If mildly elevated cholesterol (210 to 250 mg percent), 1 point. If higher (over 250), 2 points.

8. Was your last electrocardiogram normal or abnormal? If there were some abnormalities in your EKG, 1 point.

Add up your risk points. If you have any score at all from any question, you have more risk of heart attack or stroke than a person who got a zero score. If you scored 3 to 5 points, you have a moderate risk. If it added up 6 to 12 points, you are at very high risk.

THE HEART TEST THAT COULD SAVE YOUR LIFE

A routine electrocardiogram does not always tell accurately whether you have a heart problem. A better test is the two-step stress test, the stationary bicycle test, or a treadmill test. In these tests,

your heart action and blood pressure are recorded while you are exercising, showing what your heart does under stress.

Not everyone needs such a test, but you should discuss having it with your doctor if:

- You have shortness of breath or occasional squeezing pressure in walking up stairs or during stress
- You have extra heartbeats or palpitations
- There is a history of early heart disease in your family
- You have high blood pressure or diabetes
- You have high cholesterol or triglycerides in the blood
- You are overweight
- You have a high-pressure lifestyle
- You smoke cigarettes
- You have been inactive and plan to take up a strenuous sport such as jogging or tennis.

A check-yourself version of the test: Climb up and down steps of a specified height a certain number of times, then take a pulse reading. The quicker your pulse returns to normal, the more fit you are. Instructions, including a record, are available from the Canadian government: Fit-Kit, Information Canada, Ottawa, Ontario K1A OS9, for $5.95 in English or French. Check with your doctor before using. Also see Chapter 24, Do-It-Yourself Medical Tests You Can Do at Home.

A NEW HEART TEST

A simple, painless alternative has been developed for some heart patients heretofore faced with having a tube inserted into the chambers of their hearts (cardiac catheterization) or having radioactive material injected into their blood.

The new method, developed at St. Luke's Hospital in St. Louis, requires the patient to lie down on a table for 10 minutes. He is hooked up to a device called an MEF (Mass Energy Force) Recorder. A supersensitive gauge measures changes in the table's position as the patient's heart beats and tells the heart's strength.

Cardiac catheterization is still considered the best test of a patient going to have bypass heart surgery. But the new procedure tells whether the patient needs the surgery and whether the heart is working well and could stand an operation. After surgery it would tell whether the operation benefitted the patient and made the heart pump better.

A thermograph test can check circulation efficiency and tell whether you are in danger of having a heart attack or stroke.

**VITAL THINGS TO KNOW
IF YOU'VE ALREADY
HAD A HEART ATTACK**

WHAT DIET CAN DO

Low-carbohydrate diets have been shown to reduce frequency and lessen severity of angina, and help to eliminate water if you have fluid retention.

Research indicates that supplements of trace metals, including zinc, copper, manganese, and selenium, and vitamins such as C and E help prevent a second heart attack and reduce angina.

Mushrooms, it has just been found, contain a chemical, *eritadenine,* which is believed to lower blood cholesterol and reduce heart attack risk.

Immediately after a heart attack, European doctors report healing speeded and mortality rate reduced if patients are given a sugar-free, starch-free, high-protein diet, and also zinc and magnesium.

ALCOHOL IS NOT GOOD FOR YOUR HEART

The general belief that alcohol is a heart stimulant is not true. Cardiologists say there is strong evidence that alcohol is actually a heart depressant, and people with heart disease should not drink at all or should limit themselves to one drink a day. For two hours after a drink they should avoid activity that might trigger a heart attack.

EXERCISE YOU CAN DO
AFTER A HEART ATTACK

If you've had a heart attack, or suffer from high blood pressure, don't lift heavy weights, shovel snow, push pianos or cars. Don't do isometric exercises or upper arm exercises. They tend to increase blood pressure.

Walking, running, bicycling, dancing, calisthenics, volleyball, and swimming are excellent exercises for the post-coronary person if the patient starts only when his physician approves, builds up to them gradually, and keeps getting tested by his physician under treadmill or other exercise conditions. As little as 20 minutes a day every other day can improve circulation, cardiologists say. Many former heart attack victims are now running regular 26-mile marathons. Dr. Thomas Bassler, who has done research on the subject, says any heart patient who builds his stamina to the point where he can run the marathon need never fear another heart attack.

CAN YOU HAVE SEX
AFTER A HEART ATTACK?

For a long-married couple, heart rates reach only 117 to 120 beats per minute for 10 to 30 seconds, about the same as climbing two flights of stairs or a brisk walk. The dangerous sex is extramarital, where anxiety, fear, and excitement run higher. A great number of heart attack deaths occur during or after extramarital intercourse.

The test: If you can walk a block or climb two flights of stairs with no problem, you should be able to have sex without any problem at all. But do not have intercourse right after a meal (wait 1½ to 2 hours). Don't push yourself if you are tired.

A physician in New York has designed an exercise program to build up stamina for intercourse after a heart attack. Three to four months after their attack, he put men through a 12-week program on a stationary bicycle. While being tested in the doctor's office, they did 3 to 5 minutes of pedaling, then 3- to 5-minute intervals of rest, for 30 to 40 minutes on three days per week.

If you have less sexual desire than before your attack or difficulty in maintaining an erection or attaining orgasm, consult with your physician. It may be due to medication you are taking, and he may be able to switch you to another kind.

HOW TO TELL IF YOU MIGHT BE DEVELOPING CONGESTIVE HEART FAILURE

Congestive heart failure occurs when the heart becomes enlarged and loses its efficiency, causing sluggishness of the circulation. Because of its inefficient pumping action, the heart fails to get all the blood back from your arms and legs, and fluid accumulates in the tissues. The signs of congestive heart failure are:

- Fatigue
- Shortness of breath, first on exertion, then at rest
- Wheezing and difficulty in breathing at night
- Swelling of the ankles and legs and feet (do you have difficulty getting shoes on or off?)
- Swollen hand and fingers (do you have difficulty getting rings on and off?)
- Puffiness of the face
- Accumulation of fluid in the lungs
- Sudden weight gain with no change in diet
- A feeling of being bloated and waterlogged.

RESEARCH NEWS ABOUT HEART DISEASE THAT YOU CAN PUT TO USE

Aspirin provides some protection against heart attack. It apparently can reduce the tendency for blood platelets to stick together and thus cuts down clogging of arteries. (But there are many side effects, and more research is needed.)

Nitrous oxide (laughing gas) relieves pain of acute heart attacks and speeds recovery. Tanks of nitrous oxide are used routinely in coronary care units in Russia, are now being tested in the U.S.

A portable heart monitor has been developed. It monitors heart activity steadily for 24 hours. The patient keeps a diary of activity, so physicians can determine the heart's response to specific activity or medications and can evaluate progress toward a normal life after a heart attack.

Oxygen for home use in handy portable cannisters instead of heavy tanks is now available. The emergency oxygen system generates oxygen from dry-packed chemicals that can sit on the shelf or in a drawer like a six-pack until needed.

Dunking in cold water helps paroxysmal atrial tachycardia (rapid heartbeat). Patients who are afflicted by frequent bouts of the problem are being taught to take a deep breath, then immerse their faces in cold (36°F) water for 15 to 30 seconds. This maneuver slows the heart rate about 30 percent, and quickly relieves the heart symptoms.

Recent research indicates there are actually five kinds of cholesterol, not just one. And Dr. William Castelli, chief of the famous Framingham study for the National Heart, Lung, and Blood Institute, says one of them, called HDL (for high density lipoprotein), apparently helps *protect* you from heart diseases. The higher the level of the friendly HDL cholesterol in the blood, the lower the risk of your having a heart attack. Women have higher levels of HDL than men (and fewer heart attacks). You apparently can get your HDL to go up with exercise—joggers and long-distance runners have high HDL levels. Dr. Castelli recommends that doctors now do tests (simple and inexpensive) on HDL in addition to routine cholesterol tests. Low-density lipoproteins or LDL's *are* predictors of heart attack and require preventive care.

Abnormalities in heartbeat during a heart attack can also be eliminated with magnesium and potassium.

NEW DRUG TO STOP HEART ATTACK DAMAGE

A nerve-blocking drug may be able to stop heart attacks from doing any damage, researchers report at the University of Minnesota. Bretylium tosylate was given to heart attack patients and heart damage and deaths were reduced when compared to patients not receiving the drug. The F.D.A. has found bretylium to be safe and effective as an anti-arrhythmia agent, but has not yet cleared it for other use.

HEART PACEMAKERS— DO THEY REALLY WORK?

The pacemakers, implanted in the chest to keep the rhythm of the heart going, do very well in prolonging life and extending usefulness, according to an analysis in the *Journal of the American Medical Association*. There was a 65 percent survival rate after five years, and all deaths but one were due to some other ailment not related to the pacemaker.

Warning: Some household appliances can cause interference with pacemaker function if they are less than a foot away from the pulse generator, according to doctors at an American College of Cardiology meeting. Electric toothbrushes or shavers can cause dangerous pacemaker interference, they said—patients sometimes complain of dizziness when they use them.

HOW TO RECOGNIZE HIDDEN STROKES

A stroke occurs when the blood supply to a part of the brain is cut off, stopping the supply of oxygen vital to brain cells.

Sometimes a person can have a little stroke (doctors call them cerebral transient ischemic attacks or TIAs), and not even know it. They may only last two minutes or so, so the person shrugs his shoulders and goes on. But they are often a signal that a full-fledged stroke could occur if nothing is done to prevent it.

Signs of a little stroke:

- Momentary numbness or weakness of an arm or leg
- Dizziness, sometimes with a whirling feeling or staggering
- Headache
- Abrupt clumsiness (jerky handwriting, for example)
- Little unexplained falls
- Temporary loss of vision
- Brief blackouts
- Short memory lapses

A SEVERE STROKE MIGHT ALSO SHOW THESE SIGNS

- Sudden, temporary weakness or numbness of the face, arm, or leg

- Difficulty or loss of speech
- Dimness or loss of vision, particularly in one eye, or double vision
- Unexplained dizziness, unsteadiness, unconsciousness
- Sudden change in personality

The most important thing you can do to prevent a stroke from happening to you is to get your blood pressure down to normal.

NEW DRUG TREATMENT FOR STROKE

Dr. George S. Allen of Johns Hopkins Medical School reports success in treating patients with brain hemorrhage using two drugs that work in opposite ways: He gives nitroprusside to relax blood vessels from spasms and gives phenylephrine to keep the blood pressure from falling dangerously low.

HOW TO REDUCE YOUR CHANCES OF HAVING A HEART ATTACK OR STROKE

STATISTICS SHOW THE FOLLOWING FACTORS MEAN MORE RISK OF HEART ATTACK AND STROKE:	HERE'S WHAT YOU CAN DO TO ELIMINATE THEM FROM YOUR LIFE:
High blood pressure	Learn if your blood pressure is normal; take medicine for it if it isn't; eliminate sugar, cut down salt.
Family history of heart disease	Be extra alert for symptoms.
Smoking cigarettes	Be a non-smoker.
Diabetes	Watch your diet; take medication.
High blood levels of cholesterol and triglycerides	If your cholesterol levels are high, decrease cholesterol and fat in your diet. (If your cholesterol is normal, you do not have to worry about cholesterol in your diet.)
Obesity	Lose weight.
Lack of exercise	Set up a regular exercise program.
Too many refined starches in the diet	Eat whole grain foods instead of refined. Eliminate junk foods.
Lack of trace minerals; vitamin deficiencies	Take vitamin and mineral supplements.
Softness of water	Do not use a water softener.
Impaired glucose tolerance	Eliminate sugar from diet.
Stress	Try to relax more and keep from overreacting to stress and tension.
Increased stickiness of blood platelets	Avoid sugar; take vitamin supplements.

You can bet 20 years of your life it does!

At Stanford Heart Disease Prevention Program, a research team was able to reduce the risk of heart attacks in the residents of two small California towns by 25 percent through a two-year education campaign.

Now Stanford has joined the National Council of YMCAs in a program to apply the same techniques nationwide. Y classes will offer advice on diet, exercise, weight control, reducing stress, and stopping smoking. The Stanford Heart Disease Program is at the Stanford University Medical Center, Stanford, Calif. 94305.

Cancer

HOW TO TELL IF YOU ARE IN A RISK GROUP FOR CANCER

More than 100,000 cancer patients die each year in the United States who should not have died. They could have been saved by earlier and better treatment, says the American Cancer Society. To improve survival and prevent these deaths, people should learn to identify whether they are especially at risk for different kinds of cancers and then to watch for the warning signs so that if the cancer appears they can get early treatment.

Look over these summarized findings and see if you are among any high-risk groups. If so, do what you can to prevent further exposure, be especially alert for warning signs, and see your doctor immediately if any appear.

SKIN CANCER

There is higher-than-average risk if:

- You are a farmer or sailor or other person with an outdoor occupation that requires frequent sun exposure
- You sun yourself excessively as a habit
- You work with coal, tar, pitch, creosote, arsenic compounds, paraffin oil
- You belong to a family prone to skin cancer

Warning signs: changes in a wart or mole; a sore that does not heal.

Best safeguard: avoid excessive sunburning.

More than 90 percent of skin cancers can be cured if found early.

LUNG CANCER

There is higher-than-average risk if:

- You work with nickel, asbestos, or chromate
- You are a cigarette smoker

The earlier you began smoking, the longer you have smoked, the more cigarettes you smoke per day, and the more you inhale, the higher risk you have.

Warning signs: persistent cough; lingering respiratory ailment, pain in one shoulder, clubbing enlargement around the fingernails.

Best safeguard: don't smoke. (If you smoke and quit, your lungs will clear in a year.)

CANCER OF THE BREAST

There is higher-than-average risk if:

- You are obese
- You are aged 40 to 44, or over age 60
- You never had children, or had your first child when over 30 years old
- You began your menstrual period early, and/or had a late menopause
- You take estrogen for the symptoms of menopause
- You have had a benign breast disease
- Your relatives have had breast cancer, especially if they had cancer of both breasts
- You have already had one episode of breast cancer

Warning signs: lump in breast, puckering or other abnormal appearance of skin.

Best safeguards: regular self-examination, an annual physical examination and a breast x-ray such as mammography or thermography if you are age 50 or are at high risk.

GASTRO-INTESTINAL CANCER

There is higher-than-average risk if:

- You are male
- You frequently consumed pickled vegetables or dried salted fish when young
- You eat highly processed foods
- You drink heavily, especially beer
- You expose your gastro-intestinal tract to cancer-causing agents
- You are or were a coal miner
- You heat or cook with coal
- Your relatives had occurrences of polyps or had stomach, colon, or rectal cancer

Warning signs: chronic indigestion; blood in the stool (actual blood or streaks); a persistent change in bowel habits involving diarrhea or constipation; tarry stools; increase in intestinal gas.

Best safeguard: proctosigmoidoscopy (visual examination of the lower colon through a lighted tube) done routinely as part of your regular physical examination.

CANCER OF THE CERVIX AND UTERUS

There is a higher-than-average risk if:

- You are a woman ages 50 to 70
- You do not have regular Pap tests or checkups
- You have had children
- You have had early sexual intercourse and frequency of sexual experience with different partners
- You had late menopause with postmenopausal bleeding
- You are obese (latest study shows fat women have two to four times more risk of endometrial cancer)
- You have high blood pressure
- You have diabetes
- You married before age 25
- You take estrogen for menopausal symptoms
- You had poor care during and after pregnancy

Warning signs: unusual bleeding, especially around or after menopause; vaginal discharge.

Best safeguard: an annual Pap test.

BLADDER CANCER

There is higher-than-average risk if:

- You are a cigarette smoker
- You work in the leather, dye, or printing industries

Warning signs: urinary difficulty; blood in the urine.

Best safeguards: be a non-smoker.

PROSTATE CANCER

There is higher-than-average risk if:

- You are a man aged 50 or more (there is an even greater risk after age 75, when prostate cancer is the most frequent cancer in men)

Warning signs: urinary difficulty; pain in the back, pelvis, or thighs; weak or interrupted urine flow; blood in the urine.

Best safeguards: every man should have a rectal and prostate examination every year. Keep zinc levels high.

CANCER OF THE MOUTH, ESOPHAGUS OR LARYNX

There is higher-than-average risk if:

- You drink heavily
- You smoke heavily
- You are vitamin deficient

Warning signs: difficulty in swallowing; hoarseness; a sore that does not heal.

Best safeguards: don't smoke or drink heavily; take vitamins.

WHO SHOULD HAVE BREAST CANCER TESTS?

X-ray or mammography of the breast for cancer should be done in women age 50 or over, according to the Department of Health, Education, and Welfare. Younger women should not be subjected to the extra x-ray unless they have a high cancer incidence in their family or a history of cancer. It is estimated that each mammography increases your chance of developing cancer by 1 percent.

Breast cancer need not be a death sentence. When diagnosed early and treated promptly, the rate of cure can be as high as 85 percent. And it is important to remember that a breast lump does *not* necessarily mean cancer—90 percent are *not*—but only a physician can make the final diagnosis. See him quickly.

Another breast cancer test, with fewer risks, is thermography.

FIVE WAYS TO TREAT BREAST CANCER

Today, a woman with operable breast cancer can be treated in one of the following ways:

Lumpectomy or partial mastectomy: removal of the tumor and some surrounding breast tissue.

Simple or total mastectomy: removal of all breast tissue, but no lymph glands.

Modified radical mastectomy: in addition to removing all breast tissue, the surgeons take out the axillary lymph nodes in the armpit.

Radical mastectomy: removal of breast, axillary lymph nodes, and muscles of the chest wall, leaving the woman with a depression below the collarbone that is very difficult to hide. Occasionally a skin graft is performed. Some patients will suffer a permanently swollen arm.

Extended radical mastectomy: in addition to breast, axillary lymph nodes, and chest muscles, the surgeon removes the lymph nodes on the underside of the breast bone.

Efforts are being made to find less mutilating, cosmetically more acceptable methods of treating breast cancer—using limited cutting without removing the breast, radiation therapy to the other breast to kill any dispersed cells there, and chemotherapy for any widely dispersed cells. Can such treatment eliminate the need for radical mastectomy? At Massachusetts General Hospital, Boston, physicians have treated women with breast cancer by limited radiation for the other breast and drug treatment. It is still too early to judge results completely, but survival rates of the women treated so far compare favorably with those of patients treated by radical mastectomy.

IF YOU HAVE HAD A MASTECTOMY

Contact your local chapter of the American Cancer Society for a booklet called *Reach to Recovery,* describing various breast forms, exercises, and other tips. Also available directly from the American Cancer Society, 219 East 42nd Street, New York, N.Y. 10017, free. While you are in the hospital be sure your physician has someone, usually a recovered mastectomy patient, visit you for advice and counseling.

PLASTIC SURGERY AFTER MASTECTOMY

In Miami a plastic surgeon has developed a technique for rebuilding the breast by taking flesh from the stomach and moving it to the chest in a series of operations. The technique works well, but the entire series can take up to a year to complete. The other plastic surgery procedure implants an envelope of silicone gel to reconstruct a breast. A completely new artificial breast has been designed by scientists at the University of Michigan.

NEW OPERATION FOR LARYNGEAL CANCER

A new surgical technique that allows a patient to speak in his natural voice five to six days after removal of his voice box because of laryngeal cancer has been performed successfully by Northwestern University Medical School surgeons. The technique is still experimental. The trachea (windpipe) is pulled up and connected to the thick muscles at the base of the tongue, where it can vibrate and produce sounds. Dr. George Sisson of Northwestern emphasizes that only some laryngectomy patients can benefit from the operation and that success depends on how much tissue was saved when the cancer was removed.

WARNING SIGNS OF CANCER IN CHILDREN

Most people don't realize that cancer is one of the major killers of children between the ages of 1 and 14. Be sure that your children have regular checkups with your doctor and watch for these signs:

Swellings, lumps, or masses in any part of the body; particularly in the abdomen and in the arms or legs.

Persistent pains in the arm or leg; difficulty in using the arm or leg.

Persistent crying of a baby or child for which no reason can be found.

Any change in the size or appearance of moles or birthmarks.

Nausea or vomiting for which there is no apparent cause.

A marked change in bowel habits.

Listlessness or a pale, anemic look.

Widening of the pupil of the eye.

HOW TO PROTECT YOURSELF FROM EXCESSIVE X-RAYS

If a doctor suggests an x-ray, ask him if it's only routine or if it is definitely necessary for diagnosis. If it's not necessary, don't have it.

Keep a record of where and when x-rays have been taken. Sometimes previous x-rays can be used instead of new exposures.

If you are told to have pre-employment x-rays to test for tuberculosis, ask to have a tuberculin or other test instead.

Don't let your dentist give you x-rays at every visit. Many dentists believe full-mouth x-rays are needed only every few years. If you go to a new dentist, ask him to obtain x-rays from your previous dentist.

Always be sure that a lead apron is placed over your chest and lap when x-rays of other parts of your body are taken. Make sure it is done for your children also.

Avoid mobile x-ray units when possible—they generally give more exposure than conventional machines.

Avoid fluoroscopy if possible. It involves greater exposure than conventional x-rays and should only be used when your doctor needs to see movement.

Keep still when x-rays are taken so retakes won't be necessary.

Children and pregnant women should absolutely avoid x-rays unless there are very strong and serious reasons.

FIVE NOT-DEADLY LUMPS AND BUMPS

The following common conditions may scare you if they appear, but they are not cancers and need not worry you. However, since they look almost like lesions that *could* be cancerous or precancerous, you should always have your doctor look at them.

Seborrheic keratoses. These lesions can occur on the trunk, face, or scalp. They are raised and warty-looking, with a brown to murky yellow color, with a little blackhead within. Some patients have many of them. When scraped off, they usually won't recur. If they don't bother you, simply leave them alone.

Skin tags (papilloma). Cause is unknown. These little outpatchings of skin typically occur in groups under the arms, on the sides of the neck, and on the cheeks. Leave them alone, or have your doctor cut or burn them off.

Syringomas. These papules also come in groups, mostly in women, under the eyes or on each side of the nose. These are tiny tumors caused by enlargement of a sweat duct. Leave them alone.

Histiocytomas. They usually occur singly near the knees, elbows, or hips. They come from skin cells called histiocytes. No problem.

Brown spots (liver spots). They usually appear with increasing age, and particularly occur in blondes and thin-skinned people. If you have a few, they can be burned off by a doctor with an electric needle. If you have a great number, they can be removed with dermabrasion or a chemical peel. Sometimes taking supplements of vitamin C and E and niacin will make them disappear.

SOME NEW TREATMENTS AGAINST CANCER THAT ARE SHOWING ENCOURAGING RESULTS

A special heat treatment is shrinking cancer tumors in more than two-thirds of advanced cancer patients. The bodies of the patients are heated to 108° with tubes of heated gas and a heated water blanket, or by radiofrequency heating. Even in those whose tumors did not shrink or disappear, there was less pain and a gain of weight after treatment, researchers say. The treatment is being used at the University of New Mexico School of Medicine, the V.A. Hospital in Brooklyn, N.Y., and in Edinburgh, Scotland, and Newcastle, England.

Vitamin C as a cancer fighter looks promising from several studies being done, including those at the National Cancer Institute in Washington and Loch Lomonside in Scotland. The vitamin C was shown to increase the body's natural defense system. Terminal cancer patients taking it lived four times longer than those who did not.

Vitamin A may be effective against some types

of cancer, too. Scientists at Vanderbilt University, The National Cancer Institute, and Albert Einstein College of Medicine have shown that vitamin A in large doses in mice aids in both preventing and treating cancers. At Emory University, Dr. Stephen Kreitaman finds patients with oral cancer usually had much too little or much too much vitamin A. In Norway men who smoke and have a deficiency of vitamin A have cancer more than men who smoke but do not have low vitamin A. Doctors in Norway recommend that smokers take regular vitamin A supplements.

A new drug treatment using platinum is proving highly effective against cancer of the testes, bringing about complete disappearance of cancer in two-thirds of patients. As part of the treatment, the patient drinks a great deal of water and a sugar called mannitol, which cuts down side effects and allows doctors to increase doses of the platinum to kill the cancer.

Giving drugs after cancer surgery to mop up any remaining cancer cells is proving useful in treatment of breast cancer in Italy. A three-drug-punch of cytoxan, fluorouracil, and methotrexate has proved especially helpful. In the United States similar treatment has increased survival rate after surgery on patients with cancer of the colon and rectum.

A bacterium by the name of BCG, long known for increasing the body's immunity to tuberculosis, now is apparently working to clear up cancer cells left in the body after surgery or drug treatment. BCG inoculations given once a week are being used in patients with several forms of cancer, including leukemia, at the Institute of Cancerology and Immunogenetics at Bellejuif, near Paris. In patients given BCG, more than a third were still free from any recurrences for 7 to 10 years when last tested. All patients who did not receive the BCG had gone back to the hospital with relapses.

A new four-drug combination treatment for advanced Hodgkin's disease has proven effective against some cases of this serious illness that had previously defied other drug treatments. According to the American Medical Association, the new combination is known as BVDS, for the first letter of the name of each drug used. The older treatment is known as MOPP.

A drug called Orgotein has been able to eliminate side effects often caused by radiation used in treating cancer, allowing larger doses of radiation to be used. So far the drug—a natural enzyme—has been used most successfully in cancers of the bladder and the cervix at Karolinska Institute in Stockholm and at the University of Innsbruck in Austria, says the World Health Organization. (The drug was also evaluated for other urologic problems by Dr. Joseph D. Schmidt, of the University of California, San Diego. He says the drug has been of benefit in chronic cystitis, prostatitis, Peyronie's disease, benign prostatic hyperplasia, and interstitial cystitis.)

Marijuana has also been shown to be effective for mitigating side effects of cancer therapy. It helps control nausea and vomiting after chemotherapy, says Dr. Norman Zinberg of Harvard Medical School.

THE BIG STEW OVER NITRITES

Nitrates and nitrites originally were put in cured meats such as bacon, lunch meat, frankfurters, bologna, salami, corned beef, and smoked fish to protect against botulism, but now research shows that when the nitrites and nitrates combine with amines naturally found in the body, they form nitrosamines which are powerful cancer-causing agents. Note: Recent research indicates vitamin C may be able to prevent this nitrosamine formation.

Bacon, untreated with additives, is available from Nodine's, in Goshen, Conn., or from Balducci's, 424 Avenue of the Americas, New York, N.Y. It has a shorter shelf life, so buy only a week's supply at a time.

THE UNDERGROUND MEDICINES FOR CANCER

Some medicines used in other countries are not approved in the United States. However many doctors consider them worthwhile and give them despite disapproval by the American Medical Association and the F.D.A. Many patients buy the medicines in other countries and bring them to the U.S. Others go to clinics in the other countries for treatment.

The major undergound cancer medicines are:

Laetrile, also called vitamin B-17 or amygdalin. It is a substance that occurs naturally in apricot pits, cherry and other fruit seeds and in cassava and kidney beans.

Hydrazine sulfate. A chemical used for rocket fuel during the 1960s, it has recently been found effective against cancer, and received an "Investigational New Drug" classification by the F.D.A., which means that certain doctors can use it experimentally.

Enzymes. These are used in conjunction with other treatments, especially in Germany and in Mexico. A few doctors use them in the United States.

Krebiozen. This is the substance developed in Illinois that aroused such controversy. It is banned from interstate shipment, and is not used very much at this time, although those involved still claim it helps.

THE MOST USED
UNDERGROUND MEDICINE

This is laetrile. Tens of thousands of people in the United States are estimated to use it. It is approved in 23 other countries. It is not considered a cure-all by the doctors who use it, who say they get about the same percentage of remissions as with other conventional treatments. However, they stress that with laetrile, there are no side effects, and even in terminal patients, it eliminates pain and gives a feeling of strength and euphoria.

Some 800 physicians in the U.S. are estimated to be now prescribing it. Most physicians who give it simply call it a food supplement instead of a cancer treatment. At the time *Whole Health Catalogue* went to press, seven states had legalized use of laetrile (Indiana, Alaska, Arizona, Washington, Texas, Florida, and Nevada). Doctors prescribing laetrile don't use it alone, but in conjunction with a total nutrition program.

The two clinics using laetrile the most are those of Dr. Ernesto Contreras in Tiajuana, Mexico, and Dr. Hans Nieper in Hanover, Germany. More specific information about where to get laetrile in an area near you can be obtained from the Cancer Control Society, 2043 North Berendo, Los Angeles, Calif. 90027.

WELL-KNOWN CANCER CENTERS

There are 19 institutions designated Comprehensive Cancer Centers by the National Cancer Institute; they provide the most advanced treatment now available in the United States against the disease. To win this designation, a treatment center must have advanced diagnostic and treatment methods, support of a strong research program, and an organized cancer detection program. They must also participate in an integrated nationwide system of prevention, diagnosis, and treatment. These designated centers also help other hospitals, and often make recommendations on treatment, especially in chemotherapy and radiotherapy. Those that have 800 toll-free telephone numbers listed have cancer hotline information centers staffed by trained volunteers who will answer, confidentially, any questions about cancer you might have. Each center also has a directory of cancer-related services and resources in the area. In addition, at each center a group of professionals provides telephone consultation services for other health professionals.

Colorado Regional Cancer Center
Denver, Colo. 80220
(800) 332-1850
Comprehensive Cancer Center of the State of Florida
University of Miami School of Medicine
Miami, Fla. 33152
(800) 432-5953
Duke University Comprehensive Cancer Center
Durham, N.C. 27710
(800) 672-0943
Fox-Chase/University of Pennsylvania Comprehensive Cancer Center
Philadelphia, Pa. 19174
(800) 822-3963; (800) 523-3586
Fred Hutchinson Cancer Research Center
University of Washington
Seattle, Wash. 98195
(800) 292-6301
Georgetown University-Howard University Comprehensive Cancer Center (two branches):
Georgetown University
3900 Reservoir Road, N.W.
Washington, D.C. 20007
Howard University Cancer Center
520 W Street, N.W.
Washington, D.C. 20059
Illinois Cancer Council (three branches):
(800) 972-0586
Northwestern University Cancer Center
303 East Chicago Avenue
Chicago, Ill. 60611
University of Chicago Cancer Research Center
2020 West Ogden Avenue
Chicago, Ill. 60612
Rush-Presbyterian-St. Luke's Hospital
1753 West Congress Parkway
Chicago, Ill. 60612
Johns Hopkins Oncology Center
601 North Broadway
Baltimore, Md. 21205
(800) 492-1444
Mayo Comprehensive Cancer Center
Rochester, Minn. 55901
(800) 582-5262
Memorial Sloan-Kettering Cancer Center
1275 York Avenue
New York, N.Y. 10021
Ohio State University Comprehensive Cancer Center
370 West Ninth Avenue
Columbus, Ohio 43210
Roswell Park Memorial Institute
666 Elm Street
Buffalo, N.Y. 14203
(800) 462-7255
Sidney Farber Comprehensive Cancer Center
Harvard University School of Medicine
Boston, Mass. 02115
(800) 952-7420

University of Alabama Comprehensive Cancer Center
    University Station
      Birmingham, Ala. 35294
UCLA Comprehensive Cancer Center
    Los Angeles, Calif. 90024
University of Southern California—LAC Cancer Center
    2025 Zonal Avenue
    Los Angeles, Calif. 90033
    (800) 252-9066
University of Texas M.D. Anderson Hospital and Tumor
    Institute
    6723 Bertner Avenue
    Houston, Tex. 77025
    (800) 392-2040
University of Wisconsin Clinical Cancer Center
    1300 University Avenue
    Madison, Wis. 53706
    (800) 362-8038
Yale University Comprehensive Cancer Center
    789 Howard Avenue
    New Haven, Conn. 06504
    (800) 922-0824

THE CANCER CLINIC THAT MANY CALL THE BEST IN THE WORLD

A clinic that is using conventional methods as well as so-called underground methods is the Janker Radiation Clinic in Bonn, West Germany. Some authorities say the clinic is getting the best results of any program around.

In addition to conventional chemotherapy and radiation treatments, the Janker Clinic uses these techniques:

Isophosphamide, a cancer drug much stronger than others but which has had many side effects. The clinic devised ways to counteract the side effects.

A high concentrate vitamin A emulsion. This is a new way to give vitamin A in strong enough doses to combat cancer, yet avoids the usual side effects of such strong doses.

Enzymes. These are used in a number of other clinics also, and are particularly good to treat cancers of the pancreas and to stabilize remissions of other cancers.

The clinic has about 100 hospitalized patients, and 150 outpatients. For the first three or four weeks intensive chemotherapy is used which gives some discomfort, the clinic director told us, but after that the patient is treated on an outpatient basis, then returns to the United States with a supply of prescribed medicines.

Diabetes

DIABETES—THE GROWING LIFE-THREATENING MENACE

Diabetes has suddenly moved up from the seventh to the third leading cause of death.

Doctors were astounded to learn last year that the prevalance of diabetes in the U.S. increased by more than 50 percent in the last 10 years and it is still increasing.

Many scientists believe the skyrocketing increase of diabetes is due to our huge increase in the intake of sugar. Diabetes invariably appears in a culture about twenty years after sugar and refined starches are introduced to the diet.

These scientists believe that hypoglycemia is actually the beginning stage of diabetes from this overload of sugar, and that treatment of the disease in its early hypoglycemia stage by changing the diet can actually prevent diabetes from occurring. (See Chapter 5 for the diet to treat hypoglycemia.)

THE TWO MAJOR KINDS OF DIABETES YOU SHOULD KNOW ABOUT

Juvenile diabetes, also called brittle diabetes, accounts for about 30 percent of cases. Despite its name, it can occur in adults as well as children. People with this form of the disease can produce no insulin of their own at all and must have insulin injections every day.

Adult diabetes, also known as maturity-onset diabetes, is usually less serious. It sometimes needs insulin injections, but often can be managed by diet alone.

PERSONS AT HIGH RISK WHO SHOULD HAVE A DIABETES TEST EVERY YEAR

Those who are:

- Overweight
- Over age 40
- Blood relatives of diabetics
- Women who have given birth to large babies (over nine pounds)

DIABETES WARNING SIGNS

If you have any of these warning signs, get tested immediately:

- Drowsiness, fatigue
- Sudden listlessness, loss of strength and energy

- Boils and carbuncles
- Intense itching
- Cuts and bruises slow to heal
- Finger and toe pain
- Excessive thirst
- Excessive appetite
- Poor vision
- Extreme weight loss
- Infected corns and bunions
- Frequent urination

THE BEST TEST FOR DIABETES

A urine test will detect most cases of diabetes. Clinistix, available at your drugstore without prescription, show whether your body is spilling sugar into the urine. Clinitest and Tes-Tape, also available at your drugstore, also give some indication of the amount of sugar being spilled. They work by changing color when exposed to drops of urine. A blood test done in the doctor's office is even more accurate.

DIET CONTROL

Several doctors, including Dr. Robert Atkins, Dr. Leon Smelos, and Dr. George Blackburn, claim excellent results in diabetics with a low-carbohydrate, no-sugar hypoglycemia diet. The American Diabetes Association recommends a higher carbohydrate diet. For a copy of both diets, see list in the right-hand column.

Diabetics should take a vitamin and mineral tablet that provides at least 15 mg of zinc per day, since insulin is a zinc enzyme.

EIGHT ESSENTIAL RULES IF YOU ARE A DIABETIC

1. Don't eat anything with sugar.
2. Eat on time, don't skip meals.
3. Exercise; physical activity helps control diabetes by increasing the use of sugar by body, even allowing diabetics to cut insulin dose.
4. Get adequate rest and sleep.
5. Take good care of your feet. Wash and dry them thoroughly daily to avoid infection.
6. Have eyes checked regularly.
7. See your doctor regularly.
8. Carry a special identification card, as shown in the back of the book.

NEW TREATMENTS FOR DIABETIC EYE PROBLEMS

Sometimes in diabetes, tiny blood vessels grow into the eyes, rupturing, so that the eyeball fills with blood and vision is blocked. This is called diabetic retinopathy.

When the bleeding first begins, doctors can use a sharply focused laser beam to get rid of the excess blood vessels. This reduces by almost two-thirds the number of eyes that go blind.

If bleeding has already blocked sight, a new operation called a vitrectomy can be performed in which the blood is removed and a clear solution put in. The new technique is being studied in 13 hospitals across the U.S. Your eye doctor can refer you to one of them.

CLINICS SPECIALIZING IN DIABETES

Cleveland Clinic
    2020 East 93rd Street
    Cleveland, Ohio 44106
Mt. Sinai Medical Center
    100th Street and Fifth Avenue
    New York, N.Y. 10029
Joslin Clinic
    15 Joslin Road
    Boston, Mass. 02215
Mayo Clinic
    200 First Street, S.W.
    Rochester, Minn. 55902
Mason Clinic
    118 Ninth Avenue
    Seattle, Wash. 98101

RECOMMENDED

Facts About Diabetes
    American Diabetes Association
    18 East 48th Street
    New York, N.Y. 10017
    25¢
        Also publishes a magazine for diabetics, the new recommended diet, and a list of summer camps for diabetic children.
Diabetes: Don't Gamble with Your Health
    Office of Information
    National Institute of Arthritis and Metabolic Diseases
    Bethesda, Md. 20014
Dr. Atkins' Superenergy Diet
    Crown Publishers
    1 Park Ave.
    New York, N.Y. 10016
    $9.95
How to Live with Diabetes
    Henry Dolger and Bernard Seeman
    W. W. Norton
    500 Fifth Avenue
    New York, N.Y. 10036
    $6.50
Feast on a Diabetic Diet
    Euell Gibbons and Joe Gibbons
    David McKay Company
    750 Third Avenue
    New York, N.Y. 10017
    $7.95
        A collection of recipes and advice.

Toward Good Control, Guidebook for the Diabetic Patient
    Ames Company
    Division of Miles Laboratories, Inc.
    Elkhart, Ind. 46514
    Free
Taking Care of Diabetes
    Superintendent of Documents
    Washington, D.C. 20402
    20¢
A Body Map
    Baptist Hospitals Foundation
    Birmingham, Ala. 35222
        200 alternate injection locations

High Blood Pressure

LIFE EXPECTANCY AND HIGH BLOOD PRESSURE

High blood pressure may be *the* leading single risk factor in causing *all* disability and death in the United States today. From 23 to 40 million people in the United States are estimated to have it.

Of these, less than 50 percent know that they have it.

There's no way to tell whether you have high blood pressure without being checked. You can feel healthy and look terrific, but still be living with the hidden time bomb doing internal damage to your body. The major complications it causes are stroke, heart failure, and kidney failure.

You can live a normal life even if you have high blood pressure, as long as you take steps to keep it down.

At all ranges, those with lower blood pressures live longer than those with higher pressures.

You can determine what your life expectancy is at any given age and at any given blood pressure in the following table:

	MEN		
	Blood Pressure	Expected Age	Loss in Life Expectancy
AGE 35	Normal	76½	—
	130/90	72½	4
	140/95	67½	9
	150/100	60	16½
AGE 45	Normal	77	—
	130/90	74	3
	140/95	71	6
	150/100	60	11½
AGE 55	Normal	78½	—
	130/90	77½	1
	140/95	74½	4
	150/100	72½	6

	WOMEN		
	Blood Pressure	Expected Age	Loss in Life Expectancy
AGE 45	Normal	82	—
	130/90	80½	1½
	140/95	77	5
	150/100	73½	8½
AGE 55	Normal	82½	—
	130/90	82	½
	140/95	79½	3
	150/100	78½	4

YOUR BLOOD PRESSURE READING

The top number is the systolic pressure—the amount of pressure when your heart is contracting. The bottom number is the diastolic pressure—it is the pressure that is constantly present in your arteries when your heart is resting between beats.

The following classifications for blood pressure are generally accepted by medical authorities:

Normal pressure: Systolic (upper number) pressure of 100-140; diastolic (lower number) pressure of 60-90.

Borderline or mild hypertension: Systolic pressure of 140-160; diastolic pressure of 90-95.

Moderate hypertension: Systolic pressure of 160-180; diastolic pressure of 96-114.

Marked hypertension: Systolic pressure above 180; diastolic pressure above 115.

HYPERTENSION

Hypertension is another name for high blood pressure. It does not mean being tense and nervous. It means high tension (pressure) of blood within the arteries.

HOW TO BRING HIGH BLOOD PRESSURE DOWN

- Exercise regularly.
- Cut salt and sugar intake drastically.
- Don't eat licorice; it raises blood pressure.
- Stop smoking.
- Take blood pressure medication.

Recent medical articles report that yoga, biofeedback techniques, progressive relaxation, and meditation have also helped many people reduce their blood pressure, often making it possible to reduce the doses of blood pressure drugs that they were taking.

High cadmium levels are associated with high blood pressure. Cadmium is found in cigarettes, tea, and coffee. Increasing zinc intake will usually reduce cadmium.

THE HIGH BLOOD PRESSURE PILLS AND HOW THEY WORK

The most used medications are the thiazides and their relatives, and reserpine, methyldopa, hydralazine. Guanethidine and diazoxide are used in extremely severe situations. Some of these act as diuretics, flushing excess fluid from the body. Others act directly on the tiny arteries, causing them to relax and thus decrease pressure on the blood. And others act on the nervous system, blocking the nerves that go to the blood vessels.

Two very effective drugs available in Great Britain, but not the U.S., are practolol and guanoxan. They sometimes work in persons who do not respond to other drugs.

WHAT TO DO IF YOU HAVE SIDE EFFECTS

Be patient for a few weeks. If you keep taking the drug, the side effects often disappear.

Have your doctor switch you to a different brand or to a different medication. Keep working to get the best medication and the best dosages and the least side effects.

Try taking the pills at a different time of day if your doctor approves.

Work on the other factors such as obesity, smoking, salt, exercise, and relaxation so you may be able to reduce dosage of pills.

If you are dizzy in the morning or when you stand up suddenly, get out of bed slowly, avoid sudden or prolonged standing, don't exercise strenuously for the first few weeks, sit down until the dizziness passes, wear support stockings. Your doctor may be able to reduce your dosage.

If your mouth is dry, you feel weak or have muscle pains, cramps, or abdominal distress, ask your doctor about taking potassium supplements.

If you have depression or other mood disturbances, contact your doctor immediately so he can change medicine.

IF YOU ARE ON BIRTH CONTROL PILLS

If you have high blood pressure and are taking a birth control pill, use another contraceptive for some months and see if your blood pressure goes down. If so, stay off the pill permanently. If your blood pressure does not come down, then you probably can, if you wish, continue taking the pill (your doctor will tell you).

All women who are just starting to take birth control pills should have their blood pressure checked about every two months for the first year.

ARE HIGH BLOOD PRESSURE PILLS SAFE FOR THE PREGNANT WOMAN?

High blood pressure in a pregnant woman is not only hazardous to *her* health, but is also hazardous to her fetus. It is important for the pregnant woman to keep her blood pressure down, but few studies have been done to determine whether blood pressure pills are safe for the fetus. Now studies in England and Ireland indicate that the pills are safe. Half a group of pregnant hypertensive women were given the blood pressure drug methyldopa, the other half were given nothing. Of the untreated group, nine lost their babies, compared to only one loss among those who took the medication. No ill effects were found in the babies whose mothers were treated.

RECOMMENDED:

The National High Blood Pressure Information Center
    120/80 National Institute of Health
    Bethesda, Md. 20014
        Brochures, films, charts, exhibits, and speakers.
High Blood Pressure: What Causes It, How to Tell If You Have It; How to Control It for a Longer Life
    Frank A. Finnerty, Jr./David McKay Co.
    750 Third Ave., New York, N.Y. 10017 $9.95

SOME CLINICS THAT TREAT HIGH BLOOD PRESSURE
Arizona Department of Health Services, Hypertension Section
    1750 West Adams Street
    Phoenix, Ariz. 85007
Cleveland Clinic, Hypertension Clinic
    9500 Euclid Avenue
    Cleveland, Ohio 44106
District of Columbia General Hospital, Hypertension Clinic
    19th and Massachusetts Avenues
    Washington, D.C. 20003
Georgia Department of Human Resources
    618 Ponce de Leon Avenue
    Atlanta, Ga. 30308
Hypertension Screening and Education Project
    2201 Steiner Street
    San Francisco, Calif. 94115
Multnomah Department of Human Services
    5022 North Vancouver Avenue
    Portland, Ore. 97217
University of Minnesota Hospital, Hypertension Clinic
    412 Union Street, S.E.
    Minneapolis, Minn. 55455
University of Mississippi Medical Center
    2500 North State Street
    Jackson, Miss. 39216
Wake County Memorial Hospital, Hypertension Clinic
    3000 New Bern Avenue
    Raleigh, N.C. 27610

Note: Measuring devices can give an inaccurate reading if the arm band is not the correct length for your arm. Be particularly alert if you are obese. The arm band should be long enough to completely encircle your upper arm.

CHAPTER 4

The Whole Health Diet—The Vital Diet to Your Health

A number of nutrition specialists, including those in the U.S. government's own Department of Agriculture, say that hundreds of thousands of lives would be saved each year with better nutrition.

Some of the nutritionists estimate that heart disease would be reduced by 25 to 50 percent, cancer would be reduced by 20 to 40 percent, the cure rate for schizophrenia would increase by 500 percent, individual IQ and mental alertness would increase, with an increase of about 10 points for persons who now have IQs of only 70 to 80, arthritis would be improved in millions, dental problems would be reduced by 50 percent. There would be significant reductions or improvements in diabetes, osteoporosis, alcoholism, eyesight, allergies, digestive problems, kidney troubles, and muscular disorders. People would live longer, and stay younger longer with less impairment and less fatigue. Their bodies would awake to total sexual fulfillment. There would be fewer birth defects and reproductive problems. People would be happier, less moody and irritable.

DO YOU OR YOUR FAMILY HAVE ANY OF THE FOLLOWING HEALTH PROBLEMS?

In an amazing number of cases they respond to simple diet changes.

- Alcoholism
- Allergies
- Anxiety
- Asthma
- Behavior problems
- Blurred vision
- Colitis
- Convulsions
- Dental caries
- Depression
- Diabetes
- Diverticulosis
- Dizziness
- Edema
- Fatigue
- Gallstones
- Gout
- Headache
- Heart disease
- Heartburn
- Hiatal hernia
- High blood pressure
- Hypoglycemia
- Indigestion
- Insomnia
- Irritability
- Leg cramps
- Meniere's disease
- Mood swings
- Painful menstruation
- Palpitations of the heart
- Peptic ulcer
- Premenstrual tension
- Prostate problems
- Sexual problems

- Shakiness
- Skin problems
- Tendency to infections such as colds, urinary tract infections, boils, abscesses, appendicitis
- Ulcers
- Underachieving

If you have any of these conditions, you might consider it worthwhile to try a nutritional approach. Obviously there are many causes for these conditions, so nutrition therapy will not help all cases. But some people find improvement great, even to the point of completely curing the problem, or to the point of being able to lower dosages of medicines they are taking; others report only a slight benefit, or none at all.

THE VITAL DIET

This diet plan has been carefully designed to take advantage of every bit of solid advice from modern nutrition researchers, to incorporate every bit of diet and nutrition research that has been shown to be able to keep you healthy and feeling good.

THE SIX STEPS THAT YOU MUST TAKE TO MAKE THE DIET WORK

1. Stop, *completely stop,* eating sugar in all forms. That means eat no sugar or food or drink containing sugar. (See list of foods containing hidden sugars later in this chapter.)

2. Stop, *completely stop,* eating refined starches. That means no white bread, white rice, macaroni, spaghetti. But you *can* and should eat high roughage whole unrefined grains such as brown or wild rice, whole wheat, and other whole grain products.

3. Eat many fruits and vegetables, as fresh as possible, instead of frozen, canned, or precooked. Eat raw, or if you cook, cook until just tender with as little water as possible.

4. Use a moderate amount of fats and oils.

5. Limit coffee, tea, and colas to no more than 3 cups per day. Limit alcohol to moderate amounts, and special occasions.

6. Take a daily supplement of vitamins and minerals as closely geared to your own needs as you can determine from what we describe to you on the following pages. Keep up these vitamin and mineral supplements on a regular basis.

YOU *MAY* EAT ANY OF THESE FOODS

- Fish of all kinds, including shellfish, molluscs, and water-packed canned fish
- Poultry of all kinds, including chicken, turkey, wild fowl (broil, bake, or roast)
- Veal, lamb, beef, pork, ham, liver and other organ meats (use lean cuts; broil, bake, or roast)
- Hard cheeses, pot cheese, farmer cheese, low-calorie cottage cheese, yogurt
- Eggs, any style
- Nearly all vegetables, including asparagus, artichokes, avocado, beans, beets, broccoli, brussels sprouts, cabbage, carrots, cauliflower, celery, chard, chives, corn, cucumbers, eggplants, greens, kale, kohlrabi, leeks, lentils, lettuce, mushrooms, onions, okra, papaya, parsley, parsnips, peppers, pumpkin, radishes, rhubarb, sauerkraut, sorrel, spinach, squash, tomatoes, zucchini
- Nuts, seeds, coconut, peanut butter
- Fruits, berries, melons of all kinds
- Potatoes with skins on (baked or boiled), brown or wild rice, yams
- Whole grain cereals, bran, wheat germ, brewer's yeast
- Whole grain breads and flour, such as 100 percent rye, stone-ground whole wheat, whole grain cornmeal, soy, whole grain buckwheat, whole grain crackers (like Triscuits)
- Any fluids without sugar (eight glasses a day) including water, milk, fresh lemonade (no sugar), cranberry, orange, and tomato juice

The larger the variety of these foods you eat the better.

YOU *MAY NOT* EAT ANY OF THESE

- Bacon with nitrites, lunch meat with nitrites, sausage with nitrites
- Cake, pie, candy, cereal with sugar, chewing gum with sugar, cookies, ice cream, jam, jelly, Kool-Aid, pastries, sweet pickles, sweet relish, syrups, soft drinks with sugar, sugar, or any food containing sugar
- White or any refined flour, white bread, soda crackers, macaroni, spaghetti, pancakes, waffles, white bread stuffing, white rice
- Hot spices
- Imitation and synthetic junk foods

The Vital Diet is an easy diet to follow. You don't have to give up all that much. The diet is simple, but it works. Try it.

After two weeks look again at the list of problems you checked over on pages 27–28 and see if the ones you were having have been improved.

TIPS FOR THE WHOLE HEALTH VITAL DIET OR ANY OTHER DIET

As in any diet see your doctor before you start, and after a few weeks see him again to see what the diet is doing to your cholesterol, triglycerides, blood pressure, and other health indicators. In any diet you should work with your doctor in using it.

Side effects can occur with even the simplest and best diets. But nearly always these happen only during the first two or three days. Stick to the new diet; by the fourth day you will feel better.

Check with your doctor whether your new diet will change the dosage of any medication you are taking. You may, for example, need less diuretics, or a lower dosage of a blood pressure pill.

Vitamins and diet work together. One often won't work without the other. Make sure you follow the Vital Diet as well as take vitamin and mineral supplements, especially those on the "Ten Most Lacking" list (pages 32–35).

No one thing works for everybody. If at any time you have a bad reaction to a change in diet or to a vitamin, simply stop using it.

THE FOOD EXCHANGE PLAN

IF YOU HAVE BEEN USING	USE INSTEAD
Meat with fat	Meat, lean
Beef or chicken pot pie	Broiled chicken
Hot dog	Tuna in water
Lunch meats with nitrites	Left-over meats of your own
Oil-packed food	Water-packed food
Hydrogenated fats or oils	Unhydrogenated vegetable oils
Oleomargarine	Sour cream or sweet cream butter
White bread	High protein, whole wheat, rye or gluten bread
Chocolate	Carob pod or St. John's bread
White rice	Brown rice, wild rice, or bean sprouts
Pearled barley	Whole grain barley
Bread stuffing	Vegetable stuffing
Refined wheat flour	Soya flour (use ½ amount wheat flour called for in recipe) or whole wheat, whole grain rye, whole grain buckwheat, cornmeal

IF YOU HAVE BEEN USING	USE INSTEAD
Sherbet	Fruit slush or fresh fruit ice
Junk cereal	Whole grain or home-cooked cereals
Coffee	Decaffeinated coffee or weak tea
Sugar	Fructose or artificial sweetener
Canned or precooked foods	Fresh foods

MAKING THE PLAN WORK AT HOLIDAY TIME

Use plenty of vegetables and greens. If you serve hors d'oeuvres, use raw vegetables.

Instead of eggnog, serve a low-calorie punch.

Instead of bread stuffing, serve a vegetable stuffing or sprouts.

Instead of pie—heaped fresh fruit.

Plan an activity after Thanksgiving or Christmas dinner, at the very least a brisk walk outdoors.

If you're going to somebody else's party, don't use it as an excuse to eat improperly. Concentrate on people and conversation.

Keep away from the candies and pastries, concentrate on meats and salads. Eat the cheese wedge, leave the cracker. Eat the fruit cup, leave the syrup.

Don't be on the clean-up squad if that makes you eat more.

If you have cocktails, dilute them with water or juices; refill your drink with ice frequently to make it last longer. Drink juice or water . . . nobody needs to know what's in your glass.

HOW TO KEEP YOUR DIET IN A FAST-FOOD JOINT

If you're in Arthur Treacher's or Long John Silver's, eat the fish, but hold the chips.

If you're in Burger Chef, Burger King, White Castle, or McDonald's, eat the hamburger and cheese, but don't eat the bun, the fries, or catsup.

If you're in Colonel Sanders' or Gino's, eat the chicken and cole slaw, but ignore the mashed potatoes and the rolls.

At the Pizza Hut, eat the pizza, but leave the crust.

At the Steak House, eat the steak and salad, and skip the rolls.

In all of them, skip the shakes and sugar sodas, and have a diet drink or iced tea with lemon.

VITAMINS AND MINERALS THE NUTRITION RESEARCHERS RECOMMEND THAT YOU TAKE

We have surveyed the recommendations of the supernutritionists and have come up with recommendations that show the range of the vitamin and mineral doses that they themselves take and prescribe for their patients.

THREE WONDER-FOOD SUPPLEMENTS YOU MAY WANT TO ADD TO YOUR DIET

BREWER'S YEAST

Contains 17 different vitamins, 16 amino acids, 14 minerals. There are some medical reports that it prevents cancer of the liver in rats and is effective in treating infectious hepatitis. It comes plain or in flavors. Stir a tablespoon into a glass of tomato juice, fruit juice, milk, or sprinkle over salad or cereal. (If you are a beginner, start with half a teaspoon or less, and build up gradually to avoid the indigestion and gas that sometimes occurs when your digestive system is not used to it.) If you are trying to lose weight, take it 15 minutes before meals.

WHEAT GERM

The heart of the seed of the wheat, wheat germ is sifted out in the manufacture of most flour. Experimental evidence indicates it will lower cholesterol, improve fertility, lower complications of pregnancy and childbirth, and improve energy levels. Many nutritionists think it may contain vita-

VITAMIN/ MINERAL	RANGE OF DAILY DOSES MOST OFTEN USED	MAKING YOUR OWN INDIVIDUAL ADJUSTMENT
Vitamin A	10,000 to 25,000 International Units	If you eat liver or sweet potatoes twice a week, you can eliminate this supplement. You need more A if you take large amounts of E.
Vitamin B_1* (Thiamine)	10 to 300 mg	Use in equal amounts as other B vitamins.
Vitamin B_2* (Riboflavin)	10 to 300 mg	Use higher amounts if you don't eat red meat or dairy products regularly.
Vitamin B_3* (Niacin, Niacinamide, Nicotinic acid)	50 to 1000 mg	Use with caution if you have glaucoma, severe diabetes, impaired liver function, or peptic ulcer.
Vitamin B_5* (Pantothenic acid)	10 to 300 mg	Use in equal amounts as other B vitamins, or more; some prefer twice as much as B_1 or B_2.
Vitamin B_6* (Pyridoxine)	10 to 600 mg	Test the higher amounts if you take estrogen or have edema or achy joints.
Vitamin B_{12}* (Cyanocobalamin)	5 to 100 micrograms	If you have dandruff, scaly eyebrows and ears, and are fatigued, you may need vitamin B_{12} injections instead of pills.
Vitamin C (Ascorbic acid)	500 mg to 4 grams	Be sure the tablet includes bioflavinoids, rutin, and hesperidin, sometimes labeled "citrus salts." Start with 500 mg. Build higher if you smoke, have canker sores, or bruise easily. Cut back dosage if diarrhea occurs. If you are diabetic or a heart patient, check with your doctor, since vitamin C may necessitate a lower dosage of pills. Be sure to take adequate amounts of vitamin B_{12} when taking C.
Vitamin D	400 to 1000 International Units	Vitamin D can be toxic. People with heart disorders should use with particular caution. Toxicity signs are unusual thirst, urinary urgency, vomiting, and diarrhea. Use lower quantities if you get a lot of sun.

*Note: No vitamin B should be taken alone, but should be taken in conjunction with other vitamin Bs. A convenient way to take it is a *Vitamin B 50-Complex*. Make sure your vitamin preparation also contains biotin, inositol, folic acid, choline, and para-aminobenzoic acid (PABA).

mins and minerals that have not been discovered yet since it gives benefits in laboratory animals beyond the benefits of known vitamins. Sprinkle on cereal, casserole dishes, meatloaf, hamburgers, fruit, use in drinks, as coating on fish and meat, on yogurt, and even as a substitute for some of the flour called for in baking. Keep tightly capped in a cool place.

YOGURT

Contains high-quality protein, calcium, vitamin B_6, and provides bacteria that will restore your normal digestive bacteria and often help digestive disorders, canker sores, and other problems.

Yogurt can be eaten plain, seasoned with herbs, mixed with fruit. Don't buy kinds that have sugar added. It can be made with whole or skim milk, goat milk, or soy milk.

WHY YOU SHOULD ELIMINATE SUGAR

Sugar has been reported to:

- Shorten the life span of laboratory animals by one-fourth
- Reduce growth rate
- Cause weight gain
- Cause bouts of fatigue
- Increase the need for certain vitamins and minerals, especially thiamine and chromium
- Increase blood pressure
- Help cause hypoglycemia and diabetes

VITAMIN/ MINERAL	RANGE OF DAILY DOSES MOST OFTEN USED	MAKING YOUR OWN INDIVIDUAL ADJUSTMENT
Vitamin E (Tocopherol)	200 to 1200 International Units	Vitamin E should be used with caution in people with overactive thyroids, diabetes, high blood pressure, or rheumatic heart disease, starting at very low dosages and building up or down gradually. Build higher if you have vascular problems or menopause symptoms. If you decide to decrease the amount of vitamin E you are taking, decrease the amount in gradual steps.
Folic acid	1 to 6 mg	The higher amounts are usually needed by women on estrogen, in persons who get canker sores, in those with decreased sexual desire, in those with arthritis, and in those who drink consistently. Often low in pregnancy.
Iodine	.1 to 10 mg	Too much can be as dangerous as the too little that can cause goiter.
Manganese	1 to 5 mg	Be sure to take if you have dizziness, tender eyeballs, poor memory.
Magnesium	2 to 800 mg	You need the higher amounts if you drink heavily, or use estrogen; lower amounts if you eat lots of nuts, seeds, and dark green vegetables, and live where the water is hard. Should be about one-half calcium intake.
Potassium	2 mg	Potassium levels may be low on low-carbohydrate diets or on diuretics.
Copper	2 mg or less	Be sure not to get too much since it can cause depression, insomnia, headache.
Zinc	1 to 30 mg	Take the higher doses if you are taking high amounts of vitamin B_6, are diabetic, alcoholic, or have chronic infections.
Iron	10 to 60 mg	Highest amounts needed in pregnant women. Should not be taken by persons with sickle cell anemia, thalassemia, or another blood disorder called hemochromatosis.
Calcium	800 to 2000 mg	Needed if your diet is low in cheese or milk or if you have hypoglycemia.
Phosphorus	Equal to amount of calcium	You need less on a high-protein diet.
Chromium	1 to 3 mg	You can take less if you use brewer's yeast regularly.

Note: Take vitamins with meals; iron between meals.

- Raise levels of cholesterol and triglycerides in the blood
- Predispose to skin problems, including acne, boils, and abscesses
- Predispose to gastrointestinal disorders and appendicitis
- Be statistically related to heart disease
- Cause tooth decay and spongy gums
- Raise the concentration in the blood of insulin, corticosteroids, and cortisol
- Increase the size of the liver and kidneys and cause changes in their cells
- Cause gallstones
- Produce atherosclerosis and thickened arteries
- Produce disturbed behavior of blood platelets and blood clotting
- Change the activity of several enzymes
- Increase acidity of gastric juice
- Decrease ability to fight infection

Eliminating sugar from your diet as completely as possible can help these problems in most people.

LOOK FOR HIDDEN SUGARS

There is sugar in: catsup, relish, soup, most canned vegetables and frozen foods, some peanut butter, canned meats, hot dogs, tartar sauce, soy sauce, table salt, and cheese dips.

Read labels. The following mean sugar: sucrose, dextrose, lactose, glucose, sorbitol, mannitol, dextrins, corn syrup, maple syrup, maltose. If the product says "cured" that means it has been cured with sugar. If it says "natural sweetener" or "nutritive sweetener" that means there is *sugar* in it; if it says "non-nutritive sweetener," that means it has *artificial* sweetener in it.

Ingredients are listed on labels in order of their ratio in the product. If sugar is listed first, the product contains more sugar than any other ingredient.

Anything labeled "fruit juice" is 100 percent natural juice. "Fruit drink" or "fruit punch" need be only 10 percent natural; the rest is usually water, sugar, flavorings.

THE TEN NUTRIENTS MOST LACKING IN THE AMERICAN DIET TODAY AND WHY YOU SHOULD BE TAKING THEM

Survey after survey has shown that in every social and economic class huge numbers of people are lacking enough vitamins and minerals. The vitamins and minerals most consistently found robbing them of good health: iron, folic acid, vitamin A, the B vitamins, vitamin C, vitamin E, magnesium, calcium, chromium, zinc.

Here are the vitally important facts you need to know about each of them.

IRON

According to surveys, at least one out of five men and women have an iron deficiency anemia; some doctors say even more. Nearly all pregnant women are deficient in iron. It is also the most prevalent nutritional disorder in U.S. children.

Common symptoms of iron deficiency are weakness, depression, dizziness, and fatigue.

Iron should *not* be taken by people who have sickle cell anemia, thalassemia, or another blood disease called hemochromatosis. If such people do get an overload of iron, it can be treated with a new drug called dihydroxybenzoic acid developed at Rockefeller University or with desferrioxamine.

FOLIC ACID

This vitamin B, which many people haven't even heard of yet, is low in at least one out of three women and men. Some surveys have shown a deficiency in *80 percent* of women.

Symptoms of folic acid deficiency: irritability, forgetfulness, weakness, fatigue, diarrhea, headache, palpitations, shortness of breath, moodiness, decreased sex drive.

People who especially need folic acid: women on estrogen-containing birth control pills or other estrogen, pregnant women, people who take large quantities of vitamin C, heavy drinkers.

In the U.S. you need a prescription for folic acid, except in very small amounts (less than .4 mg), and the largest pill you can buy even *with* a prescription is 1 mg. In Canada and several other countries you can buy the 5-mg size over the counter without a prescription at about one-tenth the cost.

Bonus from folic acid: It often increases sex response (some people call it frolic acid). Women taking estrogen for menopause find they can reduce or even eliminate estrogen, and still have no menopause symptoms if they take from 1 to 5 mg daily, experimenting to see what lowest dosage in that range gives them the desired response.

Folic acid should only be given with caution in patients with seizure disorders, and always with vitamin B_{12}.

VITAMIN A

The most common worldwide vitamin deficiency is of vitamin A. About one-third of the people in the world are deficient in vitamin A, surveys show. The problem is becoming worse since vitamin A is being destroyed by pesticides and food additives in increasing numbers.

You should suspect vitamin A deficiency if you have trouble seeing at night, or develop boils, dry rough skin, dry brittle hair, have increased susceptibility to infections, or dry itching eyes with swollen red lids and sensitivity to glare.

Vitamin A enhances the body's immune response and so helps fight infections. It helps prevent stress ulcer (serious bleeding from the stomach in patients undergoing surgery or other physical stress), so many physicians recommend that extra vitamin A be taken when a person has severe fever, bleeding, burns, injury, or surgery.

Don't take more than 10,000 units of vitamin A per day without seeing your physician for approval and frequent surveillance.

THE B VITAMINS

Research reports indicate that various B vitamins will:

- Improve mood, reduce irritability and tension
- Improve concentration
- Help eliminate side effects of estrogen
- Help smokers reduce their dependency on nicotine
- Allow reduced dosages of tranquilizers
- Help relieve the fatigue of hypoglycemia
- Help alleviate symptoms of schizophrenia

The B vitamins should be in balance with each other, so if you take more of one B vitamin you should be sure to have other B vitamins also.

B vitamins are available in vitamin-B-complex capsules without prescription, and in wheat germ, bran, brewer's yeast, and in liver, heart, and kidney meats.

WHO NEEDS VITAMIN B$_{12}$ SHOTS?

Most people don't, but the people who do have a deficiency of B$_{12}$ often have a great relief of fatigue for several weeks after taking the shots. If you do not respond to the shots, it means you have no B$_{12}$ deficiency.

People who often have a B$_{12}$ deficiency: vegetarians, women taking birth control pills, people who take large amounts of vitamin C, or the drug dilantin, or who consume alcohol in large quantities.

B$_{12}$ is usually given by injection instead of in capsules because in some people it is difficult to absorb.

VITAMIN C

The need for vitamin C is increased during and following serious illnesses, injury, intestinal bleeding, burns, surgery, or other physical or emotional stress situations. In severe burns or injuries vitamin C levels may fall rapidly to zero. Giving vitamin C shortens convalescent time and decreases wound problems, so many doctors recommend that extra C be taken during illness or stress, *especially before and after surgery*.

Vitamin C levels are especially low in women on birth control pills, in cigarette smokers, in people who take a great deal of aspirin. Vitamin C deficiency can be one of the causes of children or adults having frequent nosebleeds and should also be suspected if you have bleeding gums and easy bruising.

Other benefits from vitamin C shown by research:

- It prevents nitrosamine formation, the cancer-producing compound formed from nitrates and nitrites in meat preservatives.
- It helps neutralize some of the damaging effects of cigarette smoking.
- It lowers cholesterol and triglycerides and aids in treatment of atherosclerosis.
- It aids healing in heart disease.
- It can sometimes alleviate low back pain.
- It is part of the orthomolecular treatment of mental disorders, especially schizophrenia

Note: Before you go in for a physical, tell your doctor if you are taking large amounts of vitamin C, since the C can interfere with laboratory test results, drastically changing results in tests for sugar in the blood and urine and giving false negative results in tests for blood in stool specimens.

VITAMIN E

There is evidence that vitamin E retards aging in cells. Cells that normally have a life span of 50 reproductions have gone through 120 reproductive cycles with vitamin E and are still alive. There is no way to prove that this would occur in humans, but most researchers in the field of aging take vitamin E themselves. "You've got nothing to lose and everything to gain," says Dr. Denham Harman of the University of Nebraska.

Meanwhile, the other things that vitamin E does:

- Combats toxic effects of industrial pollutants, cigarette smoke, smog, and polyunsaturated fatty acids

- Has an anti-clotting effect, helping prevent blood clots after surgery
- Speeds wound healing
- Improves circulatory conditions, especially to the legs
- Has been reported of benefit in treating cysts of the breast
- Helps some skin conditions
- Helps combat hot flushes of menopause
- Helps normalize blood sugar

Note: Vitamin E can cause weight gain in some people. And it should be used with caution only on your doctor's approval if you have high blood pressure, diabetes, or a history of rheumatic fever.

MAGNESIUM

Magnesium is necessary for the absorption of other nutrients. Deficiencies occur especially in people who are heavy drinkers, use diuretics, have kidney disease, take estrogen pills, or have high intakes of vitamin D or high fat intake.

Marginal deficiencies can lead to atherosclerosis, depression, irritability, dizziness, muscle weakness, convulsions, high blood pressure, sweating, cold hands and feet, and upsets in heart rhythm.

Experimental research indicates the following about magnesium:

- It is important for a healthy heart (people have fewer heart attacks where there is hard water with magnesium in it)
- It helps protect against atherosclerosis
- It speeds recovery when given to patients with angina or even heart attacks
- It helps correct inflammation of the intestines

Note: it is important for magnesium to be balanced with the proper amount of calcium (one part magnesium to two parts of calcium). This is the proportion found in the mineral supplement dolomite, and in most general vitamin-mineral capsules.

CALCIUM

A part of aging for about one in four women and one in eight men is a form of bone deterioration called osteoporosis. The bone weakness causes the fractures that occur so often from minor falls in older people, as well as "dowager's hump," and back pain. The osteoporosis can usu-

ally be reversed by adding calcium to the diet, which increases bone density.

According to the U.S. Department of Agriculture, three out of every ten families has calcium intake below the recommended minimum. You probably get enough calcium if you drink a quart of milk a day or eat 30 ounces of cottage cheese or 4 ounces of hard cheese. Otherwise researchers believe you should take calcium supplements as a lifelong habit. They are obtainable in any drug and health store.

Bonus benefits from calcium supplements:

- Decrease in cholesterol
- Decrease in irritability and fatigue
- Help to hypoglycemia
- Elimination of radioactive strontium from the body
- Help for leg cramps

CHROMIUM

Nutrition researchers say almost everyone following the American diet probably is deficient in chromium, especially if they eat sugar, which causes a loss of chromium.

Chromium is believed to be important in the prevention of heart disease. It is also essential for the utilization of insulin, thus important to combat hypoglycemia. You find chromium in brewer's yeast, nuts, shellfish, and chicken. Supplement tablets are available in health food stores.

ZINC

Low zinc levels are found in patients with leg ulcers, diabetes, alcoholism, schizophrenia, cystic fibrosis, and chronic infections.

Zinc supplements are proving extremely beneficial in the following areas:

- Revitalizing an impaired sense of taste
- Speeding up healing of wounds, skin ulcers, burns, surgical incisions, sometimes shortening healing time needed after surgery by a third to a half
- Working with vitamin A to prevent stress ulcers
- Treating psychiatric patients, including schizophrenic children, and people with depression, poor memory, and disorientation, especially when used with manganese and vitamin B_6
- Alleviating prostatitis when used early enough
- Lowering high blood pressure

- Stimulating growth and sexual maturation in some dwarfs (some dwarfism is caused by zinc deficiency)

A special clue to low zinc levels is white spots on the fingernails.

HOW TO TELL EXACTLY WHAT VITAMINS AND MINERALS YOU ARE DEFICIENT IN

The most accurate method at present is by hair analysis. You put a small sample of your hair cut close to the scalp in an envelope and send it to a laboratory, where it is analyzed by computer techniques to tell you what you have too much of or too little of that can be causing your symptoms. Your doctor can order a hair analysis as well as a diet analysis for you from Bio-Medical Data, P.O. Box 6118, Chicago, Ill. 60680. They will send back a report on your body levels of 15 minerals with recommendations for any needed restructuring of your diet.

HOW TO GET YOUR VITAMINS AND MINERALS NATURALLY

The best sources for:

VITAMIN A

- Livers
- Fish-liver oils
- Desiccated liver
- Eggs
- Kidneys, other organ meats
- Milk, cream, butter, cheese, other whole milk products
- Whole-milk yogurt
- Oysters
- Greens, green leafy vegetables
- Sweet potatoes, carrots, squash, other yellow vegetables
- Green and yellow fruit, such as peaches, papayas, mangoes

VITAMIN Bs

- Whole grains
- Rice polishings
- Wheat germ
- Peanuts, other nuts
- Bran
- Brewer's yeast
- Soybeans
- Beans
- Peas

- Eggs
- Liver, kidneys, other organ meats
- Oysters
- Pork
- Poultry
- Milk
- Greens
- Sprouted seeds and grains

VITAMIN C

- Citrus fruits and juices
- Tomatoes
- Acerola (Barbados cherries)
- Rose hips (fruit of rose plants)
- Berries
- Bananas
- Liver
- Shellfish
- Currants
- Green peppers
- Broccoli
- Mustard, collards, other greens

VITAMIN D

- Fish-liver oils
- Livers
- Desiccated liver
- Eggs
- Milk, butter, cream, cheese, and whole milk products
- Whole-milk yogurt

VITAMIN E

- Whole grains
- Whole cereals
- Seeds
- Vegetable seed oil
- Nuts
- Nut oils, such as peanut oil
- Wheat germ oil
- Wheat germ
- Seed sprouts

LECITHIN

- Vegetable oils
- Seeds
- Whole grains
- Nuts
- Lecithin granules

IRON

- Liver
- Yeast
- Blackstrap molasses
- Kidneys, other organ meats
- Eggs
- Bran
- Rice polishings
- Wheat germ
- Nuts
- Seeds
- Beans
- Peas
- Fish eggs
- Shellfish
- Cocoa
- Parsley
- Dark green vegetables

CALCIUM

- Milk and milk products
- Eggs
- Vegetables
- Fruits

POTASSIUM

- Seaweed (kelp)
- Eggs
- Blackstrap molasses
- Seeds
- Nuts
- Fish
- Potatoes
- Vegetables
- Fruits

PHOSPHORUS AND MAGNESIUM

- Seeds
- Nuts
- Eggs
- Milk and milk products
- Fish
- Poultry
- Beef
- Pork
- Yeast

TRACE MINERALS

- Whole grains
- Seeds
- Yeast
- Liver, kidney, other organ meats
- Wheat germ

- Brown rice
- Rice polishings
- Blackstrap molasses
- Meats
- Poultry
- Fish, fish eggs
- Eggs
- Milk and milk products
- Seaweed (kelp)
- Fruits
- Vegetables
- Fruit and vegetable juices

IODINE

- Apples with skin
- Beets
- Cranberries, fresh
- Carrots, raw
- Cauliflower, raw
- Desiccated liver
- Fish
- Oatmeal
- Oranges
- Shellfish

ON THE VITAL DIET YOU SHOULD ALSO STAY SLIM THE REST OF YOUR LIFE

The Whole Health Vital Diet is low in carbohydrates and high in nutrition, so if you stay on it regularly, you should feel good and you should attain and keep your ideal weight.

Weigh yourself before you start the diet, then weigh yourself at two-week intervals. Do not weigh yourself in between since any temporary daily fluctuations might discourage you from realizing your eventual ideal weight.

IF YOU WANT TO LOSE WEIGHT FASTER— TRY FASTING

Little used in the United States, fasting is popular for losing weight in Europe.

A typical fast: you eat nothing whatsoever for four days—no food, no fruit juices, no coffee, no diet sodas. You drink at least 10 glasses of water each day, and take your regular high potency vitamin-mineral supplements, and a protein-sparing supplement available under many labels at most drugstores. (You take the powdered protein mixed with water five times a day.) On the first day of the fast, you will probably feel hungry, restless, lightheaded, and may have difficulty in falling asleep or may even feel nauseated. But by the end of day two you should feel very well, with no hunger pains.

In four days you should lose about 12 to 15 pounds. And most people find also that their blood pressure is lower, their allergies improved, their complexion clearer, their cravings for cigarettes, alcohol, and junk foods gone.

Caution: Work with your doctor because fasting could affect the dosages of any medications you are taking or some other factor of health. For example, antihistamines could make you more drowsy than usual, you will probably need less of any diuretic, you would want to use an aspirin substitute rather than aspirin on an empty stomach.

After four days, return to the regular Whole Health Vital Diet.

OTHER TIPS IF YOU WANT TO LOSE FASTER

Don't take diet pills. When your body tries to readjust later, you can have a rebound with increased hunger and weight gain again.

Use up more calories by exercising more. Typical number of calories used: 350 calories per hour of bicycling, dancing, or running, 190 for walking, 360 for swimming, and 600 for cross-country skiing. The number of calories used will vary depending on how vigorously you pursue the activity.

Consider joining Weight Watchers, TOPS, or other diet group. Being part of a group often helps you stick to the diet better and get results faster. Check your telephone book for local chapters of Weight Watchers, Diet Control Centers, TOPS Club, The Diet People, Dieters Community Center, Obesity and Weight Control Centers, Buxom Belle.

Work with a doctor who is a specialist in weight control. You can ask your regular doctor to refer you to someone, or you can write to the American Society of Bariatric Physicians, 333 West Hampden Avenue, Englewood, Colo. 80110, for the name of a physician specializing in weight control who lives in your area.

Be careful of medications that can be diet-killers. Some medications can interfere with the success of a diet. You may have to consider discontinuing them or finding a substitute, with your doctor's consent and advice, naturally.

The most troublesome is estrogen, as used to treat menopause or in birth control pills. If you are taking the Pill and are overweight ask your doctor about switching to a non-estrogen brand or to another form of contraceptive. Some doctors believe that hormones injected into cattle to fatten them can cause fat in *you*. Try avoiding beef, and see if you lose faster.

If you are taking any medication, read the instructions inserted with the package and see if weight-gain is listed as a possible side effect. Also ask your doctor if your medication could be a factor in having difficulty in losing.

Sauté the low-calorie way. Instead of using a lot of oil, use a heavy skillet and sprinkle with salt or just rub it with enough sesame seed oil, safflower oil, or sunflower oil to prevent the food from burning.

A new bread might help. This is *not* ordinary bread, but a bread with wood cellulose added to give it 25 times more fiber content than ordinary bread. The bread has the same advantages as a high-fiber diet using bran—helping with weight loss as well as helping protect against heart disease and cancer of the colon. One kind—Fresh Horizons—is made by ITT Continental Baking Company. Other brands are made by Campbell-Toggart, John J. Nissen Bakery, Sunbeam, and W. E. Long Companies.

If you drink, it may be the alcohol that keeps you from losing. One ounce of 100-proof spirits usually counts 20 grams of carbohydrates; or if you count calories, it contains about 100 calories per ounce. Sweet cocktails and sweet wines like sherry and port are very high in both calories and carbohydrates. French wines average about 70 calories for four ounces, have fewer calories and less sugar than California wines. The least fattening white wine is French Alsace Riesling. The least fattening red wine is claret.

Eat your biggest meals in the morning; your smallest meals at night. A very recent study shows that when you eat is important. Morning calories go to energy, while the same calories at night go to fat.

Begin each meal with a liquid. Drink a liquid that helps satisfy you, but is not fattening. Even a glass of water helps take the edge off appetite.

HOW TO FAT-PROOF YOUR CHILD

Don't be a fat mother. Keep slim before pregnancy; don't gain more than you should during pregnancy.

Breast feed. The baby will only take what she or he really wants and needs. If you bottle feed, don't insist your baby finish the bottle. When he acts full, don't push him.

If he is already overweight, dilute his formula with water.

Don't start the baby on high calorie and high carbohydrate solids too soon.

Buy baby food without sugar, or make your own.

Don't always keep your baby in a stroller. Let her creep, crawl, and climb.

As your child grows up, don't have candy, cookies, Cokes, other junk food in the house. Keep lots of fresh fruits, vegetables, and healthy snack food around instead.

Get your family as active as possible. As your child loses weight, he will become more agile, gain more self-confidence, and soon become interested in sports activities and outdoor skills.

FREE COOKBOOKS GOOD FOR YOUR HEALTH

Send a postcard with your name, address, and zip code for any of the following:

The Chicken Cookbook
P.O. Box 307
Coventry, Conn. 06238
128-page paperback of prize-winning chicken recipes
Prize-Winning Recipes from the Golden Harvest Kitchens
General Nutrition Corp.
418 Wood Street
Pittsburgh, Pa. 15222
96 pages of natural grain and cooking-from-scratch recipes
Chesapeake Bay Recipe Brochures
Seafood Marketing Authority
Annapolis, Md. 21401
Four booklets with seafood recipes
How to Feed Your Family Better for Less
Carnation Company
Box 350B
Pico Rivera, Calif. 90665
Booklets with recipes and hints for cooking with dry milk

Secrets from Del Monte Kitchens' Tomato Recipes
Del Monte Kitchens
Consumer Concerns
P.O. Box 8111
Clinton, Iowa 52732
Economic dishes from eggplant italienne to tomato-cheese pie
Quick and Easy Lamb Recipes for Busy Women
Lamb Education Center
200 Clayton Street
Denver, Colo. 80206
Dozens of saving lamb dishes
Idea Guide for Weight Watchers Frozen Meals
Box 2299
G.P.O.
New York, N.Y. 10001

INEXPENSIVE CALORIE AND CARBOHYDRATE COUNTERS

Calories and Weight
U.S. Department of Agriculture Information Bulletin 364
Superintendent of Documents
U.S. Government Printing Office
Washington, D.C. 20402
$1.00
Calorie Guide to Brand Names and Basic Foods
Barbara Kraus % New American Library
1301 Avenue of the Americas
New York, N.Y. 10019
$1.25
Carbohydrate Guide to Brand Names and Basic Foods
Barbara Kraus % New American Library (see address above)
Home and Garden Bulletin No. 72
U.S. Government Printing Office
Washington, D.C. 20402
30¢
Lists calories, carbohydrates, protein, and fat contents of foods.

CHAPTER 5

Special Diets That Can Help Specific Medical Problems

ARE UNSUSPECTED FOOD ALLERGIES MESSING UP YOUR LIFE?

Allergies can make you sniffly, headachy, forgetful, anxious, confused, or can cause gas, belching, pain in your joints, or even severe behavior disturbances that mimic psychiatric problems. (One doctor says any psychiatrist who does not test for food allergies in emotional illness is neglecting his patient.)

Start observing what you eat to see what foods cause these reactions. Particular trouble-makers are corn, wheat, chocolate, milk, eggs, and red and yellow dyes added to beverages, chewing gum, cereal, gelatins, and pills. One woman had migraine headaches for years, but got rid of them after she stopped eating all products with yellow dye. Dr. Ben Feingold has had some success with hyperactive children, simply by removing all foods with artificial flavors and colors from their diets, often seeing results in just a few weeks.

The most effective way to discover food allergies, whether to an additive or to a food itself, is to go on a fast (under a doctor's supervision) for four or five days, with nothing but water. Then foods are slowly added back to the diet, starting with raw vegetables and fruit, checking for reactions until the allergy-causing foods are found.

If you know you are allergic to a particular food, avoid related foods.

IF YOU ARE ALLERGIC TO:	ALSO AVOID:
Lettuce	Chicory, endive, escarole, artichoke, dandelion, sunflower seeds, tarragon
Buckwheat	Rhubarb, sorrel
Cashew	Pistachio, mango
Chocolate	Cocoa, cola
Orange	Lemon, grapefruit, lime, tangerine, kumquat
Mushroom	Yeast, molds, antibiotics
Avocado	Cinnamon, bay leaves, sassafras
Watermelon	Cucumber, cantaloupe, pumpkin, squash
Onion	Garlic, asparagus, chives, leeks, sarsaparilla
Plum	Cherry, peach, apricot, nectarine
Strawberry	Raspberry, blackberry, dewberry, loganberry
Walnut	Pecan, hickory nut, butternut
Oyster	Clam, abalone, mussel
Lobster	Shrimp, crab
Fish	All true fish, either freshwater or saltwater, including canned

If your child is allergic to wheat and other cereal, try poi, the Hawaiian carbohydrate made from taro root.

If you are allergic to aspirin, also be careful of substances now found to be related: apricots, blackberries, strawberries, raspberries, currants, grapes, raisins, limes, nectarines, peaches, plums, prunes, vinegar, ice cream, chewing gum, soft drinks.

If you are allergic to corn, avoid bath powders, starch, glue on envelopes and stamps, paper cups and plates.

WAYS TO REDUCE BLOOD CHOLESTEROL LEVELS WITHOUT GIVING UP EGGS

1. Eliminate all sugar from your diet.
2. Eat no refined carbohydrates; keep carbohydrates generally low.
3. Eat lots of fruits and vegetables for their natural pectin, recently shown in England to be very effective in lowering cholesterol levels.
4. Eat whole fiber foods.
5. Take extra amounts of vitamin A.
6. Take vitamin B_3 and B_6.
7. Take vitamin C.
8. Take lecithin (it actually dissolves cholesterol).
9. Take choline.
10. Take inositol.
11. Take calcium and magnesium orotates.
12. Take pangamic acid.
13. Take chromium.
14. Take manganese.
15. Take para-aminobenzoic acid (PABA).
16. If you still need further help, take supplements of bran, pectin, and guar gum.

Very few doctors in the United States use these methods except those who specialize in nutrition medicine, yet they are amazingly effective in reducing cholesterol levels and are completely safe.

One nutrition specialist, Dr. H. L. Newbold, reports in *Dr. Newbold's Revolutionary New Discoveries About Weight Loss* that his serum cholesterol was a very high 312. After taking B vitamins for several weeks, it fell to 213. When he added vitamin C, it fell further to 190. When he added two heaping tablespoons of lecithin two times a day plus one tablespoon of safflower oil two times a day, the cholesterol level went down to 165.

OLD FOLK-REMEDY VINDICATED?

Do garlic and onions really help your heart? Doctors at a medical school in India say they compared a group of people who regularly ate garlic and onions to a group who ate neither, and found lower cholesterol levels in the garlic-onion eaters.

STRESS CAN RAISE CHOLESTEROL, TOO

Accountants' cholesterol levels rise around April 15, then drop again. Levels of flyers rise when they go on combat duty.

FOUR SIMPLE HEALTH CHANGES THAT COULD SOLVE YOUR DIGESTIVE PROBLEMS

If you frequently get indigestion, heartburn, belching, bloating, gas, abdominal pain, cramps, constipation or diarrhea, you should see your doctor to determine the cause. But it may be as simple as your diet.

The following diet steps can eliminate many of these symptoms.

Analyze what in your diet seems to bring on the attacks: fat, sugar, caffeine, milk? (Milk intolerance is especially common in blacks.) When you suspect a food or drink, eliminate it from your diet for a week or two, and see if there is a difference.

Try eliminating all sweets and starches and substituting a high-fiber diet, with whole grain bread, whole grain cereal, fruit and vegetables, or a few tablespoons of miller's bran each day mixed with your food.

Try eliminating alcohol from your diet.

Analyze what in your lifestyle might be bringing on tension. Determine what would be best for you to help relieve stress: exercise, yoga, meditation, hypnosis, simply talking to yourself in tight situations.

A DIET TO MASTER HYPOGLYCEMIA

CHECKING FOR HYPOGLYCEMIA

Are you frequently fatigued?

Do you have anxiety attacks with cold clammy hands, racing pulse, and nervousness?

Do you have fatigue, headaches, or shakiness that seems worse when you are hungry and often goes away after eating?

Do you have episodes of feeling edgy or depressed or have dizzy spells, lightheadedness?

Do you eat a lot of candy bars and drink Coke, frequently craving sugar?

You may have hypoglycemia, or low blood sugar. These symptoms aren't *necessarily* the result of hypoglycemia, but the possibility is worth checking with a 5- or 6-hour glucose tolerance test at your doctor's. (For an at-home test, see Chapter 24.)

It would seem logical to treat low blood sugar by eating sugar. But this is wrong. If you eat sugar, it stimulates the pancreas to pour insulin into the blood which lowers the sugar level in the blood to less than it was before.

THE RECOMMENDED DIET FOR TREATING HYPOGLYCEMIA

Don't eat any sugar or refined carbohydrate. (But you and diabetics can use a sugar called fructose or levulose which does not stimulate insulin response like regular sugar. You can buy it in grocery stores in Europe, your druggist can order it in the U.S. from Miller Pharmacal, P.O. Box 299, West Chicago, Ill. 60185.)

Stay away from caffeine and nicotine, which also trigger insulin release and lower blood sugar.

Eat some protein every three hours, as part of every snack and meal. Protein, whether it's meat, nuts, cheese, or eggs will cause a slow release of sugar and energy, without the wide up-and-down fluctuations that cause the symptoms of hypoglycemia.

Take one high-potency vitamin-mineral supplement every day.

THE PROBLEMS YOUR CHILD IS HAVING COULD BE DUE TO HYPOGLYCEMIA

Children can be hypoglycemic, too.

The symptoms are paleness, attacks of inattention, staring into space, listlessness, headaches, uncoordination, rapid heart beats, sweating, even convulsions. The child may be hyperactive, aggressive, destructive, or may be lethargic and apathetic.

Sometimes simply eliminating candy, cookies, cake, and soft drinks, in addition to giving vitamin and mineral supplements, eliminates the symptoms.

Use protein snacks like cheese, nuts, or eggs, between meals.

THE NEW DIET THAT IS HELPING ALCOHOLICS BEAT THE PROBLEM

Reports are coming in of alcoholism being successfully treated with special diet. Thousands of long-term alcoholics who had failed in all other treatment have been able to stay sober for the first time.

Here is the nutritional program that Dr. H. L. Newbold of New York reports is having success:

- Eating a meal or snack that contains some protein every three hours
- Keeping carbohydrate intake low; cutting out refined starches

- Eating no sugar whatsoever, or any foods or drinks with sugar
- Vitamin B$_{12}$ injections
- Calcium pantothenate, 200-1000 mg at bedtime
- Vitamin A, 10,000 units daily
- Vitamin D, 400 units daily
- B vitamins, including 500 to 1000 mg thiamine three times a day
- Vitamin E, 200 units at breakfast and lunch
- Vitamin C, 500 mg four times daily
- Brewer's yeast, one heaping tablespoon two times daily (can be put on cereal or dessert)
- Lecithin granules, two heaping tablespoons twice daily (good on fruit)
- Safflower oil, one or two tablespoons daily (can be put on salad)
- Dolomite, two or three teaspoons at bedtime, or one teaspoon three or four times during the day, whichever makes you feel best
- Folic acid, 5 mg daily or more
- Glutamine, five 200 mg capsules three times a day (be sure to take *glutamine*, not *glutamic acid,* which won't help at all)

Persons suffering from alcoholism should also be given tests for food allergies, and eliminate any allergy-producing foods from the diet.

A LOW PURINE DIET FOR PEOPLE WITH GOUT

FOODS	INCLUDE	AVOID
Breads	Whole grain	White, refined
Cereals	Whole grain	Sugared
Soups	Milk soups made with vegetables	Bouillon, broth, consommé
Meat, fish, eggs, or cheese	Fish, fowl, shellfish, meats (except those listed), eggs, cheese	Kidney, liver, meat extracts, sweetbreads, roe, sardines, anchovies, gravy, broth, bouillon
Potato or substitute	White potato with skins, sweet potato, wild rice, brown rice	Fried potato, potato chips, macaroni, spaghetti, white rice
Vegetables	All vegetables (except those listed)	Asparagus, beans, lentils, mushrooms, peas, spinach
Desserts	Fruits, non-sugar gelatins	Mince pie, sugars, and refined starches
Sweets	None	All
Beverages	Carbonated beverages, coffee, milk, tea	Sugared sodas
Miscellaneous	Spices, cream sauces, nuts, salt, condiments	Alcohol, gravy, yeast

NUTRITION AIDS TO REDUCE PREMENSTRUAL TENSION AND MENOPAUSE IRRITABILITY

The following diet and diet supplements used daily has helped many women:

- Vitamin A
- Vitamin B complex
- Vitamin C
- Calcium
- Vitamin E
- Lecithin granules
- Wheat germ
- Frequent protein
- No sugar even if you crave it

To determine your best dosages, see Chapter 4.

THE SPECIAL DIET EVERY WOMAN WHO TAKES BIRTH CONTROL PILLS SHOULD BE ON

If you take birth control pills that contain estrogen or you take estrogen for menopause or other reasons, you need extra supplements of the following:

- Vitamin B_6
- Vitamin B_{12}
- Niacin
- Folic acid
- Vitamin C

Taking the supplements not only restores the normal balance of vitamins and minerals in the body, but often alleviates symptoms of nausea, dizziness, depression, and swelling that estrogen users frequently have.

A DIET TREATMENT FOR PEOPLE WITH KIDNEY FAILURE

This diet was reported by Dr. William E. Mitch of Johns Hopkins University Hospital at a recent meeting of the American College of Physicians. He said the diet can slow, and sometimes even stop, kidney deterioration apparently in about one-third of patients with progressive kidney disease. It was even effective in some patients who had less than 6 percent of their kidney tissue functioning and in patients who had been having dialysis on kidney machines. It is impossible at the moment to tell which patients will respond to the diet and which will not, Dr. Mitch said. When it works, it can postpone the day when a patient needs artificial kidney treatments.

- Protein intake is restricted to a maximum of 15 to 25 grams per day.

- Calories are restricted to 14 calories per pound of body weight per day.
- 10 grams of amino acids are given.
- Vitamin supplements are given, with large amounts of the two B vitamins: pyridoxine and folic acid.

IF YOU ARE ON A LOW SALT DIET

LOOK OUT FOR THE SECRETLY SALTY SUBSTANCES

Foods that are high in sodium that you might not think of include: milk and milk products, almost all canned and frozen foods and TV dinners, smoked meat, bacon, frankfurters, lunch meats, sausage, smoked fish, processed cheese (unless low-sodium dietetic), mustard, all relishes and pickles, cooking wine, Worcestershire sauce, catsup, meat extracts and tenderizers (unless low-sodium dietetic), sauerkraut, pickles, or olives prepared in brine, breads and rolls with salt toppings. Check the labels!

Also don't use snuff or chew tobacco (they contain salt), don't eat licorice (it causes retention of salt and water in body), stay away from soul food (it's high in salt), rinse fish before cooking (it's often packed in salt water), and don't add monosodium glutamate or baking soda to food when you cook.

Stay away from seltzers like Alka-Seltzer and Bromo-Seltzer. They are *very* high in sodium.

Ask your health department about the amount of sodium in your local water supply. If it's high, use bottled water. Don't use a water softener, which usually adds sodium to the water.

IF YOU HAVE BEEN UNABLE TO DRINK MILK

A great number of blacks and Orientals have a condition called lactose intolerance that makes them sick when they drink milk. (Almost 70 percent of blacks and 90 percent of Orientals have it.) Other people simply get indigestion from milk. If you are one of these, try eliminating ordinary milk and milk products from your diet. Instead try a new milk called SAM (Sweet Acidophilus Milk). This milk has cultures of *Lactobacillus acidophilus* added, the same bacterium that makes yogurt work. It seems to be especially helpful for infants who are sensitive to milk and older people who have become intolerant. It will also work, as yogurt does, to prevent fungus infections and gastrointestinal upsets in people taking antibiotics. The milk is available in both low-fat and 3 percent homogenized forms from French Bauer-Cedar Hill Farms, Kroger, CincinnatiFarm, Royal Crest of Dayton, Trouth & Cloverleaf of Kentucky. More dairies will have it soon. Other fermented milks are kumiss and kefir.

IF YOU HAVE A HYPERKINETIC CHILD

Try giving him two cups of coffee per day. It often produces the same effect as medicines that are being used, without the side effects. Try eliminating all artificial flavors and colorings from the diet. (Also see Chapter 16.)

VITAMIN C FOR THE COMMON COLD

This treatment is controversial. It seems to work in some people, not in others. If you want to try for yourself, be sure to do the following:

1. Take the vitamin C *at the first sign of a cold*.

2. Insist that the druggist give you vitamin C with bioflavonoids.

3. Take 1500 mg (three 500-mg tablets) every four hours as long as you have symptoms (2000 mg if you are bigger than average).

4. Also take vitamin A (about 20,000 units per day) to enhance the action of the vitamin C.

5. Do not immediately stop taking the vitamins when your symptoms stop, but gradually decrease the dosage over several days until you are down to your regular maintenance level. (If you stop too soon, just as with antibiotics, your symptoms will bounce back.)

A MASTER COMPENDIUM OF OTHER PROBLEMS AND THE VITAMINS AND MINERALS THAT HAVE BEEN SHOWN TO HELP THEM

Again we stress that these are not the only answers for these problems, but they are nutritional treatments that have proven successful in clinical practice of the innovative doctors who use a nutritional approach to medical problems.

IF YOU HAVE:	THIS OFTEN SEEMS TO HELP:
Acne	Zinc; vitamin A
Bleeding gums	Vitamin C
Boils, abscesses	Vitamin A; eliminate sugar
Canker sores	Vitamin C complex with bioflavonoids; folic acid
Chalky teeth	Calcium lactate or calcium glycerophosphate

IF YOU HAVE:	THIS OFTEN SEEMS TO HELP:
Circulatory problems, especially legs	Vitamin E
Constipation	Yogurt; whole grains; magnesium
Cracking of skin around corners of the mouth	Vitamin B complex
Cysts of the breast	Vitamin E
Dandruff, scaly eyebrows and ears	Vitamin B_{12} injections; eliminate sugar
Dowager's hump	Calcium; magnesium; vitamin B_6
Dry eyeballs when wearing contact lenses	Vitamin A
Dry skin or dry vaginal membrane	Vitamin A; iron
Easy bruising	Vitamin C
Gum ulcers	Vitamin B; vitamin C
Hair problems	Wheat germ; vitamin E; B vitamins including PABA, biotin, pantothenic acid; lecithin; folic acid; iron
Heat rash	Vitamin C
Hemorrhoids	Vitamin B_6
Indigestion	Yogurt
Insomnia	Choline; inositol; lecithin; calcium
Joint pain	Calcium; vitamin D; vitamin B complex; vitamin C; folic acid
Kidney stones	Vitamin B complex
Leathery skin	Vitamin A; vitamin E
Leg cramps at night	Vitamin E; calcium; vitamin C; magnesium
Loss of sex drive	Folic acid; vitamin E; zinc
Low back pain	Calcium; vitamin C
Menopause symptoms	Vitamin B complex; vitamin E; calcium; folic acid
Muscle weakness	Magnesium
Nausea and edema of pregnancy	Vitamin B complex
Nausea after surgery	Vitamin B complex
Nervousness	Vitamin B complex; zinc
Oily skin	Vitamin B complex
Premenstrual tension	Vitamin B complex
Psoriasis	Vitamin A

IF YOU HAVE:	THIS OFTEN SEEMS TO HELP:
Puffy skin	Vitamin B complex
Rough skin	Zinc
Seasickness	Vitamin B_6
Skin ulcers	Zinc
Stretch marks	Zinc, vitamin B_6 often prevent further development
Sun-sensitivity	PABA capsule taken before exposure
Surgery, injury, stress	Vitamin A; vitamin C; vitamin E; zinc
Taste impairment	Zinc
Tension	Vitamin E; vitamin C; lecithin; B complex; zinc

IF YOU HAVE:	THIS OFTEN SEEMS TO HELP:
Tingling or numbness of fingers	Vitamin B_6
Tongue swollen, burning, or tingling	Vitamin Bs

If you have an iron or vitamin B_1 deficiency, do not drink much tea. It interferes with absorption of iron and B_1.

If you are over 65, have kidney problems, are taking a diuretic or digitalis, you may need extra potassium. Eat extra amounts of bananas, oranges, raisins, baked potatoes, squash.

CHAPTER 6

The No-Formal-Exercise Program for People Who Don't Have Time to Exercise

Exercise *can* make a difference. And scientific studies prove it. A University of California study showed that young adults who exercise regularly were 14 times less likely to have a heart attack or circulatory or lung disease than those who did not exercise.

At the University of Toronto men and women all over age 60 who began to exercise regularly were found in only seven weeks to have a level of fitness of persons 10 to 20 years younger.

At his clinic in Dallas Dr. Kenneth H. Cooper claims that with exercise diabetics were able to reduce medication, and stomach ulcers, cardiovascular problems, and lung ailments improved, insomnia disappeared, and subjects had less fatigue.

There are two major kinds of exercise: conditioning exercises to tone your muscles, improve your posture, and increase your flexibility; and endurance exercises which strengthen your heart, blood vessels, and lungs.

But you don't have to have a formal boring calisthenics program to get your exercise. A new German Sports Federation fitness program, for example, has just been designed with exercises for men and women who spend most of their time behind desks, in cars or jets, or sitting in front of a TV. They estimate a 10 percent increase in strength in one week, a 40 percent increase in three months.

Our *Whole Health Catalogue* No-Formal-Exercise Program for People Who Don't Have Time to

Exercise is for more than strength. It also builds flexibility, tone, and stamina. And like the German Sports Federation program you can do the exercises while in bed, in the shower, watching TV, at the office, or waiting for a bus.

BE-SAFE RULES FOR ANY EXERCISE PROGRAM

Before you start on your exercise program, check your present fitness level. Take the Simple Test for General Fitness and the Stool-Step Test for Heart-Lung Fitness in Chapter 24.

If you are in bad condition, work up gradually to stress the muscles, lungs, and heart and improve their efficiency. Check with your physician before starting any vigorous exercise or sports program.

Before you start each exercise session do some warming up with stretching or breathing exercises, or walk briskly for one minute.

Breathe deeply when exercising; never hold your breath.

Drink enough water, with one glass always before you begin strenuous sports or exercise. Don't believe the old wives' tale about not drinking when exercising. It's good to replace water loss.

When you start any exercise program, do each exercise just a few times. As you gain strength and stamina each day, you can increase the number.

Check your pulse occasionally when exercising. It's good to get it up to about 120 so you know you're giving your body a workout, but it should not be over 120 five minutes after you stop. If it is, you're overextending yourself.

You should stop what you are doing any time you have cramps, pain or tremor in the legs, difficulty in breathing, a pounding heart, pains in the chest, nausea, or if you simply feel worn out.

When you finish exercising, always taper off slowly. Perhaps walk slowly for a few minutes. Don't stand quietly in one spot—you can become dizzy and faint.

Don't exercise if you have a cold or fever or any respiratory problems.

EXERCISES TO DO WHEN YOU'RE STILL IN BED

Lie flat on your back. Stretch arms out toward the headboard. Like a lazy leopard, stretch right arm out as far as possible, and right foot. Relax. Now stretch left arm and left foot. Relax.

While lying on your back, raise right leg slowly, keeping it straight. Hold it high to the count of 10. Lower it slowly. Repeat with left leg. Do only 2 or 3 times to start, later build up to more. Good for lower abdomen.

While still on your back tighten your buttocks muscles as hard as you can. Hold for count of 5. Relax. Repeat 2 to 3 times to start; later build up to 10 to 20.

Still on your back (what exercise program ever let you lie on your back in bed for so long?), fold your arms on your chest, raise your head and shoulders slowly. Hold for 10 seconds. Relax. Repeat 2 to 3 times. Increase gradually to 10 times, and as you increase strength, advance the exercise to a full sit-up. Good for upper abdomen.

Turn over on your stomach. Hook your toes over end of mattress, keep arms at side. Slowly raise chest and shoulders as high as you can; hold for 5 seconds. Lower slowly. Do 2 to 3 times to start; later build up to 20 and don't hook your toes on mattress for support. (Another variation of this is to hold on to a towel behind the back, and arch the back to stretch head, chest, arms, and legs up and back. Hold 5 seconds and relax.)

EXERCISES TO DO AFTER YOUR SHOWER

Stand straight. Grab a bath towel at each end and hold in front of you at arm's length. Keeping arms straight, raise towel overhead, then bring towel down behind back as far as you can, keeping elbows straight and towel stretched. Do 10 times.

Stand on toes and reach for the ceiling with arms. Stretch all muscles. Come back down. Repeat 5 times.

For waistline, stand with legs apart, hold a towel high over head. Bend to the right and then to the left, keeping arms straight and bending at the waist. Do 5 times. Repeat, but this time pull with one arm and resist with the other. Do 5 times.

For arms and chest, roll up a bath towel and then twist it with all your strength as though trying to wring every last drop of water from it.

EXERCISES TO DO WHILE SITTING WATCHING TV

Sit straight, legs and feet together, abdomen pulled in. Raise both arms over head. Reach right hand toward the ceiling, stretching high as you can. Relax. Do with left arm. Relax. Repeat through one commercial.

Still sitting straight, with abdomen in, raise one arm over head with palm facing body. Bounce body to other side six times while curving arm over head. Repeat with other arm. Repeat, standing up.

Sit with feet apart, arms overhead, with fingers interlocked and palms facing toward ceiling. Bend over and touch hands to toes of right foot. Come all the way back up. Touch hands to left foot. Do for one commercial.

WHENEVER YOU'RE HOME

Go barefoot. An orthopedic surgeon says it strengthens muscles and helps prevent corns, bunions, flat feet, and ingrown toenails.

WHEN TALKING TO YOUR CHILDREN

The same orthopedic surgeon says if you regularly sit cross-legged on the floor, it will exercise the ball-and-socket hip joint and prevent osteoarthritis of the hips.

WHILE TALKING ON THE TELEPHONE OR WAITING FOR THE KETTLE TO BOIL

Put your foot and ankle up on the countertop, while keeping that leg straight. With little bounces, lower your head toward raised leg. Do 5 times, then change legs.

WHILE WATCHING TV

Sit on floor, back erect, extend arms to side. Rotate fists and arms in little circles. Back 10 times, forward 10 times, and back 10 times.

WHEN PICKING THINGS UP

Bend down from the waist, hanging loosely. Hang arms to the floor and bounce gently up and down as you pick things up.

WHEN STRETCHED OUT ON THE COUCH

Raise one leg, keeping leg straight and toes pointed. Alternate raising each leg as high as you can for as many counts as you can.

WHILE READING ON THE FLOOR

Do the same thing but lie on your stomach. Lift one leg as high as you can, with toes pointed and buttocks tightened. Alternate legs.

WHEN YOU'VE BEEN SITTING TOO LONG AT YOUR DESK

Grasp arms on sides of chair and lift yourself up off the chair seat. Sit back down and relax. Repeat several times.

Sitting in your chair, straighten your legs and hold them off the floor to the count of 10.

Put your arms out, palms down, place the back of your hands against the underside of the desk top or center drawer. Try to lift the desk by pushing up for 5 seconds. Relax.

Stand about 3 feet from your desk, put your hands on the edge of the desk and do 5 to 10 push-ups.

Sit forward in chair, legs slightly apart and feet flat on floor; clasp hands behind head at neck. Bend forward on diagonal and try to touch right elbow to left knee in bouncing motion. Relax. Repeat with left elbow to right knee. Do 5 times; work up to 10.

OR DO THE BLADE

Sitting or standing, put your arms behind your back, clasping your hands together. Keep your arms straight, squeeze your shoulder blades together as hard as you can and try to make your elbows touch. Hold for a count of 5. Relax and wiggle your shoulders. This stretches vertebrae, takes pressure off nerves, relieves tension.

IF YOU'RE SITTING AND WAITING OR IN A BORING MEETING

If you're in an armchair, push your arms down against the chair arms as hard as you can to the count of 10. Relax. Do 10 times at first, work up to 25. Firms upper arms and chest.

Tighten your buttocks muscles as hard as you can one at a time, then together for a count of 5 each.

Tighten your abdominal muscles, pulling in toward your spine. Hold to a count of 5.

Press feet hard onto floor for a count of 5.

Tighten the muscles of one leg, hold, then let them relax. Do the other leg.

Tighten your back muscles and draw your shoulders down and back. Hold for 5. Relax.

THE TOTAL-EXERCISE SPORTS THAT WILL GIVE YOU THE HIGHEST FITNESS BENEFIT

Best for heart, lungs, and overall condition are these: *Running, brisk walking, tennis, swimming, bicycling, skating, skipping rope,* and *skiing.* They condition your entire body.

With rope skipping, for example, volunteers at Lankenau Hospital in Philadelphia were shown to have 168 percent increase in endurance after jumping rope *only 5 minutes a day for 6 weeks.*

Interval running is even better than jogging. Start running about half as fast as you think you can. Run this half-speed for about 200 yards or 30 seconds (less if you are in poor condition). Then walk for about the same time. Keep repeating, alternating walking and running for about 15 minutes or as long as you want to spend at it. Increase your distance and speed every day. (Don't jog or run downhill; it puts excessive strain on the knees. Walk when you come to a downhill slope.)

Steady swimming for 15 minutes will give you the same equivalent fitness as 15 minutes of running. Good for all muscles and heart and breathing also.

Endurance exercise for building up heart and lungs should be done at least three times a week for maximum benefit.

WARMING-UP

Before starting total-exercise sports always do:

The overhead stretch. Rise on toes, reach arms from side to above head. Stretch toward the ceiling.

Jumping jack. Stand at attention; jump, spreading feet and legs outward; at the same time swing arms out and up and clap over head. Jump back to starting position. Do 10 times.

A good warm-up exercise for stretching legs before tennis is a fencer's stretch. Put right foot about 3 feet ahead of left, with right knee bent, and left leg straight. Lean both hands on bent right knee and stretch left leg back as far as possible. At start, simply stretch and maintain balance as long as possible. Later add a gentle rocking motion.

CHAPTER 7

Specific Exercises for Specific Problems

TO IMPROVE BREATHING

Get a straw and fill a glass about half full of water. Take a deep breath and blow through the straw as slowly and steadily and as long as you can. Breathe in with little short breaths. Repeat 5 to 10 times.

TO IMPROVE POSTURE

Lie down on your back on a bed or on a bench with your head at the edge. Hold your arms up pointing straight toward the ceiling. Inhale and slowly lower your arms over your head toward the floor. Your head may go over the edge. Hold for a moment. As you exhale, raise your arms again to point to the ceiling.

Stand with your back to a wall, about 6 inches from the wall. Bend your knees slightly, push your spine against the wall, stretch your head up and your shoulders back and down. Hold to a count of 5. Now keep your spine against the wall, and slide it along as you push yourself back up.

FOR LOW BACK PAIN

Lie on the floor on your back. Bend your knees and rest your feet flat on the floor about 12 inches apart and as close to your buttocks as comfortable. Tighten the buttock muscles, pull the abdomen in and flatten your back against the floor. Hold for a count of 10. Relax. Repeat for 1 to 2 minutes, at least once a day.

Lie on the floor on your back. Bring your knees to your chest and, using your hands, bring your knees in so you can feel your spine touch the floor. Hold for 5 seconds. Do 5 times.

Or lie on your back on the floor, your right ankle over your left knee, and push knee down. Then reverse.

Don't do any exercises that require arching of the back or backbends.

TO STRENGTHEN ABDOMINAL MUSCLES

Lie flat on your back with your spine pressed to the floor. Pull in your abdominal muscles as tightly as you can.

Sit on the floor, knees bent, with your feet hooked under a piece of furniture. Lean back slowly; at about one-fourth of the way, hold your position for 10 to 15 seconds; do the same at the halfway point; and at three-fourths. Then relax backward onto the floor. Do only 2 times at first; more with training. If your abdominal muscles begin to quiver, relax before going through all positions.

TO STRETCH OUT YOUR VERTEBRAE AND UNPINCH NERVES

Clasp hands behind your back with the palms touching. Try to make elbows touch each other. Hold for several seconds, several times till your back feels relaxed. Do whenever your back feels tight. This straightens and stretches vertebrae in the spinal column and takes pressure off nerves, several chiropractors have told us. It also strengthens chest muscles.

A STRETCH FOR BURSITIS

Lift a broomstick overhead, holding it with both hands about 12 inches apart. Without lowering your elbows, drop the forearms backward so the stick is behind your head. This puts traction on the bursa. Do every morning and every night.

FOR PAIN IN UPPER LEGS

Leg pain resembling sciatica can often be caused by flat feet. Stand on a rolling pin with both feet. Holding on to something, roll back and forth as far backward and as far forward as possible. Do 6 to 10 times. This lifts the bones of the arch and releases pressure on the tibial nerve that causes the leg pain. Do not walk around after the exercise, but keep weight off feet.

TO IMPROVE STRENGTH IN HAND, WRIST, AND ARM AND TO EASE ARTHRITIS

Get a 2- to 3-inch rubber ball. Squeeze it tightly; release. Do this over and over until your wrist and fingers become tired.

TO IMPROVE FINGER DEXTERITY

Lay a sheet of newspaper flat on a table. With one hand only, grab and crumple the paper into a ball.

TO STOP HAND CRAMPS

Get circulation going to the fingers again by shaking your hands vigorously and rotating the wrists around slowly.

TO FIRM UP BREASTS AND STRENGTHEN UPPER TORSO

Sit cross-legged on the floor, arms at chest level, palms of your hands together, elbows bent. Push the heels of your hands together as hard as you can. Hold for a count of 5. Relax.

Grab your left elbow with your right hand and your right elbow with your left hand. Pull your arms together as hard as you can. Relax. Repeat 5 to 10 times.

Sit in a chair at a table. Make fists, with arms stretched straight out in front of you, push your fists down with all your strength. Push for 5 seconds. Repeat 25 to 50 times.

TO FIRM AND STRENGTHEN UPPER ARMS

Clasp arms below elbows. Push strongly as though trying to push your skin up to your elbows. Relax. Do 10 times.

CHAPTER 8

How to Stop the Killing Habits So You Can Live Your Longest

Smoking

CREATING YOUR OWN SMOKING WITHDRAWAL PROGRAM

Select Q-Day for quitting and make preparations for it in one of two ways:

1. Chart your smoking habits by making a daily record of cigarettes you smoke and under what circumstances. Note those you need the least, and eliminate them right away.

2. Or, until Q-Day, force yourself to increase your smoking, even double it, so your body is in complete revolt. Then stopping is a relief.

When Quitting Day comes you can quit gradually or quit "cold turkey."

One gradual elimination system is to limit cigarettes at first to only one an hour, and then extend the non-smoking time hour by hour. Or smoke only one-half of each cigarette.

Once you've decided whether cold turkey or slow-and-gradual is best for you, then do it *immediately*.

HELPFUL TRICKS

Read through this list, mark items you think will be most helpful to you. Then do them.

Throw away your cigarettes immediately; give away your lighter and matches; put away the ashtrays.

Use substitutes: water, juices, fruit, celery, carrots, nuts, clove, ginger, gum.

Brush your teeth, use mouthwashes and cough drops frequently.

Each day put aside the cost of a pack of cigarettes. Then buy something for yourself. Two packs a day for 21 years cost more than $5000.

Switch from a brand you like to a brand you don't like.

Before you light up, ask yourself if you really need that cigarette, or are you just acting from habit.

Make it an effort to get at your cigarettes. Wrap them in paper; place them in a tightly covered box; buy only one pack at a time; at work give them to an associate or put them in another room.

If you're right-handed, try smoking with your left.

Avoid smoking areas. Go to no-smoking sections at movies, on trains or planes. For the first few weeks, see less of friends who smoke.

When you need a cigarette, keep an unlighted one in your mouth, but don't light it.

If you feel like you need a smoke, take a shower.

Get plenty of sleep the first few weeks to cut down nervousness.

Do deep abdominal breathing when you crave a cigarette. Sometimes the craving will go away in just a few minutes.

For the first few weeks cut down on coffee and alcohol if you associate them with smoking.

Strenuous physical activity or long walks can be helpful in working off tension.

Reward yourself: give yourself all the things you like best—except cigarettes.

Check with your doctor on using anti-smoking drugs.

Try hypnosis. Be sure to use a qualified professional hypnotist.

Join a smoking withdrawal clinic or other group for quitting smoking.

HERE'S WHAT CIGARETTES CAN ACTUALLY DO:

- Increase likelihood of lung cancer, bladder cancer, and stroke
- Decrease visual perception and increase likelihood of blindness
- Increase serum cholesterol, triglycerides, and other fatty acids
- Decrease hearing ability, sense of taste and smell
- Decrease sex drive and response
- Cause skin to wrinkle 20 years beyond your chronological age
- Increase frequency of allergies, asthma, bronchitis, and emphysema and decrease wind needed for sports
- Cause release of adrenalin
- Increase heart rate
- Increase blood pressure
- Cause spasm of coronary arteries as well as narrowing and thickening
- Trigger the heart into uncontrolled muscle contractions, called ventricular fibrillation
- Increase sticking-together of blood platelets, making it more likely for clots to form
- Increase likelihood of an aneurysm (dangerous thinning and bulging of an artery wall)

RECOMMENDED:

Helping People to Stop Smoking Cigarettes
    A kit for groups to establish programs.
    American Cancer Society
    P.O. Box 218
    Fairview, N.J. 07022
    Free
Smoker's Self-Testing Kit
    (HEW publication No. 72-7506) 10 cents.
    Superintendent of Documents
    U.S. Government Printing Office
    Washington, D.C. 20402
    10 cents
Seventh Day Adventists Smoking Clinics
    Seven day plan. Free. Check with local chapter of American Cancer Society for dates in your area.

Smokenders
    See your telephone directory for local chapter to help you quit.
The Bad Habits Clinic
    This clinic at Duke University in Durham, N.C., uses the technique of "flooding" to cure people of smoking. The person lights a cigarette and must inhale once every six seconds until he or she can't do it anymore. After about one week, clients can no longer stand even to be around anyone else who smokes. The clinic program costs $150. The method also helps people who have fears of snakes, flying, and other problems.

Other material on smoking, and fighting it, is available from:

GASP (Group Against Smoking Pollution)
    P.O. Box 632
    College Park, Md. 20740
ASH (Action on Smoking and Health)
    2000 H Street, N.W.
    Suite 301
    Washington, D.C. 20006
National Interagency Council on Smoking and Health
    419 Park Avenue South
    New York, N.Y. 10016
American Cancer Society
    19 West 56 Street
    New York, N.Y. 10019
American Heart Association
    7320 Greenville Avenue
    Dallas, Tex. 75231
American Lung Association
    1740 Broadway
    New York, N.Y. 10019

WITHDRAWAL SYMPTOMS AND SIDE EFFECTS WHEN YOU QUIT

The first 48 hours are the critical period. If you have shortness of breath, tightness in the chest, visual disturbances, sweating, headaches, gastrointestinal complaints, are shaky, irritable, or depressed, don't let it alarm you. Your body is simply readjusting. These symptoms will pass.

A point to remember is that scientists have found that periods of craving last only 3½ minutes, then go away. You only have to fight the craving for that long.

THE RIGHTS OF NON-SMOKERS

More evidence is turning up on the harmful effects of tobacco smoke on innocent bystanders. Children whose parents smoke, for example, are found to have twice as much respiratory illness and more frequent asthma and allergies than others do.

Because of this, the majority of states have now passed anti-smoking laws that forbid smoking in various public places. In Minnesota and New York, smoking is forbidden in *all* public places.

Say NO when someone asks if they may smoke.

Bonus: Many insurance companies will give discounts on life and/or disability insurance to persons who don't smoke. Guardian Life gives 10 percent off if you also are not overweight. Farmers Insurance gives a 15 percent discount on auto insurance, and Hanover gives 5 percent on homeowners' insurance. For free list of other companies offering discounts, write: Institute of Life Insurance, 277 Park Avenue, New York, N.Y. 10017, and enclose a self-addressed envelope.

IF YOU ABSOLUTELY INSIST ON SMOKING

We didn't even want to include this section because smoking cigarettes is probably the worst thing you can do to your health except for walking in front of a truck. But if you really are stupid enough to persist, here is how the cigarettes rate in their relative abilities to kill you.

TAR AND NICOTINE CONTENT OF CIGARETTES
RANKED FROM LOW (1) TO HIGH (128)

NF—Non-Filter (All other brands possess filters)
M—Menthol
PB—Plastic box
HP—Hard pack

RANK (TAR)	BRAND	TYPE	TAR (MG)	NICOTINE (MG)
30	Alpine	King, M	14	0.9
35	Alpine	100mm M (HP)	15	0.9
34	Belair	King, M	15	1.1
47	Belair	100mm, M	17	1.2
9	Benson & Hedges	Reg. (HWP)	9	0.6
36	Benson & Hedges	King (HWP)	15	1.1
66	Benson & Hedges 100's	100mm	18	1.2
68	Benson & Hedges 100's	100mm, M	18	1.2
126	Bull Durham	King	30	2.0
111	Camel	Reg., NF	23	1.5
85	Camel Filters	King	19	1.3
1	Carlton 70's	Reg.	1	0.1
3	Carlton	King	4	0.3
2	Carlton	King, M	3	0.3
115	Chesterfield	Reg., NF	25	1.5
124	Chesterfield	King, NF	29	1.8
77	Chesterfield	King	19	1.4
73	Chesterfield	King, M	18	1.3
84	Chesterfield	101mm	19	1.4
118	Domino	King, NF	26	1.3
101	Domino	King	21	1.2
27	Doral	King	14	1.0
28	Doral	King, M	14	1.0
39	DuMaurier	King (HWP)	16	1.1
107	Edgeworth Export	King (HP)	22	1.7
95	Edgeworth Export	100mm	20	1.4

RANK (TAR)	BRAND	TYPE	TAR (MG)	NICOTINE (MG)
110	English Ovals	Reg., NF (HWP)	23	1.7
123	English Ovals	King, NF (HWP)	29	2.1
74	Eve	100mm	18	1.3
53	Eve	100mm, M	17	1.2
121	Fatima	King, NF	28	1.8
16	Frappe	King, M	11	0.5
71	Galaxy	King	18	1.2
116	Half & Half	King	25	1.8
125	Herbert Tareyton	King, NF	30	1.8
86	Home Run	Reg., NF	19	1.6
8	Iceberg 10	King, M	9	0.6
31	Kent	King (HP)	15	0.9
38	Kent	King	16	1.0
69	Kent	100mm	18	1.2
72	Kent	100mm, M	18	1.2
6	King Sano	King	6	0.3
7	King Sano	King, M	7	0.3
97	Kool	Reg., NF, M	20	1.2
48	Kool	King, M	17	1.3
26	Kool Milds	King, M	13	0.9
54	Kool	100mm, M	17	1.2
62	L&M	King (HP)	18	1.3
79	L&M	King	19	1.3
88	L&M	100mm	19	1.4
76	L&M	100mm, M	19	1.3
57	Lark	King	17	1.2
81	Lark	100mm	19	1.3
19	Life	100mm	12	0.8
120	Lucky Strike	Reg., NF	28	1.7
108	Lucky Filters	100mm	23	1.7
10	Lucky Ten	King	9	0.7
12	Lucky Ten	100mm	10	0.8
109	Mapleton	King	23	1.3
58	Marlboro	King (HP)	17	1.1
67	Marlboro	King	18	1.2
29	Marlboro	King, M	14	0.9
56	Marlboro	100mm (HP)	17	1.2
64	Marlboro	100mm	18	1.2
25	Marlboro Lights	King	13	0.9
112	Marvels	King, NF	24	0.9
5	Marvels	King	6	0.2
4	Marvels	King, M	4	0.2
78	Montclair	King, M	19	1.4
22	Multifilter	King (PB)	13	0.9
21	Multifilter	King, M (PB)	12	0.9
70	Newport	King, M (HP)	18	1.2
61	Newport	King, M	17	1.2
103	Newport	100mm, M	21	1.6
83	Oasis	King, M	19	1.3
98	Old Gold Straights	Reg., NF	20	1.3
114	Old Gold Straights	King, NF	24	1.5
60	Old Gold Filters	King	17	1.1
104	Old Gold 100's	100mm	22	1.4
122	Pall Mall	King, NF	28	1.8
11	Pall Mall Extra Mild	King (HP)	10	0.7
13	Pall Mall Extra Mild	King	10	0.7
102	Pall Mall	100mm	21	1.5
55	Pall Mall	100mm, M	17	1.3
32	Parliament	King (HP)	15	0.9
33	Parliament	King	15	0.9

RANK (TAR)	BRAND	TYPE	TAR (MG)	NICO-TINE (MG)
63	Parliament 100's	100mm	18	1.2
40	Parliament Charcoal Filter	King (HP)	16	1.0
44	Parliament Charcoal Filter	King	16	1.0
82	Peter Stuyvesant	King	19	1.4
94	Peter Stuyvesant	100mm	20	1.4
106	Philip Morris	Reg., NF	22	1.4
119	Philip Morris Commander	King, NF	27	1.7
96	Picayune	Reg., NF	20	1.6
117	Piedmont	Reg., NF	25	1.5
127	Players	Reg., NF (HWP)	31	2.2
113	Raleigh	King, NF	24	1.5
41	Raleigh	King	16	1.1
49	Raleigh	100mm	17	1.1
23	Raleigh Extra Mild	King	13	0.9
59	Redford	King	17	1.3
80	St. Moritz	100mm	19	1.3
65	St. Moritz	100mm, M	18	1.1
75	Salem	King, M	18	1.3
93	Salem	100mm, M	20	1.4
42	Sano	Reg., NF	16	0.5
51	Silva Thins	100mm	17	1.2

RANK (TAR)	BRAND	TYPE	TAR (MG)	NICO-TINE (MG)
43	Silva Thins	100mm, M	16	1.2
90	Spring 100's	100mm, M	20	1.2
100	Tareyton	King	21	1.4
99	Tareyton	100mm	21	1.5
20	Tempo	King	12	0.9
17	True	King	11	0.7
18	True	King, M	12	0.7
52	Twist	100mm, lemon, M	17	1.3
14	Vantage	King	11	0.9
15	Vantage	King, M	11	0.9
37	Viceroy	King	16	1.1
50	Viceroy	100mm	17	1.2
24	Viceroy Extra Mild	King	13	0.8
45	Virginia Slims	100mm	16	1.1
46	Virginia Slims	100mm, M	17	1.1
128	Vogue (black)	King (HWP)	31	1.3
105	Vogue (colors)	King (HWP)	22	0.9
91	Winston	King (HP)	20	1.3
89	Winston	King	19	1.3
87	Winston	100mm	19	1.3
92	Winston	100mm, M	20	1.4

Courtesy of Federal Trade Commission and National Clearinghouse for Smoking and Health

Alcohol

HOW TO TELL IF YOU COULD BE A PROBLEM DRINKER

	YES	NO
Have you ever decided to stop drinking for a week or so, but only lasted for a couple of days?	___	___
Do you wish people would mind their own business about your drinking—stop telling you what to do?	___	___
Have you ever switched from one kind of drink to another in the hope that this would keep you from getting drunk?	___	___
Have you had a drink in the morning during the past year?	___	___
Do you envy people who can drink without getting into trouble?	___	___
Have you had problems connected with drinking during the past year?	___	___
Has your drinking caused trouble at home?	___	___
Do you ever try to get extra drinks at a party because you do not get enough?	___	___
Have you missed days of work because of drinking?	___	___
Do you tell yourself you can stop drinking any time you want to, even though you keep getting drunk when you don't mean to?	___	___
Do you have blackouts?	___	___
Have you ever felt that your life would be better if you did not drink?	___	___

Courtesy: Alcoholics Anonymous

If you answer YES to four or more questions, you are probably in trouble with alcohol.

WHAT ALCOHOL CAN DO

Alcoholics have an overwhelming incidence of cirrhosis of the liver, high blood pressure, stomach and duodenal ulcers, asthma, diabetes, gout, strokes, heart disease, pancreatic disease, malnutrition, anemia, and automobile accidents. In addition, alcohol produces headaches, diarrhea, insomnia, and irritability, reduces the production of testosterone and makes anesthesia more risky.

Alcoholism shortens life by 10 to 12 years.

DRIVING

Most people believe a few drinks won't affect the ability to drive. The fact is when alcohol hits the brain, first it depresses judgment and social restraint. Next it alters simple muscular movements, reaction time, and vision. Then it attacks balance, perception, and coordination. Finally it leads to stupor, coma, and possibly death.

It takes approximately *one hour* for your body to rid itself of one drink.

HOW MANY DRINKS CAN YOU SAFELY HAVE?

When your blood alcohol level reaches .06%, the probability of causing an accident is twice that of the no-alcohol level; at .10 the probability is six to seven times greater, and at .15 it is twenty-five times greater. The following chart shows how much of any kind of drink it takes to cause these changes.

AMOUNT PRODUCING .06%
(TWICE THE NUMBER OF ACCIDENTS) IN:

DRINK	120 LB. PERSON	180 LB. PERSON
Malt	1 12-oz. bottle	2 12-oz. bottles
Beer	2 12-oz. bottles	3 12-oz. bottles
Wine	2 3-oz. glasses	3 3-oz. glasses
Liqueur	2 1-oz. glasses	3 1-oz. glasses
Fruit brandy	2 2-oz. glasses	2 2-oz. glasses
Straight rum, vodka, Scotch, whiskey	2 1-oz. glasses	3 1-oz. glasses
Martini, Manhattan	1 3½-oz. glass	2 3½-oz. glasses
Highball with Mix	1½ 8-oz. glasses	2 8-oz. glasses

AMOUNT PRODUCING .10%
(SIX TIMES THE NUMBER OF ACCIDENTS) IN:

DRINK	120 LB. PERSON	180 LB. PERSON
Malt	2½ 12-oz. bottles	3 12-oz. bottles
Beer	2 12-oz. bottles	2 12-oz. bottles
Wine	3 3-oz. glasses	3 3-oz. glasses
Liqueur	4 1-oz. glasses	5 1-oz. glasses
Fruit brandy	3 2-oz. glasses	5 2-oz. glasses
Straight rum, vodka, Scotch, whiskey	4 1-oz. glasses	5 1-oz. glasses
Martini, Manhattan	1½ 3½-oz. glasses	2 3½-oz. glasses
Highball with Mix	3 8-oz. glasses	4 8-oz. glasses

If you have blackouts from drinking, it means you are in a severe stage of alcoholism. The term "blackout" refers not to passing out, but to forgetting events happening during a drinking episode.

HOW TO JUDGE YOUR DRINKS FOR ALCOHOL CONTENT

ALCOHOLIC BEVERAGES	PERCENT OF ALCOHOL
BEER	
Malt	7%
Ale	5
Regular beer	4
WINES	
Fortified: Port, Muscatel	18
Natural: Red/White, Champagne	12
LIQUEURS	
Strong: B & B, Cointreau, Drambuie	40
Medium: fruit brandies	25
STRAIGHT SPIRITS	
Brandy, Cognac, rum, Scotch, vodka, whiskey	45
COCKTAILS	
Strong: Martini, Manhattan	30
Medium: Old-Fashioned, Daiquiri, Alexander	15
HIGHBALLS	
With sweet and sour mixes, tonics	7

ALCOHOL AND THE PILL

Did you know that alcohol affects women who take birth control pills more than those who don't take them? Researchers at the University of Oklahoma found that women, on or off the Pill, felt the effects faster than men, and the effects lasted longest in the women on the Pill.

IF YOU ARE THINKING OF JOINING A.A.

There is a chapter in every city. Look in the phone book.

The basic A.A. approach to the problem of staying sober: The A.A. does not swear off alcohol for life; he never takes pledges not to take a drink tomorrow; he only worries about staying sober *now*, this current 24 hours.

OTHER SERVICES AVAILABLE

- National Council on Alcoholism
- Church and religious organizations
- Company and labor union programs
- Salvation Army
- State hospitals
- Mental health clinics
- Local mental health association or alcoholism information center
- Al-Anon and Al-Ateens for the relatives and friends of the alcoholic

They're all in the telphone book.

Many companies now have programs to help alcoholic employees, in fact, 25 percent of the largest corporations do. They have a success rate estimated at about 70 percent, with many people gaining promotions and raises after participating.

TWO AIDS TO QUITTING

A special diet has been of great help in many programs for alcoholics. The key points: low carbohydrate, high protein, high in vitamins B_3 and B_6 and C and supplements of magnesium. See Chapter 5 for details.

Learning techniques of muscle relaxation is helping many alcoholics to quit. At the Center for Alcohol Studies at the University of North Carolina, alcoholics learn the techniques of progressive muscle relaxation from a recording and find they have less need to turn to chemicals for relief from the pressures of daily living. At the University of Maryland, scientists found if muscles were tense, subjects relaxed more playing tennis, swimming, or bike riding than they did with cocktails.

A NEW PRODUCT—IT WILL MAKE YOU STOP WANTING TO DRINK

The Research Pharmacal Company has a product called Alkonil that is showing much success for the alcoholic who wants to quit. It is a tablet made up of glutamine (one of the amino acids), niacin, and other ingredients that is being used successfully to relieve the cravings for alcohol. (It also appears to be working in drug addicts, schizophrenics, candyholics, and coffeeholics, some of the investigators say.)

Write to: Research Pharmacal Company, P.O. Box 97, Capitola, Calif. 95010.

A SOBER-UP PILL

Scientists at the University of California have tested a group of drugs called amethystic agents which reportedly reverse the effects of alcohol in the brain by up to 50 percent within 30 minutes. The pills are not yet commercially available.

A WAY FOR FAMILIES TO DEAL WITH AN ALCOHOLIC

This method was designed by the Johnson Institute of Minneapolis.

1. Stop nagging the alcoholic; stop protecting him. He must be left on his own to deal with the consequences of his drinking.

2. Two or more family members or friends who have witnessed his drunken behavior (including children) each prepare a written list of particulars about the alcoholic's behavior, citing specific events in detail, with names, dates, and places.

3. They confront the alcoholic, preferably the morning after a drinking bout, but when he is completely sober, each reading from his list of occurrences. They ask him to enter treatment.

4. If the alcoholic refuses to enter a drying-out hospital treatment, then they ask him to pledge abstinence and join Alcoholics Anonymous, with the agreement that if he drinks again he will enter treatment immediately.

5. If this confrontation fails, the team tries again later, constantly presenting reality to the drinker.

WOMEN—THE HIDDEN ALCOHOLICS

Women alcoholics are not as noticeable as men, do not seek help as often and agencies have more trouble finding them and assisting them. To help bridge this gap, there is new booklet *Alcohol Abuse and Women* that tells a woman how to decide if she needs help and how to get it. Free from the National Clearinghouse for Alcohol Information, Box 2345, Rockville, Md. 20852.

How to Accident-Proof Your Family

TODAY'S TOP HAZARDS AROUND THE HOME

ESTIMATED INJURIES PER YEAR ACROSS THE NATION

Bicycles and bicycle equipment	372,000
Stairs, ramps, landings	356,000
Nails, carpet tacks, screws, thumbtacks	275,000
Football equipment and apparel	230,000
Baseball equipment and apparel	191,000
Basketball equipment and apparel	188,000
Architectural glass	178,000
Doors (other than glass)	153,000
Tables (nonglass)	137,000
Swings, slides, seesaws, playground climbing apparatus	112,000
Beds	100,000
Chairs	68,000
Chests, buffets, bookshelves	68,000
Power lawn mowers	58,000
Bathtub and shower structures (except doors)	41,000
Cleaning agents, caustic compounds	35,000
Swimming pools and associated equipment	32,000
Cooking ranges, ovens, and equipment	25,000

From: Consumer Product Safety Commission

THE TWELVE MAJOR FACTORS BEHIND MOST ACCIDENTS AND HOW TO PREVENT THEM

CAUSE	CURE
Fatigue, sleepiness	Take breaks to prevent fatigue
Anger, emotional upsets	Take time to calm down if you are upset
Lack of skill	Read instruction manuals; learn the proper and safe way to do things; get someone to show you if you don't know how
Equipment in disrepair	Check equipment regularly; keep things in shape and neatly stored
Daydreaming, not concentrating	Vary routine to fight monotony
Being too young or too old for the job	Don't let elderly people or young children do dangerous jobs; protect and train them
Hunger, let-down from low blood sugar	Eat snacks to fight let-down or take fructose tablets
Extreme heat or cold	Do inside jobs when weather is so bad it distracts you
Alcohol, medication	Don't operate machines or do dangerous jobs if you have been drinking or taking medication
Working too fast	Don't rush a job; don't operate machines if you are tired or tense or don't feel well
Panic in an emergency	Learn first aid to cope with emergencies; be prepared for the unexpected
Taking chances	Don't show off; don't think an accident can't happen to you

SAFETY-PROOF YOUR FAMILY WITH THIS CHECKLIST:

Enlist the entire family in safety. Teach children safe handling of tools and equipment, and to watch out for hazards.

Discuss the following safety procedures with your family (their answers should be yes to each question):

Does your family use ladders rather than chairs or boxes to reach heights?

Do cooks in the family turn pot handles *away* from front of stove?

Do family members know to slam down a pan lid to smother a grease fire, or throw on baking soda, never to put water on a grease fire?

Do the drivers in the family know never to run an automobile in an enclosed space, even for a few minutes? To shut off the engine if they sit in a parked car for more than a few minutes unless windows are open? To keep the exhaust system in good repair?

Do hunters in the family know to treat every gun as if it were loaded, keeping muzzle pointed in a safe direction? To never load a gun unless intending to shoot it at something? To open bolt when leaving gun unattended? To keep safety on, but don't trust it?

Do family members know to keep safeties, guards, and shields in place on machinery? And to always shut off power when adjusting, servicing, or unclogging machines?

Do they know not to let machines run unattended? To shut off motor when leaving job temporarily?

Do they know not to refuel hot or running engines? And not to smoke when refueling?

Do children know to keep away from machines?

On hazardous jobs, does everyone know not to wear loose clothing?

Is the family careful to read labels on chemicals, and to follow the directions, to use gloves and respiratory devices when needed, to ensure good ventilation when working with toxic fumes?

Is everyone careful not to burn discarded chemical containers and not to pour chemicals on the ground or into a stream?

Do they know not to cut the lawn when the grass is wet and slippery?

Do children know about the dangers of running into streets?

Do they know not to stand near swings?

Do they know that guns, bows and arrows, darts, and slings should only be used with adult supervision?

Now make a tour together of the house and yard with a pencil and following list. Check off all the things that need correction. Correct them.

- Are paths and sidewalks clear?
- Are porches, railing, and steps in good repair?
- Are chemicals and poisons stored in original containers, properly labeled, where children cannot get to them? Are insecticides or cleaning solutions in the kitchen or laundry where children can't get them? Are matches out of children's reach?

- Are flammable liquids (gasoline, oil, paint, etc.) stored outside? Are combustibles (paper, cloth, leaves, rubbish) away from heat and electrical equipment, including light bulbs? Are any piles of oily rags lying around?
- Are there smoke alarms and fire extinguishers in the house?
- Are tools sharp and in good repair, stored in a safe place, unable to fall on anyone?
- Is the stepladder solid with all rungs and steps repaired?
- Are screens securely fastened and high windows protected so small children can't fall out?
- Do stairs have a handrail? Is lighting on stairways bright enough? Is lighting controlled from both top and bottom? Are stairs free of junk and clutter?
- Are toys, tools, bicycles, or other items put away so they won't be tripped over?
- Are there carpets in the bathroom to prevent slipping? Are all electrical appliances far away from water?
- Are medicines where children can't get them? How about guns and ammunition?
- Are flues and chimneys working and unclogged?
- Have furnaces and heating appliances been inspected, cleaned, and adjusted by qualified service personnel? Do the furnace and water heater have adequate air, with louvered door if they are in an enclosed space?
- Are space heaters of the type that don't tip over easily; do they have a safety switch to turn them off if they tip over? If gas, are the heaters adequately exhausted and is there enough fresh air?
- Check wires for frays or cracks. Make sure electric cords don't run through door jambs or anywhere else where they are exposed to constant chafing.
- Do large glass areas have furniture or planters in front of them, or decals to reduce the possibility of walking through the glass?

DON'T LET CHILDREN GO UNATTENDED NEAR:
- Bodies of water
- Excavation projects
- Underground holes or shafts
- Empty buildings and new construction sites
- Railroad property

OTHER WAYS TO SAVE YOUR CHILD'S LIFE

Use proper seat belts and restraining devices in the car no matter what age your child is. A survey by the Insurance Institute for Highway Safety showed *93 percent* of child passengers under age 10 had no seat belt, infant car seat, or other device.

If a child is under the age of 2, do not hold him on your lap. He has no protection against a crash. If you are thrown forward, the child could be crushed between you and the dashboard. Put him in a *well-anchored* car seat or bed.

The next time you paint the basement stairs, put some sand in with the paint to make the steps more slip-proof. Add even more safety by painting the top and bottom steps a bright color.

Outside put tape that glows in the dark on all poorly lit steps and install lights where you can.

Mark all pill bottles, cleaning solutions, and other poison containers with a big red nail polish **X** and explain to your child what it means.

Every time someone in your family has an accident, as soon as possible sit down with your children and discuss what caused the accident and what could be done to prevent it.

Also see *Poison!* (page 164).

BIKE RIDING CAN BE DANGEROUS TO YOUR HEALTH

Bike deaths and injuries are becoming increasingly common, says the U.S. Consumer Private Safety Commission. Most accidents, it says, come from improper braking, double riding, striking bumps or ruts, or the cyclist disregarding traffic laws.

BIKE RIDER'S SAFETY RULES
- Observe all traffic regulations—red and green lights, one-way streets, and stop signs.
- Keep to the right and ride in a single file. Keep a safe distance behind all vehicles.
- Have a white light on front and a reflector on rear for night riding.
- Wear white or light-colored clothes at night.
- Have a bell or horn and use it.
- Always ride at a safe speed and be in complete control.
- Give pedestrians the right of way.
- Look out for cars pulling out into traffic from curbs and driveways.
- Keep a sharp lookout for sudden opening of doors on parked cars.
- Ride in a straight line. Do not weave in or out of traffic or swerve from side to side.
- Always use proper hand signals for turning and stopping.

- Slow down at all intersections and look to right and left before crossing.
- Never carry other riders. Carry no packages that obstruct vision or prevent control.
- Never hitch on other vehicles.
- Keep your bicycle in good running condition.
- Park your bicycle in a safe place where no one will fall over it.

WHAT TO DO IN A CAR EMERGENCY

If your gas pedal sticks	Tap it once or twice to see if it will spring back. Pull it up with your toe or have front seat passenger pull it up.
If your brakes fail	Try pumping the brake. If this doesn't work, put car in low gear and apply emergency brake.
If you lose steering	Apply brakes immediately and use horn or headlights to warn other cars.
If your car catches fire	Use fire extinguisher, or if one is not available, throw dirt on fire. If fire is in the rear where it could reach gas tank, abandon it immediately.
If the engine overheats	Pull off the road, let the engine cool. Look for the trouble, but do not remove radiator cap until engine is cool.
If you have a blowout	Don't slam on brakes. Grip wheel firmly and apply brakes slowly.
If the hood pops up	Don't stop suddenly, which could cause a rear-end collision, but signal immediately as you ease car to right or left off road.
If your electrical system fails	Immediately and completely pull off the road since none of your warning lights will work to warn approaching cars.

Note: Not wearing a seat belt can result in loss of injury compensation from insurance in a traffic accident, warns the Motor Vehicle Manufacturers Association. It reports that 14 states now allow defendants in auto-injury claims to seek reduction or total elimination of compensation if the claimant wasn't wearing a seat belt.

RECOMMENDED:
Safety Now
  Murl Harmon
  P. O. Box 567
  Jenkintown, Pa. 19046
  Free
  Catalogue of safe equipment and products for children.

Finding a Way to Manage Stress

ARE YOU OVERTENSE?

The National Association for Mental Health says there are a number of ways to tell if you are reacting excessively to stress. They suggest you ask yourself these questions:

1. Do minor problems and disappointments upset you?
2. Do you find it difficult to get along with people; are people having trouble getting along with you?
3. Do the small pleasures of life fail to satisfy you?
4. Are you unable to stop thinking about your anxieties?
5. Do you fear people or situations that never used to trouble you?
6. Are you suspicious of people, mistrustful of your friends?
7. Do you have the feeling of being trapped?
8. Do you feel inadequate, suffer the tortures of self-doubt?

If you answer *yes* to most of the questions, you may be suffering from excessive anxiety and tension.

TAKE THE STRESS TEST EVERY DAY— CHECK YOURSELF FOR TENSION

Everybody has tension once in a while when things go wrong, but some people are tense almost all of the time without knowing it.

Watch when you are working or solving problems whether you have a relaxed use of energy or are tight and hurrying for no good reason. Tension clues to look for are: butterflies in the stomach, eyes fluttering, eyestrain, tight neck or jaw muscles, chin jutted out, biting or grinding teeth, sweating palms or cold hands, irritability, high pulse rate, moving too brusquely with muscles tight, irregular shallow breathing or sighing respiration, tight strained voice, shoulders hunched, toes or fingers tightly curled, spine rigid, forehead tight, sometimes with a headache beginning.

When you feel these signs coming on, try to take a few deep breaths and purposefully relax.

HOW MUCH STRESS CAN MAKE YOU SICK?

Drs. Thomas Holmes and Minoru Masuda, psychiatrists at the University of Washington in Seattle, have devised a scale to help predict illness that comes from too much stress. They find that any change, good or bad, can produce stress. And if the stress is severe enough, it may be related to whether you develop a disease, when you develop it, and how severe it is. The doctors assigned point values to stressful events in peoples' lives, then found that major illness often followed a cluster of many stress-related changes that occurred in one year.

These are the life events that appeared to affect health, with the point values the scientists assigned for them.

LIFE EVENT	VALUE
Death of spouse	100
Divorce	73
Marital separation	65
Jail term	63
Death of close family member	63
Personal injury or illness	53
Marriage	50
Fired from work	47
Marital reconciliation	45
Retirement	45
Change in health of family member	44
Pregnancy	40
Sex difficulties	39
Gain of new family member	39
Business readjustment	39
Change in financial state	38
Death of close friend	37
Change to different line of work	36
Change in number of arguments with spouse	35
Mortgage over $10,000	31
Foreclosure of mortgage or loan	30
Change in responsibilities at work	29
Son or daughter leaving home	29
Trouble with in-laws	29
Outstanding personal achievement	28
Wife begins or stops work	26
Begin or end school	26
Change in living conditions	25
Revision of personal habits	24
Trouble with boss	23
Change in work hours or conditions	20
Change in residence	20
Change in schools	20
Change in recreation	19
Change in church activities	19

LIFE EVENT	VALUE
Change in social activities	18
Mortgage or loan less than $10,000	17
Change in sleeping habits	16
Change in number of family get-togethers	15
Change in eating habits	15
Vacation	13
Christmas	12
Minor violations of the law	11

In the persons studied, 79 percent became severely ill within a year if the changes occurring in life totaled over 300 points.

If your score is beyond the dangerous 300 mark, you should consider postponing some major moves, especially negative ones, until your score becomes lower and your life less stressful.

WHAT CAN YOU DO TO DEAL WITH YOUR TENSIONS?

Try to calm down your sense of time urgency and excessive hostile feelings. Learn to substitute excellence of values for quantities of things, appreciating nature, reading, music, meaningful personal relations, instead of having *things*. Put priorities on your time and energy. Learn to say no when you don't really want to do something or it isn't beneficial to you or someone else. Practice listening to people more, stop half-listening to your family while thinking of business problems; give them your entire attention.

Give yourself a frank self-evaluation as to capabilities and goals, what you really want in life, and what you are capable of. Learn to devote your time and energies to the goals and to major problems rather than to unimportant trivia.

Organize your day for the things you really want or need to do. Try to delegate some of your jobs and authority.

Don't meet minor happenings as though they were all major crises. Solve a problem and let it go.

Eliminate unnecessary events so you are not always struggling against time. Don't be in a frenzy to have all tasks immediately finished.

Consciously use slowdown maneuvers, such as deep breathing, to overcome your sense of time urgency.

Try to work in an environment that promotes peace.

Allow time for self-contemplation and exploration.

Learn to live day by day, rather than always for the future, and find some enjoyment and beauty in each day. Try the Buddha philosophy of paying attention to the here and now, savoring eating when you're eating, concentrating only on driving when you are driving, not on something else in the past or future.

When something worries you, talk it out, don't bottle it up. When things go wrong, escape from the problem for a while: go to a movie, play a game with your child, take a walk. But make it only a short escape, then come back and deal with your difficulty.

If you feel pent-up with anger or frustration, cool off by doing something physical: gardening, cleaning out the garage, tennis.

If you often are obstinate and defiant, frequently getting into quarrels, learn to give in occasionally. Stand your ground on what you know is right, but do so calmly. If you yield a little, others may too, and you can achieve a practical solution without tension.

When a work load seems unbearable, divide it into a series of tasks, take one thing at a time and work your way out of it by steps. Don't try to be a superman, trying to be perfect in everything. Give the best of your efforts and ability, but don't take yourself to task if you can't achieve the impossible.

Try cooperation instead of competition. You don't always have to edge out the other person on the highway or win a discussion. Stop being a threat to others and they may stop being a threat to you.

MAKE YOUR SLEEP WORK FOR YOU

When you have a tough problem, think about the pros and cons *before* you go to sleep and direct your subconscious to work on the problem *while you sleep. You'll often wake up with the logical answer!* (Be sure to keep a pad and pencil next to your bed so you can jot ideas and answers down.)

REDUCE STRESS BY ORGANIZING YOUR LIFE

If your life is full of conflicting demands, if you rush here and there but never seem to get anything done, simplify and organize. Ideas that work for your personal life or running your office or home:

List your personal goals for the next six months, then make an action list of the things you need to do to reach those goals. Keep your list in front of you as you organize your day.

Think about how you spend your days. What are you doing that doesn't need to be done? Eliminate all busy-busy nonessential tasks.

Get up and into the day right away instead of wandering around staring out the window for three cups of coffee. Take advantage of those super-productive early morning hours.

Keep a list of what you need and want to do that you keep in a handy-at-all-times place so you can easily add to it whenever you think of things. Keep a separate ongoing list for grocery shopping items. Every night before you go to bed, look at your calendar for engagements for the next day and at your do-it list and plan your day.

Mark your lists with stars or underline priority items so for sure you will get these done rather than spend limited time on lower priority items.

Be a perfectionist on important things, but not on low-priority items. You don't need to iron sheets.

Learn to concentrate on a task when you do it. Don't let your mind wander to other problems while you're doing this one.

When you read the mail, read each piece only once and act upon it immediately.

Don't spend whole evenings watching television. Watch only the programs really important to you and use an hour in the evening for pleasure or to get a small job done.

Always carry a notebook or file cards with you for jotting down notes when you think of things.

Carry books, pencil and paper, or small projects with you so you can take advantage of any waiting time.

Use commuting time to plan or read.

Get help for jobs you can afford to delegate.

Learn how to say *no* to things you don't want to do.

INSTANT RELAXERS

The dangle. Stop in the middle of whatever you are doing. Stand with legs apart, bend at waist. Shake your arms and hands loosely. Let your head hang, and sway from side to side. Rise slowly.

Sitting-in-a chair dangle. Sit with arms relaxed at the sides. Breathe out slowly while dropping your head. Sink your chest, and bend forward until your head is above or between your knees. Contract the abdominal muscles firmly during the last part of the bending. Breathe in gradually while raising the body so that your hips straighten first, followed by the back, shoulders, neck, and finally the head.

Head roll. Drop chin to chest. Rotate head to right and pass chin to shoulder. Circle head back and around and pass over left shoulder to make complete revolution. Repeat in opposite direction.

Head tilt. Keep shoulders down. Tilt left ear to left shoulder several times in bouncing motion. Tilt right ear to right shoulder several times.

Back stretch. Lie on back on floor. Push spine flat into floor. Release, go limp in all muscles, breathe deeply. Repeat several times. Remain limp and breathing deeply.

The head lift. Curl your fingers around the sides of the neck, meeting in back. Lift straight upward and forward as though you were trying to lift your head off your shoulders. Turn your head slightly from right to left while you continue lifting.

The slantboard. Buy a slantboard, or make one with an ironing board propped up securely on a wooden box or chair 15 inches high. The chair should have its back to the wall so it can't slide. Lie on the slantboard with feet elevated and spine straight for 15 minutes at a time.

Try a neck massage. Close your eyes and massage all about your neck, finding the areas that are most tense and concentrating on them. Then starting at the top of your neck at the base of the skull massage on both sides of the spinal column at once in firm small circles. Let your head and neck go limp. Work slowly down from the skull along the vertebrae to the shoulders. Then slowly run your fingers along the hairline, first very firmly, then very lightly. Next gently run fingers along eye sockets, then down cheekbones and along jaw bones. Leave eyes closed and lie still for several minutes feeling the relaxation.

And don't forget the values of a good hot tub or shower.

WAYS TO REV UP YOUR CIRCULATION TO HELP FIGHT FATIGUE AND STRESS

Don't take a taxi, walk; don't take an elevator, climb; jog; skip rope; run; play tennis, golf, any sport; dance; climb; swim. Have a massage. Use a shower massager; alternating hard shower spray from hot to cold. Do a headstand or shoulder-stand for as long a time you can, using a towel or pillow to cushion your head.

When you're sitting for a long time at your desk or on a trip, make it a point to get up and stretch periodically, and don't let the chair seat press at the back of your knees where your femoral artery is.

RELAXATION TECHNIQUES TO FIGHT TENSION WITHOUT A PSYCHIATRIST

Train yourself to move more slowly when you work. When you feel yourself getting tense, breathe deeply several times and consciously let your muscles go limp.

If you can, lie down and let your thoughts drift while counting from 1 to 10, or imagine a series of numbers painted languorously in the sky, or picture yourself drifting slowly on a cloud, or swimming through soft waves in a balmy, blue sea.

Or lie on your back completely relaxed. Imagine you are a sponge, arms limp and away from the body, shoulders relaxed, legs apart and loose. Press your neck and back into the sofa, floor, or bed. Close your eyes, breathe deeply through your nose, relax each part of your body, while still thinking of your body as a sponge, relaxed and limp, but soaking up strength and tranquility.

Learn abdominal breathing. It can be done lying flat on your back, or with knees bent and drawn up, or sitting in a chair. Place one hand on your abdomen and one on your chest, so you can feel that you are breathing with the abdomen alone, not with the chest. Inhale deeply through the nostrils and expand the abdomen without pulling the air up to the chest. Keep your shoulders and chest relaxed. Exhale slowly through the nostrils while pulling the abdomen to the back of the spine.

Try a sighing breath. This yoga technique will rapidly quiet the mind. It can be done anywhere; standing, sitting, waiting for a bus. Instead of pacing, inhale deeply through the nostrils to the count of 8, then with lips puckered (as if cooling soup) exhale very slowly through the mouth to the count of 16 or as long as you can. Concentrate on the long sighing sound and feel the tension dissolve. Repeat at least 10 times.

Cassette tapes may also help:

Relaxation Tape, Dick Sutphen
Valley of the Sun Publishing Co.
Box 15232
Phoenix, Ariz. 85018
$10.00

Deep Relaxation, Dan Golerman
Psychology Today
595 Broadway
New York, N.Y. 10012
$7.95

HAVE SOMEONE GIVE YOU A RELAXING MASSAGE

Use mineral oil or vegetable oil, talcum or body powder. The floor with some padding and a sheet is better than a bed, which gives too much.

Lighting should be dim.

Your massager should have fingernails short, hands freshly washed, and jewelry removed.

Strokes should be smooth, steady, without jerkiness. The entire area of your body being massaged should be completely and systematically covered.

Your massager should always try to have one hand touching you, without breaking contact once it is established.

Your massager should let fingers and hands explore the anatomy of the area they are massaging, feeling the shape of your underlying structures.

Weight rather than muscle should be used to apply pressure.

If a massage must be brief, have your massager concentrate on the back, head, neck, and feet—usually the most relaxing and beneficial places.

To work on a tense spot, a wide area should be massaged around it first, then your tense spot massaged using strong pressure.

ENJOYING IT MORE

Keep your body as limp as you can. Do not try to help. Let yourself be completely taken care of.

Leave your arms loosely at your side.

Close your eyes.

Focus your attention on your breathing and concentrate on the encounter of the touch.

When the massage is over, lie still with your eyes closed for a while.

SOME KINDS OF MASSAGE STROKES

Strokes can be with the palm, heel, or edge of hand, fingers, or even one finger or thumb, and can include the following:

- The hands slipping over the skin
- The hands not slipping over the skin, but making the superficial skin tissue move over the deeper underlying tissue
- Superficial light stroking which should be slow, gentle, and smooth
- Deep stroking toward the heart, in the direction of venous flow of the blood
- Lifting and squeezing the tissue
- Rolling with the palms
- Kneading the tissue with alternating compression and relaxation
- Raking the skin with the fingers
- Moving fingertips with deep pressure in tiny circles

- Drumming with the fingertips
- Large sweeps with the forearms
- Light slapping with hands cupped
- Defining the inner anatomy, following the contour of each bone and muscle

RELAXING WITH YOGA

Remove or loosen any tight clothing. Lie on your back, close your eyes. Breathe in deeply (through the nose) and raise your arms over your head. Hold your breath and stretch, tensing all muscles. Then go limp and exhale slowly (through the nose), dropping your arms to your side.

Now lie limply, and take another long, deep breath. Exhale as far as you can, releasing your breath very slowly.

Starting with your feet, tense your muscles then let go. First the toes of your right foot. Tense; relax. Then the toes of your left foot. Now move gradually to tense and relax the ankles, calves, knees, and thighs until your legs feel loose and free. Think of waves of relaxation spreading into your abdomen, chest, and shoulders; then all along your spine and back. Feel the muscles begin to loosen. Tense abdominal muscles, relax. Tighten your buttocks and relax. Now let arms and hands become limp. Relax fingers one by one. Close and open fists, first right hand, then left. Relax the muscles in arm. Shrug shoulders, then relax. Relax up along the sides and back of neck.

Tense facial muscles then relax. Let jaw sag with lips slightly parted. Yawn. Feel scalp loosen. Let eyes relax and rest. You feel the relaxation gradually enveloping your entire body. You feel completely relaxed.

Now lie still and become aware of the steady, slow beating of your heart and of your breath as it flows in and out. Breathe in deeply, breathing in energy from around you. As you breathe out, more and more tension leaves you. You no longer feel confined by your body.

You concentrate more and more on the flow of your breath. You feel a state of peace all around you, relaxed peace.

LEARN MEDITATION

The meditation state is a state of alpha, your brain putting out alpha waves as it does in the first moments of falling asleep. It's a quiet state of inner reflection. To experience meditation, find a quiet environment. Sit in a comfortable position. Close your eyes. Take deep, slow, long breaths. Feel a calming influence coming over and into your body. Breathe rhythmically and quietly. Let your muscles relax, let your mind blank to nothing . . . drifting. Don't work at it, just let it happen. Let your mind wander as it wishes. Observe it, but don't try to control it. Or in some meditation techniques you keep saying one meaningless word or phrase over and over to keep your mind from wandering. Now and then you will enter into brief deep interludes of retreat. If you are completely relaxed, you are experiencing meditation.

Practice the technique for 10 to 20 minutes twice a day, but not within two hours after any meal.

The technique helps decrease the activity of the sympathetic nervous system and thus can reduce tension and anxiety, slow respiration and heart rate, lower blood pressure, decrease occurrences of irregular heartbeats, alleviate asthma, and help smokers and alcoholics quit.

Actually there are many ways to meditate. Some are passive, such as TM, concentrating only on a word or phrase. Others involve concentrating on the respiration, as in yoga or Zen meditation; or you can sometimes focus your gaze on a lighted candle, a leaf, or on still water. Some are basically designed to produce a sense of calmness and inner harmony, a peace and serenity that wipes away tension. Others are designed for you to try to experience a union of the body's energy with the vaster energies of the universe.

You can learn of meditation classes in your area by checking the yellow pages under "Meditation," checking for classes at universities or local Y's, or even asking a minister or priest who often is in touch with groups.

STRESS CONTROL THROUGH BIOFEEDBACK

With biofeedback a person learns to control the autonomic functions of his body by monitoring body functions on a machine that uses meters, sounds, or flashing lights to tell him the effect he is producing on muscle tension, skin temperature, heart rate, blood pressure, or other functions. The person simply imagines the change he wants to produce, and lets it happen, and the machine tells how strong an effect was produced. In many large cities, biofeedback laboratories are open to the public, such as the Stress Transformation Center, 78 East 79th Street, New York, N.Y.; and in other cities, persons must be referred by a psychologist or physician. Your physician should know if there

is a center in your area. In addition to being used to learn to fight stress, the biofeedback technique has proved effective in treating headaches, high blood pressure, ulcer, Raynaud's disease, insomnia, phobias, anxiety states, asthma, epilepsy, heart arrhythmias, and speech problems.

Another stress center. The director of the Cardiac Stress Management Training Program at Colorado State University, Richard Suinn, says the six-session breaking-the-cycle-of-stress program consists of the following:

Learning to identify the early warning signals that stress is beginning (such as tightening of neck and shoulder muscles, teeth clenching, queasiness, frowning).

Learning relaxation with regular sessions at home, using music, deep muscle relaxation, or meditation.

Imagining stressful situations and mentally figuring ways to solve them with the least amount of stress.

Using the relaxation and problem-solving techniques during the day whenever stress builds up.

Taking better control of the environment by scheduling appointments more realistically, setting priorities, managing demands from others.

Results at the clinic show people cannot only reduce their stress cycle, but in the process usually lower high cholesterol levels and sometimes lower blood pressure.

STRESS AND DIET

Your diet can definitely affect whether you tend to be tense or tranquil.

To find out the specific effect of diet on your personality, you should undergo four diet experiments. Do each at a separate time so the results from one do not affect the other.

1. Eliminate caffeine totally from your diet. No coffee, tea, cocoa, colas, or other caffeine drinks, or caffeine medications such as headache pills, for one week. If you find you're less nervous and less tense, caffeine may be something you should eliminate permanently from your diet. Try adding one cup or glass a day back to your diet and test its effect to determine just how much caffeine you can tolerate without becoming tense. No one should have more than four cups a day. Also to cut down caffeine, try decaffeinated coffee; throw out the first cup of tea from a tea bag, and use the second, which will have less caffeine.

2. After you have tested caffeine, try eliminating sugar from your diet, completely avoiding table

sugar and all foods and drinks that have any sugar in them. Run this test for a week also and see if it eliminates your tensions. If so, eliminate sugar permanently from your diet. (If you miss it, use fructose, the sugar diabetics can use that is readily available in Europe and slowly becoming available in this country.)

3. Take vitamin and mineral supplements, making sure they contain choline and inositol, the natural tension alleviators. See if these don't make a further difference.

4. If none of these steps seem to be the key to your tension and anxiety, then try the hypoglycemic diet as described in Chapter 5. One of the symptoms of hypoglycemia is anxiety, tension, and periodic irritability, and the hypoglycemic diet does wonders at eliminating the symptoms if this is the cause.

STRESS AND YOUR ENVIRONMENT

The weather can affect your emotions greatly. A falling barometer, for example, can mean depression and difficulty in solving problems; so when you know the barometer is going down, postpone important decisions, drive extra carefully, watch your emotions, and prepare for an off-day. Low atmospheric pressure may cause forgetfulness, and thunderstorms may induce hyperactivity. Intense cold increases incidence of heart attacks, duodenal ulcer attacks, and migraine headaches.

For more information: Public Affairs Pamphlet, 381 Park Avenue South, New York, N.Y. 10016, No. 533, 35¢.

Light, too, can have a profound effect. John Ott, specialist in medicine and lighting, says many problems, including hyperactivity in children, are being linked to fluorescent lighting and insufficient ultraviolet light. In a Florida radio station when fluorescent lights were installed, people became irritable, jumpy, rebellious, quit without explanation. When UVT lights were installed, things returned to normal.

Make sure your windows and your eyeglasses are UVT (ultraviolet transmitting). You can obtain UVT bulbs and "Daylight white" tubes for your home from most stores (made by Duro-Test Corporation). Simply ask your regular dealer for them. They are readily available. The International Commission on Illumination says the UVT light increases activity of the sex glands, decreases tooth decay, and increases children's ability to concentrate and learn.

Smog, too, says Dr. Leroy Schieler, pollution expert, can cause nervousness, irritability, depression, and other mental problems, as well as nausea and fatigue. In fact, he says, constant smog can affect the mood of an entire population of a smog area and for long periods. Some researchers even speculate there is a connection between some airborne chemicals like hydrogen sulfide and the high suicide rates of communities that have such pollutants.

HIDDEN LEAD POISONING

It is not just slum children eating lead paint who get lead poisoning. The poisoning is spreading like wildfire through the population. We're getting it in the air we breathe, from car exhausts, from contaminated food, and even from some hair dyes that are dangerously high in lead content. Some doctors are finding that patients with crippling arthritis-like symptoms are really suffering from unsuspected lead poisoning and many people who suffer from extreme irritability really have subclinical cases of lead poisoning that have never been diagnosed.

You can be tested for lead and other toxic metals by sending in a hair sample for analysis. See Chapter 4.

NOISE—WHAT IT CAN DO TO YOU

Noise pollution has been shown to cause deafness, irritability, heart disease, high blood pressure, ulcers, fatigue, and sexual dysfunction. How does it do it? Ear surgeon Dr. Samuel Rosen explains: "Adrenalin is shot into the blood stream, heart rate increases, blood vessels constrict and there are reactions in the intestines. The symptoms persist . . . and outlast the noise. You may forgive the noise, but your body never will."

AN EXPERIMENT TO SHOW
NOISE CAN MAKE YOU NASTY

Two scientists set up this experiment. An actor gets out of a car with two armfuls of books, apparently moving into a new house. As a pedestrian passes by, he drops the books.

Under normal conditions, 80 percent of people passing by stopped to help. When a noisy lawnmower was going, the number of people who stopped to help dropped to 15 percent. The test was run 1,000 times with the same results.

Says one of the scientists: "If you think you have been unusually unreasonable to someone, look around; maybe you should turn down the television set or move away from that air conditioner."

NINE WAYS TO CUT DOWN NOISE

1. Make sure windows are tight-fitting and properly caulked.

2. Use storm windows, double track or double glazed windows.

3. Use drapes at windows, the thicker the better.

4. Use acoustical materials on inside home surfaces, such as cork or acoustical tiles.

5. Use carpeting with a pad on floors.

6. Use carpeting on walls.

7. Use cork or other insulation around dishwashers, air conditioners, other electrical noise-makers.

8. Run closets along walls of rooms next to noisy rooms, such as bath or laundry.

9. Plant trees and shrubs between your house and the street or other noisy area.

How to Get a Good Night's Sleep Without Resorting to Pills

FOURTEEN INNOVATIVE STEPS TO BREAK THE INSOMNIA HABIT WITHOUT USING PILLS

1. Get more exercise during the day. But don't exercise just before going to bed.

2. Live by your natural rhythms. Don't go to bed until sleepy.

3. Eliminate noise with carpeting, drapes, other sound-conditioning; use ear-plugs if necessary. Make sure the bedroom isn't too hot or too cold. Most people sleep best between 60 and 65 degrees. See if you need a new mattress, or a firmer one, or softer.

4. Have a snack that's not sweet. Milk is especially good. Don't drink coffee, tea, or cola at night.

5. Don't drink too much alcohol. It will rob you of dream time and make for a poor night's sleep.

6. Take inositol, which is a B vitamin. A 2000 mg tablet taken at bedtime acts as a natural sleeping pill. (It will also lower your cholesterol.) Calcium supplements may also help. Second choice: Take an aspirin. It seems to promote sleep. (Don't take it, however, if you have an ulcer or other bleeding tendencies.)

7. Establish a go-to-bed ritual, whether it's brushing your hair, checking the doors, hugging a teddy-bear, or saying a prayer.

8. Make your room absolutely dark.

9. Don't play the radio all night. Research shows it keeps you from a deep sleep. If you like music to go to sleep by, have an automatic timer to turn it off.

10. Don't let problems get to you. Pick one and think it through. Let the rest wait until tomorrow.

11. Think of something pleasant that happened during the day.

12. Use progressive relaxation, yoga, breathing exercises, or biofeedback training for relaxation.

13. Purposefully stay up all night. Don't let yourself go to sleep even when you want to. (This seems to help patients who have insomnia because they are depressed; in those who are not depressed, it only makes them tired.)

14. Sleep less. Maybe you don't have insomnia, you simply are lucky enough to need less sleep than others. The clue is how you feel the next day.

FOUR EXERCISES TO GO TO SLEEP BY

1. Create a picture in your mind. A soft, silent, snow scene; a pastoral painting of horses grazing along a meadow; a bird drifting through a sunset sky; a leaf floating on a pond.

2. Think of downward movement. Picture yourself floating down like a feather from a cloud, or imagine going down a long, long staircase or riding down an elevator, going deeper and deeper.

3. Close your eyes and relax your body as completely as you can, starting from your toes and relaxing every muscle right up to your scalp, letting yourself sink deeper and deeper into relaxation. Then count slowly from 10 down to 0, painting the numbers slowly on a cloud or visualizing them going down a staircase. Tell yourself that when you reach 0 you will be asleep.

4. Talk yourself to sleep. Tell yourself your eyelids are growing heavy, heavier, heavier; that

your entire body is becoming very relaxed; that you are relaxing more and more, deeper . . . and deeper . . . your eyelids are heavy . . . and heavier; that you are completely relaxed from the top of your head . . . to the tips of your toes; that you are getting sleepier and sleepier . . . sleepier and sleepier . . .

NEW NATURAL SLEEP PILLS

A natural substance called L-tryptophan is now available as an over-the-counter substance in most health food stores. It's a non-addictive non-hangover pill with no side effects. Dr. Clinton C. Brown, of Johns Hopkins University, used doses of 1½ grams of the L-tryptophan and found subjects took half as long to fall asleep and slept 45 minutes longer than usual. L-tryptophan is found naturally in high-protein foods like meat, milk, and cheese, and could be the reason people sleep better if they take a glass of milk before they go to bed.

Also see step 6, page 65, for information on inositol. Magnesium also is a natural tranquilizer.

BUT YOU MAY NOT BE LOSING AS MUCH SLEEP AS YOU THINK

Dr. William C. Dement at the Sleep Disorder Clinic at Stanford University studied patients who complained of insomnia. He found consistently that most subjects underestimated the amount of time they slept, and overestimated the amount of time it took for them to get to sleep. If they complained of taking an hour to go to sleep, most actually fell asleep within fifteen minutes. But usually the insomniacs woke up many more times during the night than they realized, Dr. Dement said, which might be the reason for their feeling of lack of sleep the next day.

RECOMMENDED:
Go to Sleep Hypnosis Tape, Dick Sutphen
Valley of the Sun Publishing Co.
Box 15232
Phoenix, Ariz. 85018

KICKING THE SLEEPING PILL HABIT

Get off the pills gradually, working with a doctor. If withdrawal is difficult, you may have to spend a few days in the hospital.

When you stop using pills, you may have nightmares and difficulty in sleeping for several months. This is a natural rebound reaction from having been on the pills. Do not go back on the pills again; the problem is temporary.

WHAT TO DO FOR SNORING THAT KEEPS YOU AWAKE

Increase the humidity in the bedroom. Dry swollen membranes sometimes cause snoring.

Check for allergies. Certain foods or pollen or pet dander may be causing swelling of tissue.

Sleep on your side. Most people snore on their backs. Prop a pillow behind the back to keep from turning over.

Stop smoking.

Cut down on heavy nighttime drinking, so that sleep is not drugged or restless.

Try some commercial devices like dilators to hold nostrils open or chin straps to keep mouth closed.

Have surgery if snoring is caused by a crooked nose, enlarged tonsils or adenoids, or nasal polyps.

STRANGE SLEEP HABITS THAT CAN RUIN LIVES

Hypersomnia is the opposite of insomnia. The hypersomniac needs an excessive amount of sleep. Left alone, he may stay in bed and sleep all day, often sleeping as much as 16 to 18 hours a day. Hypersomniacs are often late to work, are branded lazy and shiftless when they really need to see a doctor.

Narcolepsy is a medical problem in which a patient has an attack of uncontrollable sleep, or even paralysis. Again the patient builds up terrible guilt feelings and embarrassment, not realizing there are medicines that can help. High selenium levels have been found in narcoleptic people. Narcolepsy disappeared when selenium levels were lowered.

Periodic sleep apnea is a condition in which the patient stops breathing in his sleep, or falls asleep suddenly and unexplainedly, even in the bathtub or in the middle of a business deal. Breathing may stop for as long as a minute and half. Some victims snore for about two minutes, then stop breathing for about 30 to 90 seconds. It occurs most frequently in obese people with thick necks, and in those who sleep on their backs.

Sleepwalking. Often sleepwalkers will not notice dangers like drop-offs, open windows, cars bearing down on them, so they *do* get hurt despite myths to the contrary.

Keep a sleepwalker's bedroom on the first

floor; put away dangerous objects and car keys; put gates at stairways and latch bedroom windows tight.

Do not shake a sleepwalker, but call his name until it penetrates his consciousness, help him realize where he is, and guide him gently back to bed. Usually a sleepwalker left alone will perform his mission and go back to bed. If episodes are frequent, or last more than ten minutes, see your doctor to try to determine the cause.

CHAPTER 9

Wending Your Way Through the Birth Control Maze, With Special Information on Sterilization, Abortion, and Hysterectomies

FINDING THE BEST BETS IN BIRTH CONTROL

Rhythm Method: This method is to have intercourse only in the days before menstruation and after, trying to guess when the woman is fertile, and avoiding that time. But a woman's egg is *not* always produced on schedule. Reliability: inaccurate.

Douching: The uterus creates suction during intercourse and the sperms stream toward the uterus within seconds. Reliability: forget it.

Withdrawal: Many women have relied on the man to withdraw at the last minute before ejaculation. Most of these women are pregnant. Reliability: not effective.

Condoms: Don't wait too long to put it on. Don't let it get torn. Don't store it in your wallet for a long time. Also an excellent protection against venereal disease, secret studies in Nevada brothels have shown. Reliability: 90 percent effective.

Jellies and Foams: A medicated cream or foam is inserted into the vagina and then melts from the body's heat. Available in both prescription and non-prescription form. You insert them a few minutes before intercourse. If an hour goes by, or prior to repeating intercourse, another application should be made. Some protection against venereal disease. Reliability: very effective.

Diaphragm: The diaphragm is like a tiny bowl. Go to a doctor or woman's center for fitting. The diaphragm should be inserted before intercourse and always be left in place for at least six hours afterward. It should never be used without a con-

traceptive cream, because it is the cream that is the insurance against pregnancy. Always examine the diaphragm for defects, especially at the edges, before and after use by putting water in it or holding it up to the light. Diaphragms have a life span of about one year. If you gain or lose more than 10 pounds, have a baby, miscarriage, or gynecologic operation, you probably need to be fitted for a new size. Reliability: 90 percent effective.

The Pill: Usually if there is a mishap, it is because a woman forgot to take the Pill on schedule. If she has nausea, breast tenderness, or bleeding between menstrual periods when she is on the Pill, she should discuss it with her doctor immediately so he can try a different brand, which often is all that's needed to eliminate the symptoms. Women who have high blood pressure or a tendency toward blood clots should use birth control pills only if followed carefully by their doctors. Always call your doctor if you have frequent severe headaches, visual disturbances, or weakness in the legs. Reliability: more than 99 percent effective.

(Some doctors claim that Valium, Seconal, and an arthritis medicine called Butazolidin can inhibit a birth control pill, making pregnancy posssible.)

See p. 42 for special diet women on the Pill should follow.

Facts on the dangers of the Pill: Here's what we know for sure. Pill-takers show a higher than normal risk of developing blood clots, which can cause stroke or heart attack. The Pill can increase blood pressure in some women. You can easily test this by having your blood pressure taken before going on the Pill and several weeks after. It can cause liver problems in some women. It can aggravate disorders of sugar metabolism, and also seems to be related to gallstones. Most of these things are more likely to occur in women over age 40 (and in women who smoke), so many doctors feel women over age 35 to 40 and smokers should use another contraceptive method. Most doctors recommend that women should not take the Pill if they have cancer of the breast or uterus, liver disease, elevated levels of blood fats, coronary artery disease, depression, past blood clot problems, sickle cell disease, migraine headaches, fibroid tumors, or epilepsy. Also be *sure* to stop taking the Pill immediately if you think you might be pregnant. The Pill will often eliminate or lessen symptoms of premenstrual tension, breast engorgement, menstrual cramps, cysts of the breasts and ovaries.

Note: If you want to become pregnant, switch off the Pill to another contraceptive method for three months to lessen chance of damage to fetus. Also switch to another form of contraception for a month before any scheduled surgery to lessen chances of postsurgery blood clots.

Intrauterine Devices: These devices, called IUDs, consist of a plastic or rubber loop or coil, sometimes coated with copper. The IUD is inserted by a physician into the uterus, where it interferes with fertilization of the egg. The loops can be left in place for years with no need for removal. Reliability: 97 percent effective, but there are many side effects.

COUPLES ARE SWITCHING METHODS

More than half of women have changed contraceptive methods in the last two years, according to a report in the *Journal of the American Medical Association.* Mostly they are moving away from the use of birth control pills to barrier methods or to sterilization.

THE ABSOLUTELY POSITIVE WAY TO BE SURE TO HAVE NO MORE CHILDREN —STERILIZATION

It has become *the* most widely used method of birth control for couples in their 30s, in fact, more than 7 million Americans already have had either a male vasectomy or female tubal ligation. The operations are legal in *every* state. If you want one and a doctor does not want to give you one, stand on your rights and insist he refer you to someone who

will do the procedure, or contact your local Planned Parenthood office, which often offers the procedures inexpensively, or contact the Association for Voluntary Sterilization, 14 West 40th Street, New York, N.Y. 10018, which will give you the name of a doctor or clinic in your area where you can have the procedure done.

For Men. The operation for men is a vasectomy, done in 15 to 30 minutes in a clinic or doctor's office.

It is simple, speedy, safe, and cheap. In the future, during intercourse, the man feels all the same pleasure and still has an ejaculation, but the ejaculated fluid has no sperm in it, so that no baby is produced.

The operation can be done either in a special visit to the doctor, or in conjunction with a hernia operation or a prostate operation already scheduled.

The operation is so simple that most men return to work the next day and resume intercourse within a week.

Note: Be sure to use another form of birth control for at least four months and until you get two negative sperm counts to make sure there is no leaking of sperm.

The New Quick Band-Aid Operation for Women. A women can have a hysterectomy (removal of the uterus). Or she can have her tubes tied off or cut in a new 10- to 15-minute operation called laparoscopic sterilization. A tiny half-inch incision is made in the abdomen. An instrument called a laparoscope is inserted in the incision, the tubes are sealed off in a few minutes, and a Band-Aid applied. The women leaves the hospital or doctor's office after resting a couple of hours. Reliability: both male and female procedures are 100 percent sure and effective.

NEW METHODS OF BIRTH CONTROL NOW BEING TESTED

These include an injectable that needs to be given two to four times a year, a nasal spray, pills to be taken the morning after, a paper pill that is like a stamp impregnated with hormone and is eaten, and a pill for men.

OVULATION INDICATOR

This new device, called Ovutimer, may improve the accuracy of the rhythm method of birth control. It enables a woman to determine her fertile and safe days by using a special probe to withdraw mucus from her cervix. The Ovutimer determines whether it is thick mucus, present on safe days, or thinner mucus, present when pregnancy can occur. Available soon.

WHERE TO CHECK FOR FREE OR LOW-COST SERVICES

100 percent guarantee. In Seattle, a birth control clinic named Population Dynamics offers a free abortion to any woman patient who becomes pregnant through failure of her contraceptive devices or of her husband's vasectomy.

Medicaid. A law requires that state welfare agencies offer family planning services, information, and supplies to all public assistance recipients. And most of the states pay for voluntary sterilization procedures as a method of contraception.

Teenagers. Some doctors and clinics will provide pregnancy testing and contraceptive information to teenagers without parental consent, some will not. You will have to check yourself. In New York students have put together a list of clinics and hospitals in the area that will give contraception, venereal disease treatment, and information about sex to young people without their parents' consent. The list is obtainable from Student Coalition for Relevant Sex Education, 300 Park Avenue South, New York, N.Y. 10010. The U.S. Supreme Court has just declared unconstitutional a New York State law that had prohibited the sale of contraceptives to persons under sixteen. It also declared unconstitutional laws that restrict advertising or display of contraceptives and that require a licensed pharmacist to distribute them.

Women's Health Centers. Many feminist health centers offer free courses in self-examination, free pregnancy screening, counseling, and gynecological advice. There is usually a 24-hour hotline to deal with emergencies. Some have their own abortion clinics, others a referral service, many have films and brochures on sex, pregnancy, nutrition, contraception, and other matters. Check the telephone book, or a local chapter of the National Organization for Women.

RECOMMENDED:
Our Bodies, Ourselves, Boston Women's Health Book
    Collective
Simon and Schuster
1230 Avenue of the Americas
New York, N.Y. 10020
$4.95

HOW TO ARRANGE AN ABORTION

It is now legal for women anywhere in the United States to obtain an abortion.

The main methods are *dilatation and curettage* (D & C) and *the suction method.* Either procedure takes as little as 10 to 15 minutes, but should be done in a hospital or an approved clinic. Most women can be back home the same evening.

Do it early! You should see a doctor within two or three weeks after you have missed a period. Through the third month, abortion is quite safe—safer than the normal delivery of a baby. But the earlier you act, the better. In fact the latest report in the *Journal of the American Medical Association* shows that an abortion done at two months' pregnancy or less is 37 times safer than continuing pregnancy and childbirth.

Jack Vaughn, former president of Planned Parenthood, says that abortion services are mostly concentrated in non-hospital clinics of large metropolitan areas. He says an estimated 250,000 to 750,000 women—mostly the poor, the young, and the residents of small towns and rural areas—still do not have access to abortions. He points out that less than 20 percent of the nation's public hospitals reported they provide abortions.

If you have a doctor you see regularly, ask him about getting an abortion. Or call the Planned Parenthood office in your community. Or call your local hospital and ask for the department of obstetrics and gynecology. Or call the city or county public health department.

A New York City Family Court recently ruled that the man responsible for the pregnancy can be compelled to pay the cost of an abortion.

AFTER THE ABORTION

Follow your doctor's instructions regarding physical activity and intercourse. You can expect some bleeding for a few days. Have a checkup two to three weeks after the abortion. *To avoid another unwanted pregnancy, get birth control information.* See your doctor, a family planning clinic or Planned Parenthood. If you are sure that you will never want another pregnancy, consider voluntary sterilization.

NEW GEL TO LET WOMEN SELF-ABORT

A British doctor has invented a simple do-it-yourself abortion medication. Dr. Morsyn Embrey of the John Radcliffe Infirmary in Oxford, England, says the abortion gel, packaged in a tube like toothpaste, would allow women to perform their own abortions at home. The gel is already in use at his hospital, he says, and has been found to be safe and effective in the first two months of pregnancy.

The vaginal gel contains the hormone prostaglandin. It is expected to be widely available in England within the next two years.

HYSTERECTOMY

Hysterectomy is the surgical removal of the uterus. When you have a hysterectomy, it means you no longer have menstrual periods and you can no longer have children. But it has no effect on sex performance at all.

The operation is usually performed through about a four-inch incision in the lower abdomen, although occasionally it is done by working through the vagina. Intercourse is usually banned for about six weeks.

The most common reasons for hysterectomy are fibroid tumors, polyps, prolonged or irregular vaginal bleeding, precancerous lesions that could be in danger of becoming malignant, a uterus that has become weakened or out of place; or if the abdomen is being opened for other reasons anyway, it is often done as a convenient sure method of sterilization.

If you are in your 40s and you have fibroid tumors, but feel strongly that you do not want to have a hysterectomy, you should know that fibroids usually shrink at menopause and often cause no trouble after that. Talk it over with your doctor, ask for a second opinion.

RECOMMENDED:
*A Guide to the Methods of Postponing or Preventing
    Pregnancy*
    Ortho Pharmaceutical Corporation
    Raritan, N.J. 08869
    Free
    A 31-page booklet, illustrated, on various methods of
    birth control.
*Birth Control: All the Methods That Work—and the Ones That
    Don't*
    Planned Parenthood Federation of America
    810 Seventh Avenue
    New York, N.Y. 10019
    25¢
    In English or Spanish.

CHAPTER 10

How to Sail Successfully Through Pregnancy and Childbirth

WHEN YOU WANT TO GET PREGNANT

Establish your fertile time. It begins on the 14th day after the first day of menstruation and lasts about a week. It takes the average man about 48 hours to regenerate an effective charge of sperm, so intercourse should be scheduled for every other day during this week. If this rough guess doesn't work, you can get scientific and practice the rhythm method in reverse. The woman should take her temperature every morning after awakening (while still in bed), and keep track of it on a chart. When the temperature goes up about half a degree, this is the fertile period. Abstain from intercourse for the week before this fertile period; have intercourse on the first day of the fertile period.

Best position: The wife remains flat on her back with her legs elevated for an hour after intercourse so that gravity will not work against the sperm.

IF YOU'RE HAVING TROUBLE GETTING PREGNANT

The most common causes of problems are:

- Inability to consummate intercourse
- Premature ejaculation
- Injuries
- Infections
- Chronic problem such as diabetes or underactive thyroid

- Anatomical problems such as undescended testes or blocked fallopian tube
- Hormone deficiencies
- An ovarian cyst
- Too weak or too few sperm
- Cervix with the wrong acidity or that has an antisperm substance
- Varicose vein of the testes
- Excessive cigarette smoking
- Tight underwear (several researchers say it can reduce a man's fertility because the pressure and heat kill sperm)

By correcting these problems, more than half of apparently infertile couples are able to conceive a child.

A SIMPLE TREATMENT THAT OFTEN WORKS

Many times a couple's infertility can be due to *a woman being allergic to her husband's sperm.* If the husband wears a condom for several months (sometimes up to six months is needed), then the woman is not repeatedly exposed to sperm, and antibody levels are reduced. Then the condom is discontinued.

Some women are infertile because some chemical is missing from their cervical mucus that is vital to making sperm effective. When their husband's sperm were bathed in cervical mucus from another woman and then used to impregnate the wife, the wives were able to become pregnant.

MEDICATIONS THAT SOMETIMES HELP

Thyroid medications, various sex hormones, vitamin B_1, and a new drug called clomiphene citrate.

ARTIFICIAL INSEMINATION

Sometimes insemination is done with the husband's sperm, sometimes with a donor's sperm, sometimes with the two mixed so no one ever knows which sperm actually impregnated the egg. The physician performing the insemination tries to match the donor to the husband in height, build, complexion, and checks the donor's family history, Rh compatibility, and freedom from disease.

FOR FURTHER HELP

Contact your local medical society, the American Fertility Society, 944 South 18th Street, Birmingham, Ala. 35205, or the local office of Planned Parenthood to find a specialist in infertility. The causes of infertility are about equally divided between men and women, so both partners must be studied together.

CENTERS SPECIALIZING IN FERTILITY PROBLEMS

Boston Hospital for Women
    221 Longwood Avenue
    Boston, Mass. 02115
New York Fertility Research Foundation
    123 East 89th Street
    New York, N.Y. 10028
Tyler Clinic Research Foundation
    921 Westwood Boulevard
    West Los Angeles, Calif. 90024
Yale-New Haven Hospital
    789 Howard Avenue
    New Haven, Conn. 06510

DO-IT-YOURSELF PREGNANCY TESTS

Nearly all family planning program physicians agree that women have a basic right to information about their own fertility as simply and confidentially as possible. A do-it-yourself kit does this. Several are available in Canada and Western Europe, but in the U.S. the F.D.A. has prohibited over-the-counter sales of the tests. Recently, however, a federal judge denied F.D.A.'s right to restrict the sales. The case is under appeal.

Do-it-yourself tests presently available outside the U.S. are Confidelle (Denver Laboratories, Toronto, Canada, $6.00) and Ova II, made in New Jersey (Faraday Laboratories, Hillside, N.J., $4.95) but sold only in Europe.

To do a test, a woman adds a few drops of urine to each of two vials—a control vial and a test vial. After shaking the vials, she compares the two for results. If the two mixtures are different in color, pregnancy is indicated. The test is based on the increased excretion of hormones during pregnancy, including estrogens, which react chemically with the reagents to produce the color change. The test seems to reliably diagnose pregnancy beginning two weeks following a missed period.

The tests are considered an initial screening to encourage medical consultation. Manufacturers' instructions advise that the test be repeated two weeks later regardless of results, and urge the woman to consult her doctor if results are positive or she has missed her period.

A NEW TEST

Dr. Lorrin Lau of Johns Hopkins University is currently at work on another pregnancy test which may be capable of even earlier diagnosis. The test uses a hair-thin capillary tube containing premeasured, freeze-dried reagents. Urine is drawn into the tube; the tube is rocked for 3 to 5 minutes and results examined.

The capillary test is not yet commercially available, but promises to be very inexpensive (it was reported in field tests to cost less than 10¢ per test).

CONTROLLING THE SEX OF YOUR FUTURE CHILD

Your baby's sex is established the instant sperm fertilizes the egg. If a sperm with an X-chromosome gets there first, you will have a girl; if a sperm with a Y-chromosome gets there first, it will be a boy. Dr. Landrum Shettles, in his book *Your Baby's Sex: Now You Can Choose*, says you can weight the odds toward the sex of your choice by the following.

For a girl: Precede intercourse on each occasion by an acid douche of two tablespoons of vinegar to one quart of water. Wife should avoid orgasm because it increases alkaline secretions. Use face-to-face position with man on top, with shallow penetration. Have frequent intercourse in the days after the menstrual period, but stop intercourse two to three days before ovulation.

For a boy: Precede each intercourse with a baking soda douche of two tablespoons of baking soda to a quart of water. Wife should have orgasm before or at same time as husband. Rear penetration is best with deep penetration at moment of male orgasm. Avoid intercourse from the menstrual period until the day of ovulation to encourage maximum count. Have intercourse as close to the time of ovulation as possible.

ESTIMATING THE TIME YOUR BABY WILL ARRIVE

Figure the date of the *first day* of the last menstrual period. Count back three months and add 7 days. (If one of the three months is February, add 10 days.) This is the theoretical date when the baby will be born. It will probably arrive within two weeks one way or the other of this.

THE ONE MOST IMPORTANT RULE TO KNOW AS SOON AS YOU GET PREGNANT

Go to your doctor right away and see her or him regularly throughout your pregnancy. Take a notebook and pencil and a list of questions you want to ask with you when you go. Write down her or his instructions (they are easy to forget later).

TO BE OR NOT TO BE A PARENT

A counseling center called a Baby . . . Maybe Service has been set up in New York City to help couples weigh whether they want to have children or not, the best times, the costs, and so on. The referral team includes specialists in obstetrics, gynecology, genetics, psychology, infertility, and adoption. Counseling costs about $35 per session. A book about it:

A Baby . . . Maybe, by Elizabeth Whelan (director of the service), Bobbs-Merrill, 4 West 58th Street, New York, N.Y. 10019.

COMMON PROBLEMS OF PREGNANCY AND EASY WAYS TO SOLVE THEM

NAUSEA

Have two soda crackers *before* you get out of bed.

At any time, take small sips of Coca-Cola, or snack soothing foods: gelatin, custard, cooked whole wheat toast with honey, mashed or baked potato, rice crackers, cream of celery or potato soup.

Eat small snacks frequently instead of three large meals.

Take 100–150 mg of vitamin B_6 along with other Bs.

GAS, HEARTBURN, INDIGESTION

Find what food is causing the problem, and eliminate it.

Try taking a tablespoon of cream 30 minutes before meals.

Don't wear tight things around your abdomen.

If the problem persists, consult your doctor. Do *not* take baking soda.

VARICOSE VEINS

Do not wear tight round-the-leg garters. Wear support stockings, putting them on while you are still in bed in the morning before fluid has a chance to build up in your feet and legs.

Elevate your feet and legs several times a day.

CONSTIPATION

Drink eight glasses of water a day. Eat plenty of fresh fruits and vegetables, and dried fruits such as prunes and apricots. Make sure cereals are whole grain. Avoid all refined starchy and surgary foods. Consult with your doctor if any stronger measures are needed such as mineral oil.

ITCHING SKIN AND VAGINA

Take a bath with baking soda or corn starch added. Do not douche unless your doctor so orders.

Consult with your doctor: an allergy or an infection may be the cause.

VAGINAL DISCHARGE

A slight vaginal discharge during pregnancy is normal. If the discharge is thick, heavy, or is accompanied by odor or itching, consult your doctor.

MUSCLE CRAMPS

Wear low-heeled shoes. Massage your legs. Walk about in bare feet.

Lie on your back, legs together loosely. Have husband push down against knee with one hand, and push up against the sole of the foot with the other hand pointing toes toward head. Release. Repeat several times.

Sometimes the baby's head presses on certain nerves and causes shooting pains. Try changing your position.

You may have a calcium deficiency. Talk to your doctor about calcium supplements.

Would you believe that one out of nine expectant fathers has morning sickness or craves unusual foods? It's a symptom of an emotional need to share the wife's pregnancy, says Dr. Arthur Colman, California psychiatrist. He suggests that the husband increase his participation in the pregnancy.

RECOMMENDED:
Preparation for Childbearing
Maternity Center Association
48 East 92nd Street
New York, N.Y. 10028
Free

WHEN TO CALL YOUR DOCTOR RIGHT AWAY

If you have any of the following, don't wait for your next checkup, but call your doctor right away:

- A constant headache that doesn't go away with food, a nap, or warm bath or shower
- Swelling of the face, hands, feet, or legs
- Blurred vision
- Bleeding from the vagina
- Fever
- Pain in the abdominal region
- Pain or burning on urination, or marked decrease in amount of urine
- A sudden gush of water from the vagina before the baby is due
- Prolonged severe vomiting that is more severe than the usual three-month morning nausea

Take your temperature before you call your doctor. Write down all the symptoms you want to tell him about before you dial so that you don't forget anything. Always tell him your name and how many months pregnant you are. He has lots of mothers to take care of and may have forgotten your due date.

TWELVE WAYS TO PREVENT BIRTH DEFECTS

1. Do not take any drugs or medicines during pregnancy unless absolutely necessary. Don't even take aspirin, antacids, or sedatives, and especially don't take tranquilizers.

2. Have your babies when you're between age 20 and 35. Birth defects are more prevalent when the woman is 18 or younger or over 35, and when the man is over 45.

3. Have an interval of at least two years between pregnancies.

4. Do not smoke cigarettes during pregnancy. Do not drink more than an occasional drink of alcohol. Keep your consumption of coffee, coke, tea, and other caffeine-containing drinks to only 1 or 2 cups a day.

5. Go to a doctor right away, go back for regular checkups, and follow his advice throughout the pregnancy.

6. Be sure you have been immunized against German measles *before* you get pregnant.

7. Keep yourself in good health, and that includes following your doctor's recommended diet and vitamin program and avoiding exposure to contagious diseases.

8. Don't eat undercooked red meat and avoid contact with cats (to avoid a toxoplasmosis infection).

9. Don't have x-ray examination or radiation treatments.

10. Watch your weight, keeping weight gain to recommended amounts, but no lower.

11. Stop at three. With every child after that there is increasing risk of malformation.

12. If a close relative has a disorder that is hereditary, tell your doctor about it and ask him to recommend a genetic counselor.

SOME MEDICAL FACTS ABOUT BIRTH DEFECTS YOU SHOULD KNOW

"Offspring of animals fed the caffeine in 11 cups of coffee had higher rates of birth defects, including cleft palate, missing fingers and toes and malformed skulls"—Center of Science in Public Interest.

"A mother's smoking may slow the breathing rate of her unborn child, lower his birth weight, and increase his chances of suffering from bronchitis and pneumonia in the first year of life"—Committee on Environmental Hazards, American Academy of Pediatrics.

"Even the alcohol equivalent of two bottles of beer will cause high concentration of alcohol in the fetus, ten times higher than the amount found in the mother. One doctor found as many as 43 percent of babies born to alcoholic mothers had birth defects or died soon after birth. He recommends that heavy drinkers either give up alcohol during pregnancy, or seriously consider having an abortion if they become pregnant"—Texas Research Institute.

"Mothers who take aspirin or other anti-inflammatory agents that affect blood coagulation are more apt to develop bleeding problems"—*Journal of the American Medical Association.*

"Any woman should challenge any physician who writes a prescription for her, asking whether she really has a condition that needs treatment. General advice is that unless a medicine is absolutely needed, the woman should say no. Even when it comes to simple things like antacids, sedatives, antibiotics, or aspirins, a woman and her fetus will be better off is she does not take them"—National Foundation Symposium on Drugs and the Unborn Child.

A MAN'S DRINKING CAN AFFECT THE SPERM

Dr. Fouad Badr, of the University of Kuwait, has found a very significant correlation between a man's drinking and birth defects in his offspring. Even a single heavy-drinking night at the time of conceiving could cause an abnormality of sperm cells, Badr says, and could cause mental retardation or physical abnormalities in the baby.

WHAT YOU NEED TO KNOW ABOUT THE RH FACTOR

If a pregnant woman has Rh negative blood, and carries a baby with Rh positive blood, her body will form antibodies which then attack her next Rh positive baby, destroying the baby's red blood cells. Result—a stillborn baby or a baby brought into life with physical or mental handicaps. The risk increases progressively with each succeeding pregnancy.

A vaccine is now available that is almost 100 percent effective in preventing the Rh sensitization.

Have a simple blood test to determine your Rh blood type. If you are Rh positive, you need not worry about any danger. If you are Rh negative, get the vaccine called RhoGAM *each time* you deliver an Rh positive baby *and* following any miscarriage. The RhoGAM should be administered within 72 hours after the delivery or miscarriage.

HICCUPS IN THE FETUS—A SIGN OF ALLERGY?

Hiccups can occur as early as 4½ months of pregnancy and are not as rare as once thought, says Dr. W. Ambrose McGee of West Palm Beach, Florida. The hiccups are related to allergy, he says, the hiccups in the fetus almost always occurring a few hours after the mother eats or drinks something she is allergic to. And usually the child later in life develops allergy problems, too.

Avoid foods that cause hiccuping. Tell the pediatrician of the fetal hiccuping so he can be on guard for later allergic signs and symptoms.

HOW MUCH WEIGHT YOU SHOULD GAIN

Doctors used to say only 10 to 14 pounds, but current opinion is that this might have contributed to the rise of infant mortality. Current recommendation is to have a weight gain of 24 to 25 pounds.

AN AMAZING DO-IT-YOURSELF EXERCISE TO TURN A BABY FROM A BREECH TO A NORMAL POSITION

If your doctor discovers by the middle of the seventh month that your baby is in a breech position, you have a 90 percent chance of turning it to a normal position by a simple exercise. It involves no risk whatsoever, says originator of the exercise Dr. DeSa Souza, obstetrician-gynecologist of Bombay, India. She reported the technique to the World Congress of Gynecology and Obstetrics as follows:

Lie on your back on a hard surface with the pelvis raised by pillows to 9 to 12 inches higher than your head. Maintain the position for 10 minutes. The position should be taken on an empty stomach twice a day; before lunch and before dinner are recommended. It should be continued at least 4 to 6 weeks, although in most cases the baby turns in 2 to 3 weeks' treatment.

HOW TO ACHIEVE COMFORT DURING PREGNANCY WHEN YOU SWEAR THERE'S NO COMFORTABLE POSITION YOU CAN FIND

The Maternity Center Association recommends the following.

1. Lie on your back with a pillow under your shoulders and head and another under your thighs just above your knees. Rotate legs and feet outward to alleviate lower back pain. (Late in pregnancy, avoid remaining flat on your back for prolonged periods. The increased weight of the uterus may cause constriction of major blood vessels, resulting in a feeling of faintness.)

2. Lie on your right side with a pillow or two placed diagonally under your head, breast, and

shoulder. Your right arm and leg should be behind you, left arm and leg in front. Allow abdomen to rest on the bed. If necessary, place a small pillow or folded towel under abdomen for support or a pillow to support left leg.

3. Lie on the floor or bed. Prop your heels on a chair, stool, or headboard so that your legs are at about a 45-degree angle to your body. This promotes good circulation in the legs and reduces discomfort from varicose veins, leg cramps, and leg fatigue.

4. When you sit, keep your back straight, slide back in the chair. Sit tall with weight evenly distributed. Your back, buttocks, and shoulders should be supported by the back of the chair. Your feet should be flat on the floor or resting on a footstool. Let your legs relax and your knees separate naturally.

5. Pelvic rocking will help relieve abdominal pressure and lower backache. It can also be resumed following birth of the baby to firm abdominal muscles. It can be done when standing, sitting, lying down, or on all fours. Tighten abdominal wall, pulling in and up, and tuck in buttocks. This rocks pelvis upward, flattening lower back as you straighten the hollow there. Then slowly relax abdomen and buttocks. Repeat the exercise 5 or 6 times maintaining a slow, rhythmic motion.

6. A modified knee-chest position will help relieve pelvic pressure, hemorrhoids, gas, cramps, and, occasionally, lower back and leg pain. Kneel, keeping your knees apart. Place your arms and head on the floor so your pelvis will be higher than the rest of your body. Tighten your abdominal muscles slightly in order to relieve the pressure of the baby on your abdominal wall. Keep your back straight. Maintain this position for a minute or two.

HOW TO PREP YOURSELF AT HOME BETTER THAN IN THE HOSPITAL

In most hospitals before delivery you are shaved of all your pubic hair by a nurse using a hand razor. Now research by Dr. Simon J. A. Powis of Northampton, England, shows that using a hair removal cream at home yourself is better. Remove the pubic hair just as you would hair on your legs, gently putting the cream on, waiting about 10 minutes, and then washing it off in the shower. Using the cream instead of hospital shaving was less irritating, reduced bacteria count more, and eliminated prickling of hair stubs during regrowth, Dr. Powis said.

HOW TO DELIVER A BABY YOURSELF IN AN EMERGENCY IF YOU HAVE TO

Check the mother's pelvic region. If the baby's head cannot be seen in the birth canal, she may still be able to make it to the hospital. If you can see the baby's head, prepare for an emergency delivery. But call the doctor or an ambulance. They may make it there before the baby delivers. Meanwhile be calm and do the following.

Have the mother wash herself well, then lie down in bed. Slip a clean towel or sheet under her hips for the baby to be delivered on. (Sheets and towels can be sterilized by ironing them with a hot iron.) In an emergency clean newspapers can be used.

Wash your own hands and arms thoroughly, lathering right up to the elbows; rinse with hot water.

If there is time, boil a pair of scissors, a large clean handkerchief, clean new shoelaces or strips of clean cloth, and an ear syringe in a pot of water for five minutes to sterilize.

As the head appears in the birth canal, stand to the side of the mother and place your hand under the infant's head, supporting it as it emerges. *Do not pull!* Let nature take its course. You are simply catching.

If the umbilical cord is wrapped around the baby's neck, gently loosen it.

If the bag of waters has not broken and the baby being born is still inside it, break the sac with a pin or the tip of the scissors.

If the baby's shoulder is caught on the pelvic bone and it has started to cry, it is all right. If it has not started to cry and breathe, and it is not delivered in the next two contractions, slide your fingers in and under the baby's shoulder and try to gently rotate the shoulder toward the face. (This assistance is almost never needed.)

Wipe baby's nose and face and inside of his mouth with the clean sterilized handkerchief, or clear his air passages of mucus by gently inserting the ear syringe into the nose or mouth, removing mucus until the baby can breathe without gurgling.

If the baby still is not breathing, hold it upside down in the air by its legs, face down, tipping its forehead back gently to let the mucus run out.

If the baby still is not breathing properly, use mouth-to-mouth resuscitation, *very* gently.

When breathing has begun, place baby on the mother's abdomen or between her thighs. Cover the baby to keep it warm. Do not stretch the cord; leave it slack.

Gently massage the mother's abdomen to help uterus contract. If the mother lets the baby nurse at her breast, it will help the afterbirth come out and will help contract the uterus. Wait for the afterbirth to come out. *Do not pull on cord,* which could cause hemorrhaging. It will come out naturally later with the afterbirth.

If the doctor or ambulance is expected, do not cut the cord. There is no hurry. If the doctor is not expected, then wait until the cord turns from blue to limp and pale, and stops pulsating.

Tie one of the sterilized shoelaces or strips of cloth tightly around the cord in a square knot halfway between the baby and the mother. Then tie the other shoelace or piece of cloth tightly about three inches from the first. Cut between the two ties with the sterilized scissors.

Cover mother and baby and keep them warm.

Do not wash the white material off the baby. It protects the skin. Keep gently massaging mother's abdomen to help her uterus contract and minimize bleeding. Massage where you feel the lump just below her navel.

If there is bleeding from the mother's torn tissue around the opening of the birth canal, hold a gauze pad or towel against it. Have her lower her legs and place them together to help stop bleeding. Stay with the mother until the doctor comes, or if the afterbirth has been expelled, she may be taken to the hospital. Let her wear a sanitary napkin for minor bleeding.

Save the afterbirth and take it to the hospital with you for the doctor to examine.

WHAT TO DO FOR YOURSELF TO BE BETTER THAN EVER AFTER CHILDBIRTH

Dr. Gideon Panter, in *Now That You've Had Your Baby* (David McKay Co.) recommends the following:

In the hospital, massage your own uterus. You can feel it as a hard lump. Massaging it helps your uterus contract back to normal size and helps prevent bleeding.

From day one after birth you can begin exercises to get you back in shape. Do the pubococcygeus squeeze and the pelvic rock (see Chapter 11), and even flat on your back you can do foot circling and pointing toes and feet up and down (improves muscle tone and helps prevent blood clots).

If you have a painful episiotomy, or a swollen perineum (the skin between the anus and the vagina), try applying an ice bag, taking a warm shower (you can take them as soon as you feel steady enough, even with the stitches still in), or shine a heating lamp (or your bedside reading lamp) on the area.

At home, in addition to the warm showers, take sitz baths (shallow baths of only 2 to 3 inches with a little salt added), and keep using the heat lamp.

To prevent constipation and development of hemorrhoids, drink two to three quarts of water, eat fruits and whole grains, and if necessary use milk of magnesia or mineral oil.

Itching of the abdomen. Dab on a lotion of phenol and camphor in olive oil and lime water. If the itching is all over the body, tell your doctor right away because it could be an allergic reaction.

Keep up your prenatal vitamin and mineral supplements, making sure you are getting enough calcium and iron. But don't drink more than four glasses of milk daily—it can give you too many phosphates and cause leg cramps. If you are resuming birth control pills, take folic acid in addition to your other vitamin supplements.

To keep from being constantly tired, get all the rest you can . . . *at least* one nap every day.

No sex for two to three weeks, then you can only have sex *outside* the vagina, so masturbation or petting is permissible. You should not have intercourse or anything *inside* the vagina until after your 4- or 6-week checkup at the doctor's to make sure that your cervix is closed and all is back to normal. The first intercourse should be done very slowly and gently and with a surgical lubricant to decrease friction. Dilation of the vagina done gently first with the fingers may be necessary to prevent pain from the first intercourse.

HOW TO SUCCEED AT BREAST FEEDING

To encourage production of milk, nurse at every feeding the first few days, including night feedings. You can use an occasional supplementary bottle later.

Hold the baby close to your body so its cheek touches your nipple, thus stimulating the rooting reflex. The range of sight for the infant is approximately 17 inches, therefore keep the baby as near to that distance from your eyes as possible—the breast is just right in order to ensure contact. If he cannot locate the nipple, insert it *and* some of the surrounding dark tissue into his mouth. Allow some breathing space for the baby by compressing the breast slightly beneath his nose.

Nurse 5 minutes on one breast, then 5 minutes

plus any extra time the baby wants on the other. Alternate the breasts with which you begin feedings to provide equal stimulation. (Keep track with a safety pin on your bra to indicate which one to start with next.)

When taking the baby off the breast, break the suction first, pressing the breast away from the corner of the baby's mouth.

Allow the baby to control the number of daily feedings, even if they come every 2 to 3 hours.

Don't worry if your milk comes slowly in the beginning. The milk will increase as your baby needs more. Avoid things that could make you tense. Make sure that you get enough rest.

A glass of wine or beer a half hour before nursing will help your milk flow freely. And relax during feedings, using pillows for support for you and baby.

While in the hospital, use the reading lamp to give your breasts a heat treatment. Focus the light on your breasts for 10 to 15 minutes, two or three times a day. Continue this at home.

Do not become discouraged if your nipples become sore during your first few days of nursing. Continue to nurse, and your breasts will become tougher.

If your breasts become engorged and swollen at first, try a warm shower or hot towels placed over the breasts. If they become painful, try ice packs or ask your doctor if you should take an analgesic. Soreness sometimes occurs because the let-down reflex is not working efficiently. Try hand-expressing your milk for a few seconds before the baby nurses. Dietary iodine will often eliminate this problem, sometimes in minutes.

Use a supplementary bottle every day in place of one nursing period. This gets baby used to accepting prepared formula from a bottle as well as milk from your breast, so that if anything happened that you could not nurse, she could be switched to a bottle with no problem.

Watch what you eat. The chemicals you take in often appear in your milk. Too much coffee can give your baby coffee nerves, making her nervous and irritable. Too much orange juice can produce colic.

Medicines, too, can pass into the milk. Don't take any medicines without your doctor knowing and approving. Anticoagulants can be life-threatening to the baby. Antibiotics may cause allergies later. Tetracycline can cause tooth defects. Laxatives, tranquilizers, sleeping pills, aspirin, can all be passed on in the milk.

Codeine, heroin, morphine, and marijuana will also be excreted in breast milk to the baby.

A NEW DEVICE TO WATCH FOR

A promising device for monitoring oxygen levels has been developed by Drs. Albert and Renate Huch, a husband-and-wife team from West Germany. It is an apparatus, the size of a coin, that can be touched to the skin of a baby still in the birth canal during delivery to see if it is getting enough oxygen. It can also tell when a baby is getting too much oxygen and thus can prevent blindness that is caused by over-oxygenation. The Huch sensor is being tested at the University of California in San Francisco and at Columbia Presbyterian Medical Center in New York. The device should also be valuable in measuring oxygen supply in heart attacks and other situations.

CHAPTER 11

How to Be Your Own Sex Therapist at Home

NEW SEX FACTS

Of couples getting married now, 80 percent have had premarital sex relations with their intended mate or with another partner.

Oral sex is practiced by 80 to 90 percent of people under age 25.

Pornographic books and movies have been shown to stimulate women as well as men.

Kinsey found that 50 to 60 percent of adolescent girls masturbate, and 99 percent of adolescent boys. Now researchers have found that most adult men and women still masturbate, even during marriage. Of women who masturbate, about 75 percent are said to reach climax in about four minutes. Researchers find that men and women who have masturbated have increased response with intercourse.

A drug has been found that when given to sex offenders can eliminate sex fantasies and desires. The drug, Depo-Provera, reduces the body's production of testosterone. A similar drug is used in Europe (under the name Androcur) to successfully treat sex offenders. Many child molesters and other sex offenders in the U.S. "have virtually begged for it," according to one psychiatrist, but institutions are not using it.

Bad weather may be good for your love life. Most people's sex urges rise when the barometer drops to 29.9 or lower, one survey found. Readings at this level or lower are usually associated with a storm or approaching storm front.

A Paris chemist, Dr. Marcel Perret, is marketing a perfume called *This*. It uses pheromones, the natural odors that have been found important in animal and human sexual attraction. (The female silkworm moth releases a pheromone so powerful that a single molecule of it will tremble the hairs on the antennae of a male moth within miles and cause it to fly upwind.)

In orgasm, the heart rate increases to 140 to 180 beats per minute (normal is 70).

Sex does not disappear with age. In one study of 250 subjects aged 60 to 90, sexual relations ranged from three times weekly to once every other month.

WHAT REALLY HAPPENS INSIDE THE EXPENSIVE SEX CLINICS

Sessions may be once a week for 12 to 15 weeks. Or in an out-of-town clinic you may stay in a motel and go to sessions every day for 12 to 14 days. Price is $2,500 to $4,000 for some well-known clinics. Those affiliated with a university or teaching hospital may run as low as $300 to $400.

You take tests, fill out questionnaires and give

medical, sexual, and psychological history. Your sexual functioning is assessed and marital relationship evaluated. You watch films on sex, many purposefully shocking to desensitize you to any squeamishness or embarrassment about sex.

The first day you are given a physical examination, usually in the presence of your mate. This is also used as an educational session, teaching each of you about the anatomy of the other. Also during this session you and your mate are checked for possible physical causes for sexual problems. Is the foreskin too tight on the penis? Are there adhesions on the clitoris? Is the vaginal tissue dry or thin? Is there high blood pressure or diabetes or hepatitis or alcoholism or other medical problems that could cause decreased sexual performance? What medicines or drugs are being taken?

You have an interview session with your counselor to talk about your feelings about sex, as well as about your specific problem, and about anxieties and stresses at the office and at home, and about general communications between you and your mate.

Later sessions probe feelings even more deeply. Sexual exercises are done both in the clinic under direction and at home, with each person taught to appreciate his own and his mate's body, to shed his inhibitions, and to learn or relearn paths of pleasure of touching and talking.

One important phase of the therapy of every sex clinic is total abstention from intercourse up until usually the tenth session.

Masturbation is encouraged.

And yes, some centers use sex surrogates. One, the Center for Behavior Therapy in Beverly Hills, reports that surrogates are especially effective with persons in their 60s and 70s.

SOME ADVICE GIVEN BY COUNSELORS

Get the TV set out of the bedroom.

Make sure you share a large bed.

Set aside at least one night a week for yourselves without the children.

Reserve at least 30 minutes each night for quiet talk alone, with clothes off and defenses down. In these sessions, husband and wife must stop blaming anything on themselves, each other, their in-laws, the children, anyone. And they must interact and talk without hostility, without putting each other into an adversary position, and without interpreting how the *other* one feels, only speaking for their *own* feelings.

THE MIRROR TECHNIQUE

You and your mate stand nude before a full-length mirror. You take a "feeling trip" over each other's body, telling how you feel about various parts.

THE SENSATE FOCUS TECHNIQUE

The couple is not allowed to have intercourse, or even orgasm, but they concentrate on developing sensual feelings. First the wife caresses her mate's entire body. Then the man caresses the woman. After general caressing sessions, they proceed to caressing nipples and genitals, guiding each other verbally and non-verbally. If after several sessions they become too sensually aroused to put off orgasm any longer, they are allowed to bring each other to orgasm manually or orally, but still are not allowed to have intercourse.

TOUCH TRAINING

This exercise is similar to sensate focus, and is geared to further increase your ability to pleasure your partner and your partner's ability to pleasure you. Many people expect their partners to automatically and instinctively know how and where to touch them. In this exercise you actually *tell* your partner. Each of you strokes the other's body in all areas and in all ways, and the receiver indicates what is especially or maddeningly pleasing. It can be done without a massage cream one night, with a cream another night.

LEARNING TOGETHER

The man should put his fingers lightly, relaxedly, sensitively upon the woman's clitoris and the area around it. The woman puts her hands on top of her husband's and moves her husband's hand freely, without thinking, into whatever areas give her pleasure. He will soon feel the places, the ways, and the rhythms that please her most.

SEX EQUIPMENT EVERY HAPPY HOME SHOULD HAVE

A bed with a very firm mattress and firm construction, so it doesn't creak, rattle, or collapse.

Bedposts are handy.

If there is room have another mattress on the floor and lots of pillows, different sizes, different shapes, different firmness, some for sleeping, some to go under, to raise, to cushion, to snuggle . . . whatever your fancy decides.

A soft extra comforter to keep from getting chilled.

A rocking chair, armless, and an extra chair and ottoman for creative positions, if there is room.

A soft rug.

Bedside drawers for lubricating creams and other paraphernalia. Strategically placed mirrors or portable ones.

Subdued lighting.

In moments of inspiration, use any piece of furniture in any room of the house.

TEN WAYS TO INCREASE COMMUNICATION AND COMPATIBILITY

1. Turn off the television set after an hour's viewing per night and talk.

2. Call your spouse from the office once in a while.

3. Go for a walk together.

4. Share the household chores sometimes, or work in the yard together.

5. Spend an evening reading together.

6. Say "I love you."

7. Make a list—separately—of the most enjoyable things you have done together and the things you haven't done yet but would like to. Compare lists, pencil the overlapping things, and do them this week.

8. Touch each other and kiss each other during the day and evening freely, so every touch and every kiss does not mean it is expected to lead on to intercourse.

9. Talk about the pressures that are bothering both of you, in relation to careers, family, aging, whatever you feel will make you become closer and more understanding.

10. Build each other's self-confidence. Don't make your partner feel inadequate. Show love and affection and be relaxed.

SOME COMMON CAUSES OF SEXUAL PROBLEMS AND NO-NONSENSE WAYS TO SOLVE THEM

If the vagina is dry, intercourse painful, or after intercourse there are friction sores, use a lubricant jelly. Vaseline is too thick; use a surgical lubricant you can buy in any drugstore, such as K-Y jelly.

If excessive fatigue is a cause for disinterest, check with your doctor about iron pills, vitamin B_{12} injections, or increasing your intake of vitamins and minerals in general.

If you just don't feel ready, have a warm bath, a drink, and a cuddle or massage.

If you are a heavy drinker, the biggest help could be to stop the booze. Prolonged drinking of alcohol causes the liver to produce excessive amounts of an enzyme that destroys testosterone, the libido hormone. Even on a short-term basis university research shows that most men after three drinks cannot achieve an erection.

If you cannot reach orgasm without difficulty even during masturbation, talk to your doctor about taking hormone pills. Testosterone for men; a combination of estrogen with a little testosterone for women. Zinc supplements often work wonders for men.

If a woman's clitoris is too small to be properly stimulated, testosterone pills in very small amounts will increase its size and so increase stimulation.

If you are shy about sex, try watching pornographic films together. Many people who thought they would be terribly shocked found after a while that they became turned on by the films, and also by talking about their reactions to the films were able to open new avenues of communication they had never before had.

Does your partner lack proper personal hygiene? Sit down and talk about it.

Does your partner not stimulate slowly enough, long enough, or at the rhythm you like best? Talk about it and possible ways to solve it.

Decreased sex drive or ability can be related to undiagnosed diabetes, hepatitis, high blood pressure, or other diseases. Have a general physical checkup.

Talk over sex problems with your gynecologist or a urologist. He may find some physical condition that accounts for your problem or your mate's—vaginal infection, hemorrhoids, some condition that surgery could correct.

Vaginal opening too tight? Have your mate lubricate his fingers well, then gently put one finger into the opening, and press the edges of the opening in all directions, especially back toward the rectum. Then he can insert two fingers and methodically press them against all the edges and walls of the vagina. He should do this in many sessions, and you should not attempt intercourse until he can easily use three fingers.

If the vagina is stretched and enlarged, try a position with the woman's legs closed and the man's legs placed outside of hers. Also strengthen vaginal muscles with the pubococcygeus exercise, described later in this chapter, doing the contractions several hundred times a day. If this does not work, vaginal plastic surgery can tighten it.

Do you handle a lot of pesticides in your job? This can cause sexual problems. Avoid them.

What drugs or medicines do you take? All of the following can affect both sexual desire and performance: sleeping pills, tranquilizers, aspirin, barbiturates, hypnotics, codeine, anti-depressants, anti-psychotic drugs, some high blood pressure drugs (but not all), anti-cholinergic drugs to treat ulcer and eye disorders. If you have decreased sex desire and ability and you take any of these drugs, talk to your doctor about lowering the dosage or taking a different kind of pill. If your doctor ordered you to take them for specific problems, don't stop taking them without his okay.

ALEX COMFORT'S EXERCISE TO CORRECT PREMATURE EJACULATION

1. In this practice exercise you are not allowed to have intercourse. Get your partner to slowly masturbate you while seated astride. Her aim will be to keep you in erection, even if she has to stroke you only once in three seconds. If you call "stop" she must stop. If on the first occasion you ejaculate at once—try again half an hour later. Do this often. In about three weeks of regular practice you should be able to hold at least a second, and probably a first erection, for a full five minutes, and this will get longer and longer.

2. Set up by agreement a session where you will not have intercourse. But you concentrate on stimulating her, learning to use your hands and your tongue. Don't forget her breasts. Having times when you specifically set out to satisfy *her* will help you to relax about your virility problems.

THE MASTERS AND JOHNSON VARIATION OF THE SQUEEZE TECHNIQUE

In practice sessions, the woman stimulates the man orally or manually to the point of ejaculation. He tells her when he has arrived at the "point of no return." She immediately squeezes his penis by placing her thumb just below the head on the side facing her, her index finger just above the ridge of the head on the side away from her, her other fingers below the ridge. She squeezes almost painfully for 8 to 15 seconds. This is repeated 4 or 5 times for several sessions.

To prevent early ejaculation in actual intercourse, when the man recognizes his "point of no return," the penis is withdrawn and she squeezes in the same manner.

OTHER AIDS TO PREMATURE EJACULATION

Hold absolutely still inside your partner, letting her feel you inside her vagina, but not moving.

Use an anesthetizing jelly available in the drugstore.

Wear a condom to decrease sensation.

Use a lubricant to cut down friction.

Have your doctor prescribe a very small amount of an anti-depressant such as Tryptizol or Tofranil to slow down orgasm.

Masturbate, using the occasion to build up awareness and appreciation of the rest of your body and slow reflexes to make your erection last as long as possible without an orgasm.

Have intercourse more often so you don't respond as quickly.

Focus on your breathing, taking a deep breath if orgasm is approaching, holding it for moment or two, then slowly exhaling.

If nervousness or insecurity is your problem, talk yourself into relaxing, and gaining self-confidence by moving as slowly as possible instead of rushing into the act anxiously.

HOW IMPOTENCE OFTEN STARTS

The man is tired or perhaps has had too much to drink and suddenly he finds he cannot produce an erection. If he laughs about it, chances are all is normal again in a few hours or perhaps a few days. But give him the idea he is getting old or losing his power and suddenly his fears build up, needlessly but relentlessly. The next time he is so worried about his performance, he turns himself off. Now he is really afraid, and a pattern sets in. What was a normal common occasion in every man he has turned into a chronic problem.

However, note: researchers have discovered that alcohol decreases production of testosterone, so heavy regular drinking can produce permanent impotence.

But there are other causes of impotence also: diabetes, multiple sclerosis, Parkinsonism, hormone deficiencies. It can be caused by a number of medicines including tranquilizers, some high blood pressure medicines, certain hormones, amphetamines.

A prostate operation does *not* cause impotence: in fact some patients say they enjoy sex more and perform even better after the surgery. It does cause the ejaculation to go back into the bladder instead of being released through the penis at orgasm, but it in no way decreases the feeling of the orgasm.

TREATMENT OF IMPOTENCE

- Investigation of what physical factors might be causing the problem and correction of them
- Counseling so patient understands that impotence is *not* something to be expected as part of middle age
- Hypnosis
- *The simplest treatment of all that all sex clinics use:* absolutely under no circumstances allow yourself to have intercourse for a time you agree upon (at least 10 days). You should lie in bed with your mate for a scheduled time each day, to explore each other's bodies, caress, kiss; but no matter how much of an erection you achieve and how great your desire, you are not to have intercourse until the agreed-upon time is up.

THE ONLY SEXUAL DON'TS WE KNOW ABOUT

Don't ever pretend to be choking anyone. Never block a partner's airway in any way.

Never blow into the vagina. It can cause air embolism and death.

Don't fool with vacuum cleaners and other household appliances. Vacuum cleaner injuries of the penis can easily occur, and air blown mechanically around the anus or vagina can cause rupture. Water inserted into the vagina under pressure can go up into the uterus.

Don't use Spanish fly. It is not an aphrodisiac but a poison that causes irritation. It has killed many people even in small doses.

Don't keep doing anything if your partner seriously says to stop.

Don't inhale anything for kicks. Anything that is strong enough to produce sexy sensations is unsafe.

SEX EXERCISES

These exercises are designed to help you have even greater pleasure in sex.

THE GLUTEAL SQUEEZE

1. Sit on the floor with your legs together and your toes pointed. Tighten your buttocks (gluteus maximus muscles), and squeeze your posterior cheeks together. Hold this for 8 counts, and then relax for 4. Repeat 10 times.

2. The woman should when she tenses her buttocks also squeeze the thighs together and contract the muscles of the vagina.

The man should try to extend and raise the penis.

SQUEEZE YOUR PARTNER

Place two chairs facing each other. Sit on the edge of one chair, your partner on the other chair. The man places his knees outside the woman's knees. He tries to push her knees together; she tries to push them apart. Now switch, with the woman's knees outside pushing the man's knees together.

THE BALL SQUEEZE

Sit on the edge of a chair. Place a beach ball between your knees, and squeeze your legs together as hard as you can for 8 counts. Relax for 4 counts. Repeat 10 times.

BACK-LYING THIGH ADDUCTION

Lie on the floor, knees slightly bent and together, arms beside head. Squeeze your legs together as hard as you can while you count to 10.

BREATHING FOR SEX

Lie on your back for this exercise, completely and deeply relaxed. Now practice slow pelvic thrusts upward in time to your breathing, with an upward swing of the pelvis with each exhalation. Use this same technique during intercourse, concentrating on your breathing, and exhaling with every forward thrust.

ARNOLD KEGEL'S PUBOCOCCYGEUS SQUEEZE

Pretend that you are going to urinate, then squeeze hard as though you were trying desperately to stop the flow. At the same time contract your muscles to squeeze your anus shut as though trying to stop a bowel movement. Start holding for the count of 5, then relaxing. Build up to the count of 10. Can be repeated a hundred times a day in any position whenever you think of it. It's good for both men and women to increase ability to have orgasm. And when done during intercourse will give new sensations and control to both man and woman. If you have trouble with this exercise, your doctor can insert a perineometer that measures intravaginal pressure and tells how much you are contracting your muscles. You can also buy an electronic device for stimulating these muscles that has proved very successful in treating orgasmic difficulties and stress incontinence. Called Vagitone, it is available through your doctor from Techni-Med in Torrance, Calif. 90510.

SPECIAL MASSAGES FOR LOVERS

Stroke the entire length of the body with feather-like long strokes.

Give a preliminary all-over massage, concentrating on the stomach, insides of the thighs, buttocks, lower back, breasts, ears, lips, backs of the neck, the palms, inside the elbows, armpits, soles of the feet, toes, and backs of the knees.

Go over the entire body with one finger.

Run one finger slowly between and around each toe.

With the fingertips, massage in tiny circles around the tip of the tailbone and the muscles around it.

Run one hand from the genitals up the spine to the back of the neck, alternating one hand and the other, always having one hand in contact with the body.

Move one finger slowly in a tiny circle on the smooth area between the anus and the genitals.

SEX AND DIET

If you have restricted your cholesterol intake too much, it can make it impossible for your body to make hormones properly, and so affect your sexual functioning.

If you have hypoglycemia, you may suffer frigidity or impotence. See your doctor for a 5- or 6-hour glucose tolerance test.

A vitamin or mineral deficiency can cause sexual dysfunction, especially deficiencies in vitamin A, E, folic acid, other Bs, and zinc. Some foods—sarsaparilla root, pollen, and hops—used in gypsy, Oriental, and Indian recipes for hundreds of years have just recently been shown by chemical analysis to contain hormone ingredients.

SEX THERAPIST GUIDE

The American Association of Sex Educators, Counselors and Therapists has compiled a booklet listing therapists certified for their educational training and clinical experience. It also includes a code of ethics by which you can evaluate unlisted therapists. Write AASEC, 5010 Wisconsin Avenue, N.W., Suite 304, Washington, D.C. 20016. $3.

Another source of help is the Sex Information and Education Council of the U.S. (SIECUS), 137-155 North Franklin Street, Hempstead, N.Y. 11550.

RECOMMENDED:

The Pleasures of Love, an album obtainable from sex therapist Dr. Don M. Sloan, New York Medical College, Fifth Avenue and 106th Street, New York, N.Y., offers lessons in sexual communication to help heighten sexuality

Sex education and childbirth films are available at the following places (send for current lists):

Multi-Media Resource Center
330 Ellis Avenue
San Francisco, Calif. 94102
Texture Films
1600 Broadway
New York, N.Y. 10023

CHAPTER 12

How to Raise a Better Child

EIGHT WAYS TO NOT BE HASSLED WHEN CARING FOR A NEW BABY

1. Breast feed so you don't have to worry about your baby being allergic to milk.

2. Let your baby suck its thumb or a pacifier as much as it wants, or even its thumb, fist, or toe. It won't hurt anything.

3. Don't give baby a bath every day. Wash its bottom when you change its diaper and wash hands and face regularly. But except for very hot days a bath and hairwash twice a week is plenty.

4. Don't sterilize the formula. Modern formulas are prepackaged and sterile-packed.

5. Don't rinse diapers. If you know your baby has a bowel movement at certain times—such as after it nurses—put diaper liners in the diaper at that time or use disposable diapers and simply throw them out. For the times you misjudge, fold the diaper inside out and hold the soiled area on the surface of the water in the toilet and flush it out.

6. Check the economics of diaper service or disposable diapers against the cost of regular diapers plus soap and water at home.

7. If your baby is teething, use a teething ring, cooled in the refrigerator. Or rub a little bourbon or paregoric gently on the baby's swollen gums as a local anesthetic when gums hurt from teething.

8. Use a playpen right from the start. Your baby will be used to it. If you start using a playpen after baby learns to crawl, it will seem like a jail to it.

THE TWO MOST IMPORTANT THINGS NOT TO SHORT-CUT ON

Love. And attention. Your baby needs them most of all. And the major reason for eliminating as many frills of baby care as possible is so you will have the time to give your baby love and attention. Babies who are held and cuddled develop faster physically and mentally. They especially love skin-to-skin contact. Sing to your baby, talk to it. Carry it with you on your jaunts about town.

CHECKUPS

Your baby should receive a physical examination every month beginning at one month and through six months. After six months, most pediatricians feel that a checkup every three months is sufficient. Immunizations—essential to protect your child from serious diseases—must be done.

NEW GROWTH CHARTS

The National Center for Health Statistics has just released new growth charts based on data from 20,000 U.S. children. The charts indicate the heights and weights within which 80 percent of U.S. children fall. If your child is above or below the average height and weight range for his age, check with your physician.

See growth patterns charted below.

IF YOUR CHILD IS VERY SHORT

Recently growth hormone from the pituitary gland has been used effectively to increase the height of children who are excessively small. The use is experimental, but is showing good results. It also is working in dwarfs with this problem (about 1 percent), if given before bones have matured, says Dr. Maurice Rafen of Tufts University School of Medicine.

The unloved child, too, may be small for his age. Doctors at the University of Virginia Hospital, Charlottesville, find if a child is removed from an uncaring home and placed in one where there is love, a growth spurt often results. If returned to the former home, the child stops growing again.

Some dwarfism can also be caused by zinc deficiency and, if so, can be corrected with zinc supplements.

A STRICTLY PRELIMINARY FINDING

The *Journal of the American Medical Association* reports a study on 44 school-age twins to test the effect of vitamin C. Half of the twins received daily doses of vitamin C for five months, half received an inert substance. An unexpected side effect: seven treated boys grew an average of about one-half inch more than their untreated co-twins. It could be a coincidence, but doctors are checking the effect on growth further.

CENTERS THAT SPECIALIZE IN TREATING GROWTH DISORDERS

Children's Hospital
    561 South 17th Street
    Columbus, Ohio 43205
Children's Hospital of Pittsburgh
    125 De Soto Street
    Pittsburgh, Pa. 15213
Kaiser-Permanente Medical Center
    280 West MacArthur Boulevard
    Oakland, Calif. 94611
Massachusetts General Hospital
    32 Fruit Street
    Boston, Mass. 02114
North Carolina Memorial Hospital
    University of North Carolina
    Chapel Hill, N.C. 27514
St. Louis Children's Hospital
    500 South Kingshighway Boulevard
    St. Louis, Mo. 63110
University of Virginia Hospital
    Jefferson Park Avenue
    Charlottesville, Va. 22901

WHAT YOUR DOCTOR SHOULD BE CHECKING FOR AT YOUR REGULAR VISITS

The American Academy of Pediatrics gives the following guidelines for what procedures you should expect from pediatric checkups and what growth developments you and your doctor should be checking for.

See table on page 88.

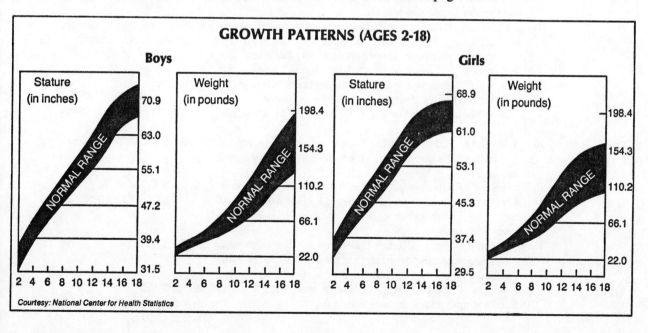

GROWTH PATTERNS (AGES 2-18)

Boys

Stature (in inches) — 70.9, 63.0, 55.1, 47.2, 39.4, 31.5
NORMAL RANGE
2 4 6 8 10 12 14 16 18

Weight (in pounds) — 198.4, 154.3, 110.2, 66.1, 22.0
NORMAL RANGE
2 4 6 8 10 12 14 16 18

Girls

Stature (in inches) — 68.9, 61.0, 53.1, 45.3, 37.4, 29.5
NORMAL RANGE
2 4 6 8 10 12 14 16 18

Weight (in pounds) — 198.4, 154.3, 110.2, 66.1, 22.0
NORMAL RANGE
2 4 6 8 10 12 14 16 18

Courtesy: National Center for Health Statistics

AGE	DEVELOPMENT LANDMARKS	PROCEDURES TO BE DONE
1 Mo.	Eyes follow to midline. Baby regards face. While prone, lifts head off table.	Diaper test for phenylketonuria (PKU).
2 Mo.	Vocalizes. Smiles responsively.	Diphtheria, tetanus, and pertussis (DTP). Oral polio. Urine screening.
3 Mo.	Holds head and chest up to make 90-degree angle with table. Laughs.	DTP. Oral polio.
4 Mo.	Holds head erect and steady when held in sitting position. Squeals. Grasps rattle. Eyes follow object for 180 degrees.	DTP. Oral polio.
5 Mo.	Smiles spontaneously. Rolls from back to stomach or vice versa. Reaches for object on table.	
6 Mo.	No head lag if baby is pulled to sitting position by hands.	
8 Mo.–9 Mo.	Sits alone for 5 seconds after support is released. Bears weight momentarily if held with feet on table. Looks after fallen object. Transfers block from one hand to the other. Feeds self cracker.	
10 Mo.	Pulls self to standing position. Stands holding on to solid object (not human). Pincer grasp—picks up small object using any part of thumb and fingers in opposition. Says Da-da or Ma-ma. Resists toy being pulled away from him. Plays "peek-a-boo." Makes attempt to get toy just out of reach. Initial anxiety toward strangers.	Hemoglobin or hematocrit determinations. Tuberculin test (Tine or intradermal).
12 Mo.	Cruises—walks around holding on to furniture. Stands alone 2 to 3 seconds if outside support is removed. Bangs together two blocks held one in each hand. Imitates vocalization heard within preceding minutes. Plays pat-a-cake.	Measles vaccine. Urinalysis.
15 Mo.	Walks well. Stoops to recover toys on floor. Uses Da-da and Ma-ma specifically for correct parent. Rolls or tosses ball back to examiner. Indicates wants by pulling, pointing, or appropriate verbalization (not crying). Drinks from cup without spilling much.	
18 Mo.	Puts one block on another. Mimics household chores like dusting or sweeping.	DTP. Trivalent oral polio.
21 Mo.	Walks backwards and upstairs. Feeds self with spoon. Removes articles of clothing other than hat. Says 3 specific words besides Da-da and Ma-ma.	
2 Yrs.	Kicks a ball in front of him with foot without support. Scribbles spontaneously—purposeful marking of more than one stroke on paper. Balances four blocks on top of one another. Points correctly to one body part. Dumps small objects out of bottle after demonstration. Does simple tasks in house.	Hemoglobin and/or hematocrit determinations. Urinalysis. Tuberculin test.
2½ Yrs.	Throws overhand after demonstration. Names correctly one picture in book, e.g., cat or apple. Combines 2 words meaningfully.	
3 Yrs.	Jumps in place. Pedals tricycle. Dumps small article out of bottle without demonstration. Uses plurals. Washes and dries hands.	As for 2 Yr. DTP booster.
4 Yrs.	Builds bridge of 3 blocks after demonstration. Copies circle and cross. Identifies longer of two lines. Knows first and last names. Plays with other children so they interact—tag. Dresses with supervision.	As for 2 Yr.
5 Yrs.	Hops 2 or more times. Catches ball thrown 3 feet. Dresses. Can tolerate separation from mother for a few minutes without anxiety.	As for 2 Yr.
6 Yrs.	Rides bicycle. Copies a square. Draws a man with 6 parts. Defines 6 simple words. Names materials.	As for 2 Yr. Trivalent oral polio. Tetanus. Diphtheria.

HOW TO PHONE YOUR PEDIATRICIAN

The American Academy of Pediatrics recommends the following:

Don't call your pediatrician outside of office hours unless your child's problem is urgent and cannot wait.

If your child is sick, always try to take his temperature before calling for advice.

Have a pencil and paper ready when you phone to write out instructions your pediatrician gives you. Make a list of the questions you want answered before you call. Have the number of the pharmacy on hand so your pediatrician can order a prescription if necessary.

Be prepared to tell the person who answers the phone exactly what is wrong. Use words which have clearly understood meanings. Instead of saying, "He has a fever," say, "He has a temperature of 102°F by rectum." Instead of saying, "He has diarrhea," say, "He has had ten large watery bowel movements in the last six hours."

Tell the age of the child, when he started to get sick, if he has a fever and if so how much, what you think is wrong with the child, and what you have done so far.

If your child has a cold or cough, be prepared to describe the cough (dry, loose, "crowing," painful) and breathing (normal, fast, labored).

Find out before you call if he has a headache, earache, sore throat, or chest pain.

If your child has a stomachache or pain, be ready to describe the location of the pain, how the child reacts to the pain, if the abdomen feels tight or rigid, if the child has been hit in the stomach, and if he has any other symptoms such as headache or vomiting.

If your child has been injured, describe the details of the accident and your impression of his general condition (alert, dazed, listless, or unconscious).

WHEN TO CALL
YOUR PEDIATRICIAN IMMEDIATELY

You should call your pediatrician at any hour of the day or night if your child has any of the following symptoms. If you cannot reach your pediatrician, call or take your child to the emergency room at the nearest hospital.

Serious accident or injury. Bleeding that cannot be stopped by direct pressure on the wound.

Unconsciousness.

Anything beyond a local reaction to insect sting or a recent injection if it occurs within 30 minutes, such as fever, joint pain, vomiting, headache, generalized hives, and tightness in throat or chest.

Breathing difficulties, such as severe difficulty getting his breath, extreme anxiousness, or turning blue.

Convulsions.

Abdominal pain lasting more than an hour or two. (Give the child nothing to eat or drink and do not administer any laxative.)

Black, bloody, or tarry bowel movement in an infant who is not taking iron.

Diarrhea in infancy. (If an infant has three or four loose watery stools, he could rapidly develop dehydration. Watch for signs of dehydration such as listlessness, fever, dry skin, and failure to urinate.)

WHEN TO CALL YOUR PEDIATRICIAN
DURING OFFICE HOURS

Fever. A temperature over 101°F for two or more hours.

Persistent headaches. If a child complains of headache more than twice a week, or if the headache is associated with nausea or vomiting.

Dizziness. If the child cannot keep his balance or constantly feels that the world is spinning around.

Persistent vomiting.

Unusual fatigue and weight loss. If fatigue persists for a number of days, is accompanied by weight loss or is associated with an activity that has never before tired the child.

Constant cough or hoarseness. Especially if it keeps the child awake at night.

Frequent sore throats and mouth breathing.

Frequent nosebleeds. If bleeding continues after simple first-aid measures or if there is frequent bleeding of the nose at night or while the child is inactive.

Sore or swollen joints. If continued pain, swelling, redness or lack of mobility, especially if there is any fever.

Frequent or painful urination; or recurrence of bed-wetting.

Enlarged lymph nodes in neck and sore throat.

Abdominal pain.

Croup.

Asthma.

Earache. If an infant rubs his ear or cries incessantly when he has a cold, especially at night, suspect an earache.

Skin changes. If a skin lesion doesn't heal in a few days; slow healing cuts or bruises; continuing rashes or itching anywhere on the body.

Puffy eyes, swollen hands and feet.

Muscle weakness. If a child was formerly active and can no longer go up and down stairs easily or run about without becoming weak.

Bed-wetting. In a child of 6 or more or in a child who previously had control.

School phobia.

Poor classroom performance.

WHAT TO MENTION TO YOUR PEDIATRICIAN AT YOUR NEXT VISIT

THE FIRST YEAR

Failure to notice moving objects.

Absence of leg kicks: If you hold an infant upright under his arms, he will normally raise and lower his legs as if walking. Failure to do so may mean a nerve or muscle problem.

Failure to hold his head up: If a baby is unable to hold his head up by 3 months, roll over by 4 to 5 months or sit up alone by 8 months.

Failure to pull himself up or toddle at 10 to 14 months.

Absence of teeth: A baby's first teeth usually should appear between 3 and 8 months.

A fat, flabby baby.

No attempt to mimic sounds or words by 1 year.

PRESCHOOL AGE (1–6)

Unusual or excessive activity: a child who is continually restless and overactive, short attention span in school and clumsiness.

Poor muscle coordination.

HOW TO PLAN YOUR CHILD'S NUTRITION

Start out right by eating properly during pregnancy.

Breast feed your baby.

Give it the vitamin and mineral supplements your pediatrician recommends.

Be sure baby food does not have sugar or salt added to it by the manufacturer.

Make your own baby food with a food blender or a simple table-model baby food grinder. (Bananas, yogurt, fruits, cooked potatoes and vegetables can simply be mashed with a fork.)

Keep cookies, candy, cake, and sugared soft drinks out of the house.

NEW HEALTHY POPSICLE

Called "Ten Plus," it is made of all natural ingredients including skim milk, orange juice, and eggs. Make your own of fruit juice also.

SIGNS YOUR CHILD MAY NEED A CHANGE IN DIET

- Failure to grow and thrive
- Too thin
- Lethargy
- Irritable
- Pale as from anemia
- Dull hair and lackluster eyes
- Sores around the mouth
- Poor eye adaptation to dim light
- Flaccid muscles
- Easy tiring
- Sore, bleeding gums
- Short attention span

If your child has such symptoms, have a doctor check him out.

BOTTLE CAVITY SYNDROME

Don't put your baby to bed with a bottle. And don't let your child walk around all day with a bottle. It causes early tooth decay called "bottle cavity syndrome."

HOW TO ACCIDENT-PROOF A CHILD IN A CAR

A baby held in the front passenger's arms occupies what safety experts call the "death seat." Don't just hold your child, use a safe car seat or car bed.

The American Academy of Pediatrics recommends that children never be unrestrained in the front seat of a motor vehicle or in the cargo section of a station wagon. They also state that children under 4 years of age, or weighing less than 40 pounds, should not be restrained by standard safety belts: the abdominal pressure in a forward crash may cause internal injuries. However, they recommend that you use the safety belt if nothing else is available, putting a small pillow between the seat belt and your child.

Advice on car seats:

It should pass actual crash tests ("dynamic testing") simulating automobile collisions.

It should give adequate head and back support.

Putting a baby or child in it and taking him out should be simple.

The straps should be very sturdy, at least 1½

THINGS TO KNOW ABOUT COMMON INFECTIOUS DISEASES

DISEASE	INCUBATION PERIOD	WHEN CATCHING	PRECAUTIONS
Chicken pox	2–3 weeks	1 day before rash to 6 days after blisters first appear	Isolate patient until 6 days after appearance of first blisters. If exposed person is taking cortisone or other steroids he should call a doctor at once.
Diphtheria	2–6 days or longer	Usually 2 weeks, sometimes 4	Isolate patient until 3 consecutive nose & throat cultures are found free of germs. Exposed person should have nose and throat cultures taken, should require a booster dose of diphtheria toxoid and be quarantined for 7 days.
Hepatitis	10–160 days	Unknown	Patient should be isolated for first week. Exposed persons should receive gamma globulin.
Influenza	1–3 days	Before onset to 1 week after	Avoid crowds during epidemics.
Measles	7–14 days	From 4 days before to 5 days after rash appears, especially during coughing stage	Isolate patient from first signs until 5 days after rash appears. Give gamma globulin to those exposed.
German Measles	14–25 days	From early symptoms for at least 4 days	Isolate patient from first signs until 5 days after rash appears.
Mononucleosis	Thought to be 4–14 days	Unknown	Laboratory tests will confirm when infection is gone.
Mumps	14–28 days	From 6 days before symptoms until swelling has disappeared	Isolate patient until swelling is gone.
Whooping Cough	5–21 days	Greatest in coughing stage, through fourth week	Isolate patient (but need not be indoors) for 3 weeks from onset of the whooping. Children who have not previously been immunized should be quarantined for 14 days after exposure and unvaccinated exposed children under age 2 should receive gamma globulin.

inches wide, and should adjust easily to the child's size.

It should not have a tubular aluminum frame.

It must be possible to fasten the child's seat to the car itself by seat belts or other devices. The kind that fit over a car seat are not safe.

HOW TO KNOW IF YOUR CHILD HAS WORMS

Your children can get worms from playing with dogs or cats, playing with dirt, eating raw meat or fish, or eating food handled by infested persons. Symptoms can vary from loss of appetite, nausea, and headache to loss of weight, fatigue, diarrhea or constipation, skin rash or cramps, or the child may have no symptoms at all except itching and sleeplessness. Usually you can see the worms in the child's bowel movement. The most common in the U.S. are pinworms, which are ⅛- to ½-inch long.

See the doctor right away for a laboratory test and for medicine to kill worms. He may want all members of the household to be treated, or at least tested.

Prevention: Don't eat raw meat or unwashed fruits and vegetables. Wash hands after playing with animals or dirt. Wash hands before eating.

NEW TREATMENT FOR BLUE BABIES

At birth some children have a heart condition in which a major blood vessel has a defect in it, so all blood doesn't get to the lungs properly for oxygen.

To live, these babies needed surgery. Now Dr. William F. Friedman of the University of California at San Diego reports that the arthritis drug indomethacin when given to the baby will trigger the blood vessel to close as it should. So far it has worked in all but one infant tried.

HANDLE WITH CARE

Never toss or bounce an infant 2 years old or younger. Jiggling, shaking, or jerking can lead to bleeding in the brain. When lifting or handling the infant, always use a hand or arm to cradle the head.

Don't swing toddlers by the ankles. Never shake an infant by the shoulders or slap its head.

Don't jerk children by the hand. Jerking a child's arm can cause a dislocation of the elbow. It usually happens to children aged 2 to 5 when they get pulled up a curb, are lifted high out of the waves at the beach, or are swung high by both arms to touch the ceiling. (The pain may be in the shoulder, the collarbone, or the wrist, but if pressure is put on the elbow, there is severe pain. Take your child to the doctor, who can snap the arm bone back into proper position.)

WHAT TO DO TO HELP BED-WETTERS

The causes are many: weak bladder muscles, irritation of a nerve, infection, pinworms, spicy foods, or fatigue. It can be a secondary symptom associated with diabetes, epilepsy, or sickle cell anemia. Or it may have psychological causes such as fear of the dark, too much stress, excitement, jealousy of a new baby, difficulty in school, harsh treatment from parents, feelings of insecurity, or frightening dreams.

Consult your family doctor or pediatrician for a thorough physical examination and medical history for possible causes.

Consider allergies. A study of 100 children who were chronic bed-wetters and who had failed to respond to conventional treatment was made. Some of the foods that commonly cause allergies were removed, and the children were started on anti-allergy medication. Bed-wetting was eliminated in 87 of the 100 children within 6 days! When the offending foods were reintroduced to the diet, the bed-wetting started up again.

If no structural defects or other physical causes are found, you can work with the physician to explore possible psychological causes.

Avoid excess intake of fluid in the late afternoon and early evening. See that the child always empties his bladder before going to bed.

Try steadily increasing the bladder capacity. Have the child force fluids during the day (just the reverse of what is usually practiced) and hold the urine as long as possible to increase bladder capacity. A prescription drug called Tofranil helps increase bladder capacity also.

Avoid cocoa, spices, salt, and sweets, especially at dinner and at night snacktime.

Remove all milk and milk products—many times the child will stop the same day.

Try giving the child magnesium supplements.

Talk the problem over with your child. Explain to him that he is old enough to tell himself when to urinate. But don't scold, nag, threaten, or suggest that there is anything shameful or dirty about wetting the bed. Give self-assurance and love. Help him have a sense of humor and faith in himself.

Encourage him to accept responsibility for his own bladder function. Have him talk to his pediatrician alone about learning to care for himself.

Let a bed-wetter older than 8 or 9 use an alarm clock and take over responsibility for his bladder by setting his own clock, waking himself up, and going to the bathroom at night.

Note: Bed-wetting can also occur in adults; 1 out of 100 military recruits were discharged for bed-wetting, according to one report.

WATCH FOR BUBBLE BATH PRODUCTS

The F.D.A. warns that bubble bath products can produce serious irritation to the skin and the urinary tract, and to the lungs if inhaled. If your child's skin becomes red or itches or if there is pain on urination, discontinue bubble bath immediately.

HOW TO TELL IF YOUR CHILD HAS A LEARNING PROBLEM

Problem children can be identified before they start school, according to Dr. Ronald J. Cantwell, pediatrician at the University of Miami School of Medicine. And every child should be checked for potential disability, he says, because early diagnosis and treatment could prevent school failure and the need for dropping out.

Dr. Cantwell outlined these points to look out for:

1. A parent, brother, or sister who had a similar problem such as a reading difficulty, repeating a grade, or dropping out

2. A child born prematurely or very small

3. A child with a history of persistent vomiting or colic, poor feeding or sleeping habits, slowness in sitting up or crawling, or a delay in walking alone

4. A child who does not put words together in phrases by age 2 or has other speech problems

5. A child who is hyperactive, has behavior difficulties, has poor coordination, or is clumsy

6. A child who in kindergarten has difficulty in coloring within the lines, is inattentive, can't print his name or count, or who has difficulty discriminating between sizes, shapes, and colors

The following is a test designed by Dr. Cantwell for pre-school checkup.

Put the child at ease and tell him you are going to play some games. Give him a tennis ball to throw and note the preferred hand. Have him kick the ball and note the preferred foot.

Then have him do the following, keeping score as you go.

1. Balancing on the preferred foot for 10 seconds.
   Steady balance—5 points
   Fair balance—3
   Poor balance—2

2. Repetitive tapping of the preferred foot for 10 seconds.
   Rapid and rhythmic—5
   Slow and less rhythmic—3
   Very slow and irregular—2

3. Walking along a line for 10 feet.
   Walks smoothly and confidently—5
   Walks a little awkwardly and more slowly—3
   Walks only with great difficulty—2

4. Catching a tennis ball from a distance of 10 feet.
   Catches three throws consecutively—5
   Catches two throws—3
   Catches one throw—2

5. Thumb-finger opposition: with preferred hand level, touch thumb with tips of second, third, and fourth fingers serially, and as rapidly as possible.
   Moves fingers smoothly and rapidly—5
   Faltering slower moments—3
   Slow and awkward movements—2

6. Count to twelve.
   Counts without error to eleven or twelve—5
   Counts to nine or ten—3
   Counts to seven or eight—1

7. Show me your nose, ear, thumb, elbow, eyebrow.
   For each correct reply—1

8. Touch the door, then pick up the pencil, then sit down in the chair.
   Three correct—5
   Two correct—3
   One correct—1

9. Print the capital letters of the alphabet.
   All correct—5
   One error—3
   Two errors—1
   More than two errors—0

10. Name days of week.
    Six to seven correct—5
    Four to five correct—3
    One to three correct—1

Add the number of points. Maximum score is 75. A score below 40 definitely requires further investigation by a doctor and by an educational psychologist to test the child's capability of doing first-grade school work.

Symptoms Checklist for Learning Disabilities, The New York Institute for Child Development, 36 East 36th Street, New York, N.Y. 10016. Be sure to specify the child's age and grade level. Free.

A BLOOD TEST FOR CRETINISM

University of Pittsburgh doctors have developed a simple blood test for detecting cretinism, a condition of too little thyroid hormone that can cause mental retardation. The ailment is hard to detect and is frequently overlooked until too late for successful treatment. Now Dr. Thomas P. Foley, Jr., reports the disorder can be detected by measuring serum levels of a hormone called thyrotropin. The test can be included in PKU screening programs.

BRAIN INJURIES TRACED TO INFANTS' FALLS

A major cause of brain injury in infants may be that a great number of them fall on their heads. Of brain-injured infants examined at Children's Memorial Hospital in Chicago, 3 out of every 4 children had fallen hard or been dropped on their heads during the first year of life. Investigators say the head injuries may be one reason for some mental retardation, learning problems, and convulsions later in childhood.

Babies most often fall when placed temporarily on adult beds, sofas, dressing tables, and counters.

A NEW PROGRAM FOR RETARDED CHILDREN

A new outpatient service at Kennedy Institute's Behavior Management Clinic in Baltimore teaches parents to apply principles of behavior therapy to retarded at home. The director of behavioral psychology at the institute meets with parents and their retarded children to pinpoint how often and under what circumstances temper tantrums, aggressiveness, and other behavior problems occur. They then decide how the parent should tackle the problem. One program is for the mother to reinforce good behavior with tokens that can be traded for treats or taken away for misbehavior. Parents are told to establish rules, stick to them, monitor the children's behavior in detail, and reward good behavior with attention.

Information about the program is available from the John F. Kennedy Institute, 707 North Broadway, Baltimore, Md. 21205.

THE BALL-STICK-BIRD SYSTEM

A new reading system has been devised that has proved effective in teaching reading skills to children who have difficulty in reading and even to retarded children with IQ's as low as 33, says Dr. Renée Fuller. A set of readers and a teacher's manual is available for parent use. Ball-Stick-Bird, Box 592, Stony Brook, N.Y. 11790. $37.

HOW TO PREVENT LEAD POISONING

See that your child gets plenty of iron, says Dr. Philip Lanzkowsky of Long Island Jewish Medical Center. He says many children eat paint and plaster because "they are intuitively searching for the iron their body lacks." Other research indicates that a deficiency in vitamin E enhances accumulation of lead in tissues; giving E reduces lead toxicity. Researchers have also shown that vitamin C helps pull out lead.

Be sure to use only non-lead paints in your house. If there is any old lead paint, scrape it off and repaint with non-lead. Do not use outdoor paint in the house. It only takes two or three paint chips a day over the weeks to cause severe illness, possible brain damage, and sometimes even death in a child.

Cases of lead poisoning have also been reported in both adults and children from sleeping in a room where dust or flakes of old paint on a ceiling drifted down on the unsuspecting sleeper. Or poisoning can occur from lead in street dust or from auto exhaust fumes.

Any normally alert child who begins to show signs of slowness, seems dull, sleepy, or cranky all the time, who complains of nausea, or who seems hard of hearing should be checked for lead poisoning immediately. (Call your local public health office and ask where you can get a free blood or urine test for lead content. See Chapter 4 for hair test.)

Note: The Pencil Makers Association says the "lead" in pencils is not really lead so will not cause lead poisoning. But you still shouldn't chew on pencils because there *is* lead in the lacquer paint on the pencil.

PAPER TOWEL CAUTION

Before you use a premoistened towel, check the ingredients listed on the package. If the towel contains benzalkonium chloride, don't use it near the mouth or eyes of children. Drs. John T. Wilson and Ian M. Burr of Children's Hospital in Nashville report in the *American Journal of Diseases of Children* that the chemical is poisonous in heavy concentration.

HOW TO GUIDE SPEECH DEVELOPMENT IN YOUR CHILD

Read stories aloud, in fun and with love.

Have your child describe and interpret pictures for you.

Take your child with you on your usual trips to the grocery store, post office, etc., explaining in simple terms what you do there.

Encourage him to learn nursery rhymes and songs, and play word games, but never ask him to recite pieces or show off his speech.

Don't make him self-conscious about his speech by praising it or criticizing it.

If he hesitates and repeats a lot when he speaks, note under what conditions he does this, then try to remove the stress from the type of situations that bother him.

Be a good listener—let him know you enjoy hearing him talk to you.

If you notice any real difficulties with speech or hearing, take him promptly to an accredited speech clinic for professional help at an early age.

STUTTERING— TWO DOCTORS' TREATMENTS

Dr. Martin Schwartz of Temple University in Philadelphia has a patient learn deep abdominal breathing, which develops a breathier, softer voice. Then instead of pursing his lips together tightly, anticipating trouble before he says a word, the patient learns to touch his lips together softly and to speak in a soft, easy tone. To remove fear, the patient is first encouraged simply to think about a telephone while talking in his new voice. Then he practices his new voice while looking at the phone. Then he touches the phone, and finally actually talks on the phone.

Dr. Irwin Rothman, also of Philadelphia, has the stutterer speak words in time with the beat of a metronome. (A portable metronome device to provide consistent practice in rhythmic speaking, now commercially available, is worn like a hearing aid.) At first the metronome is set at approximately 70 beats per minute, one syllable of speech to each beat; later, as the patient gains facility, he speeds up his speech, and uses the metronome in progressively more stressful situations.

TELLTALE SIGNS OF VARIOUS DRUGS

Marijuana. Red eyes. In early stages person may be stimulated and animated; later may be sleepy or stuporous. Odor like burned alfalfa or rope may cling to clothes.

LSD. Dilated pupils. Person may wear sunglasses indoors to protect eyes. Person may seem normal, sit around in a dreamlike state, or become agitated.

Amphetamines, pep pills. Appetite may be suppressed. Person may be restless and nervous, may become very talkative or have delusions. Mucous membranes may be dry, so person may have bad breath and lick lips frequently.

Barbiturates, depressants. User may appear drunk but have no odor of alcohol. With a small amount person may be relaxed, sociable, and good-humored. With large amounts may have thick speech, clumsy movements, drowsiness, and poor judgment.

Heroin, other narcotics. Person usually appears sleepy and lethargic, may seem very intoxicated. Pupils of the eye may be constricted, not responding to light. Needles or equipment may be found hidden. Often wears long sleeves even on hot days to hide needle marks on arms.

But don't jump to conclusions if you think you detect any of these symptoms. There may be other explanations. And don't snoop around sniffing a child's clothes or inspecting his eyes or accusing him of drug use. Such actions could lead to the child's use of drugs out of rebellion or lead to a deep gulf of mistrust and hostility.

WHAT YOU CAN DO

Keep cool.

Learn the facts about drugs, and see that your children know them.

If your children are becoming involved with drugs and cannot or will not stop, obtain professional counsel and assistance.

TREATING A BAD TRIP

Make contact with the person. This can be done physically by holding hands or hugging. If it is a severe bad trip, this may be the only way contact can be made. If verbal contact can be made, keep reassuring the person that he is in good hands, and ask questions to try to determine what was taken, how long ago, how much.

Get professional help at a hospital emergency room or at a local drug treatment center.

If the person has taken a hallucinogenic drug, there will be alternating periods of lucidness and intense drug reaction. Time these cycles. If the cycles are becoming more frequent, the person is in the early part of the trip and will probably get worse. If the cycles become less frequent, the person has already peaked and is coming down.

The area in which treatment takes place should be quiet, away from large groups of people, and have dim lighting.

Have the person try deep breathing.

Many people on bad trips are fearful of abandonment; if you have to leave the room for a few minutes, introduce someone else and remain long enough to be sure that contact is made with the new person before you leave.

EMERGENCY STEPS TO TAKE IN TREATING ANY DRUG OVERDOSE

Make sure that there is an adequate airway, giving mouth-to-mouth resuscitation or oxygen if necessary.

Try to determine what drug was taken, in what dose, what contaminants were present, how the drug was taken, and when.

If the drug was taken orally within the hour and

A SPECIAL COMPENDIUM OF DRUG FACTS

ILLICIT (PROHIBITED) DRUGS
(Manufacture and distribution prohibited except for approved research purposes.)

	SLANG NAMES	WHAT THEY ARE	HOW TAKEN
HALLUCINOGENS	LSD, Acid	LSD-25 is a lysergic acid derivative. Mescaline is a chemical taken from peyote cactus. Psilocybin is synthesized from Mexican mushrooms.	In tablet, capsule, ampul (hypodermic) form or in saturated sugar cubes.
HEROIN	Snow, Stuff, H, Junk, and others	Heroin is diacetylmorphine, an alkaloid derived from morphine. A white, off-white, or brown crystalline powder.	May be taken by any route, usually by intravenous injection.
MARIJUANA (*Cannabis*)	Joints, Sticks, Reefers, Weeds, Grass, Pot, Indian hay, Locoweed, Mu, Giggle-smoke, Mary Jane	Marijuana is the dried flowering or fruiting top or leaves of the plant Cannabis sativa l., commonly called Indian Hemp. Usually looks like fine, green tobacco. Hashish is a preparation of cannabis.	Marijuana smoked in pipes or cigarettes. Hashish is infrequently made into candy, sniffed in powder form, mixed with honey for drinking or with butter to spread on bread.

LEGITIMATE DRUGS
(Essential to the practice of medicine; legitimate manufacture and distribution are confined to ethical drug channels.)

AMPHETAMINE	Bennies, Co-pilots, Footballs, Hearts, Pep pills	Amphetamines are stimulants, prescribed by physicians chiefly to reduce appetite and to relieve minor cases of mental depression. Often used to promote wakefulness and/or increase energy.	Orally as a tablet or capsule. Abusers may resort to intravenous injection.
BARBITURATES	Red birds, Yellow jackets, Blue heavens, Goof balls	Barbiturates are sedatives, prescribed to induce sleep or, in smaller doses, to provide a calming effect.	Orally as a tablet or capsule. Sometimes intravenously by drug abusers.
COCAINE	The Leaf, Snow, Speedballs (when mixed with heroin)	Extracted from the leaves of the coca bush. It is a white, odorless, fluffy powder that looks like crystalline snow.	Orally or intravenously, alone or with heroin. Or coca leaves are chewed with lime.

IMARY EFFECT	HOW TO SPOT ABUSER	DANGERS
ll produce hallucinations, exhilaration, or depression, and apparently rarely may lead to serious mental changes, psychotic manifestations, suicidal or homicidal tendencies.	Abusers may undergo complete personality changes, "see" smells, "hear" colors. They may try to fly or brush imaginary insects from their bodies, etc. Behavior is irrational. Marked depersonalization.	Very small quantities of LSD may cause hallucinations lasting for days or repetitive psychotoxic episodes, which may recur months after injection. Permanence of mental derangement is still a moot question. Damage to chromosomes has been demonstrated.
ike morphine in all respects, faster and shorter acting.	Morphine-like.	Like morphine; dependence usually develops more rapidly. Dependence liability is high.
feeling of great perceptiveness and pleasure can accompany even small doses. Erratic behavior, loss of memory, distortion of time and spatial perceptions, and hilarity without apparent cause occur. Marked unpredictability of effect.	Abusers may feel exhilarated or relaxed, stare off into space; be hilarious without apparent cause; have exaggerated sense of ability.	Because of the vivid visions and exhilaration which sometimes may result from use of marijuana, abusers may lose all restraint and act in a manner dangerous to themselves and/or others. Accident prone because of time and space sense disturbance.
ormal doses produce wakefulness, increased alertness and a feeling of increased initiative. Intravenous doses produce cocaine-like psychotoxic effects.	An almost abnormal cheerfulness and unusual increase in activity, jumpiness and irritability; hallucinations and paranoid tendencies after intravenous use.	Amphetamines can cause high blood pressure, abnormal heart rhythms and even heart attacks. Teen-agers often take them to increase their "nerve." As a result, they may behave dangerously. Excess or prolonged usage can cause hallucinations, loss of weight, wakefulness, jumpiness and dangerous aggressiveness. Tolerance to large doses is acquired by abusers.
mall amounts make the user relaxed, sociable, good-humored. Heavy doses make him sluggish, gloomy, sometimes quarrelsome. His speech is thick and he staggers. Sedation and incoordination progressive with dose, and at least additive with alcohol and/ or other sedatives and tranquilizers.	The appearance of drunkenness with no odor of alcohol characterizes heavy dose. Sedation with variable ataxia.	Sedation, coma and death from respiratory failure. Inattentiveness may cause unintentional repetitious administration to a toxic level. Many deaths each year from intentional and unintentional overdose. Potentiation with alcohol particularly hazardous. The drug is addictive, causing physical as well as psychic dependency, and withdrawal phenomena are characteristically different from withdrawal of opiates.
ral use is said to relieve hunger and fatigue, and produce some degree of exhilaration. Intravenous use produces marked psychotoxic effects, hallucinations with paranoid tendencies. Repetitive doses lead to maniacal excitation, muscular twitching, convulsive movements.	Dilated pupils, hyperactive, exhilarated paranoic.	Convulsions and death may occur from overdose. Paranoiac activity. Very strong psychic but not physical dependence and no tolerance.

(Chart continues on next page)

LEGITIMATE DRUGS (*continued*)

	SLANG NAMES	WHAT THEY ARE	HOW TAKEN
CODEINE	Schoolboy	A component of opium and a derivative of morphine, in most respects a tenth or less as effective as morphine, dose-wise.	Usually taken orally, in tablets, for pain; or in a liquid preparation, of variable alcohol content, for cough. Can be injected.
METHAMPHETAMINE	Speed, Crystal	Stimulant, one of the amphetamines.	Orally, as tablets or in an elixir, or intravenously.
MORPHINE	M, Dreamer, and many others	The principal active component of opium. Morphine sulphate: white crystalline powder, light porous cubes or small white tablets.	May be taken by any route; its abusive use is mostly by intravenous injection.

From American Social Health Association: "A Guide to Some Drugs Which Are Subject to Abuse."

if the patient is still conscious, make him vomit to empty the stomach as much as possible.

Take the person to the emergency room of the nearest hospital.

Take a sample of the drug along if it is available.

FREE OR NEARLY FREE BOOKS ON CHILD CARE
Your Child from 6 to 12
    Superintendent of Documents
    U.S. Government Printing Office
    Washington, D.C.
    65¢
Your Child and Household Safety
    Dr. Jay M. Arena
    Chemical Specialties Manufacturer's Assoc.
    1001 Connecticut Avenue
    Washington, D.C. 20036
    50¢
A Medical Emergency Guide; also *Your Child's Safety*
    Metropolitan Life Insurance Co.
    1 Madison Avenue
    New York, N.Y. 10010
    Free
Communicative Evaluation Chart from Infancy to Five Years
    Ruth M. Anderson, Madeline Miles, Patricia A. Matheny
    Educators Publishing Service
    75 Moulton Street
    Cambridge, Mass. 02138
    50¢

Enjoy Your Child—Ages 1, 2 and 3
    James L. Hymes, Jr.
    Public Affairs Pamphlet No. 141
    Public Affairs Committee
    381 Park Avenue South
    New York, N.Y. 10016
    35¢
Childhood
    Dr. Lee Salk and Eda LeShan
    Blue Cross Association
        For a free copy call your local Blue Cross office.
The Natural Baby Food Cookbook
    Margaret Kenda and Phyllis Williams
    Avon Books
    959 Eighth Avenue
    New York, N.Y. 10019
    95¢
Test Your Child's I.Q.
    Victor Serebriakoff and Dr. Steven Langer
    David McKay Co.
    750 Third Avenue
    New York, N.Y. 10017
        Includes standardized I.Q. test for children of all age levels.
    $7.95
Successful Toilet Training
    T. Berry Brazelton, M.D.
    Baby Talk Magazine
    66 East 34th Street
    New York, N.Y. 10016
    55¢

PRIMARY EFFECT	HOW TO SPOT ABUSER	DANGERS
Analgesic and cough suppressant with very little sedation or exhilarant (euphoric) action. Dependence can be produced or partially supported, but large doses are required.	Unless taken intravenously, very little evidence of general effect. Large doses are morphine-like.	Occasionally taken (liquid preparations) for kicks, but large amount required. Contribution of the alcohol content to the effect may be significant. Degree and risk of abuse very minor.
Effects resemble amphetamine but are more marked and toxicity greater.	Extreme restlessness and irritability; violence and paranoid reaction possible.	Excessive psychotoxic effects, sometimes with fatal outcome.
Generally sedative and analgesic (rarely excitatory). The initial reaction is unpleasant to most people, but calming supersedes and may progress to coma and death from respiratory failure.	Constrictive pupils. Calm, inattentive, "on the nod," with slow pulse and respiration.	Man is very sensitive to the respiratory depressant effect until tolerance develops. Psychic and physical dependence and tolerance develop readily, with a characteristic withdrawal syndrome.

Baby Feasts from Family Meals; also *Osterizer Guide for Feeding Baby Better*
    Oster Corp.
    5055 North Lydell Avenue
    Milwaukee, Wis. 53217
    Free and 50¢, respectively
Feeding Your Baby During His First Year; also *Food Before Six; A Feeding Guide for Parents of Young Children*
    National Dairy Council
    111 North Canal Street
    Chicago, Ill. 60606
    Both Free
Keeping Yourself Together: A TA Primer for the Single Parent
    Kathryn J. Hallett
    1005 Dunn Road
    St. Louis, Mo. 63031
    $1 plus postage
        A pamphlet for the single parent on using transactional analysis in situations arising after death, divorce, or desertion.
Beautiful Junk
    Superintendent of Documents
    Government Printing Office
    Washington, D.C. 20402
    40¢
        Ideas for making toys out of boxes and other throwaway materials.

Inexpensive material on organizing Day Care Centers is available from the following groups:

Women's Action Alliance
    370 Lexington Avenue
    New York, N.Y. 10017
Office of Child Development
    U.S. Department of Health, Education and Welfare
    P. O. Box 1182
    Washington, D.C. 20013
The Day Care and Child Development Council of America
    1401 K Street, N.W.
    Washington, D.C. 20005
"Lullaby from the Womb"
    Capitol Records, The Capitol Tower
    P. O. Box 2391
    Hollywood, Calif. 90028
    Record $6.98; Cassette $7.98
        Dr. Hajime Murooka, a Japanese physician, has recorded the gurgling, boomping noises within the womb of an expectant mother. Soothing music for babies and parents.

13

Slowing the Clock of Age

When Arthur Rubinstein was 80, someone told him he was playing the piano better than ever. "I think so," he agreed. "Now I take chances I never took before. Now I let go and enjoy myself!"

"Youth is not a time of life; it is a state of mind; it is not a matter of rosy cheeks, red lips and supple knees; it is a matter of the will, a quality of the imagination, a vigor of the emotions; it is the freshness of the deep springs of life. . . ."—Samuel Ullman

SPECIAL NUTRITION NEEDS OF OLDER PEOPLE

The first step in slowing down the aging process is to put body chemistry in balance. The best way—nutrition!

Special vitamins and minerals the older person should be sure to have in adequate amounts are these:

Calcium, which is necessary to counteract bone deterioration and prevent bone symptoms that often mimic arthritis. It can also help prevent receding gums and help tighten loose teeth, and if dentures are worn can help prevent the jaw bone from changing shape due to lack of calcium.

Vitamin C, which has anti-oxidant properties believed to help delay aging. Vitamin C is necessary for production of collagen in the joints and also reduces atherosclerosis.

B vitamins, especially niacin, which counteract

tendencies to blood clotting and so give extra protection against heart attacks and stroke.

Pantothenic acid, the vitamin found in royal jelly that prolongs the life of the queen bee and which when fed to mice and rats was shown to increase their life span by another one-third.

Inositol and choline, which help the body form lecithin, which reduces cholesterol levels, prevents fatty infiltration of the liver, and is important to brain tissue.

PABA (para-aminobenzoic acid) which is part of the molecule in Gerovital, known for years in Europe to fight symptoms of aging.

Also see the Whole Health Vital Diet in Chapter 4.

NEW NEWS ABOUT VITAMIN E

Vitamin E, which protects blood vessels and repairs blood vessel damage, is also an anti-oxidant, and has extended life of cells in laboratory experiments, but whether it works in humans to extend life has always been controversial. But there is evidence that a deficiency of it will cause premature aging, and Dr. Jeffrey S. Blank and a team of researchers at the University of Puget Sound found that vitamin E definitely prolongs the productive life of human red blood cells. The vitamin-E-enriched blood cells can carry nourishment far more efficiently to the tissues, Dr. Blank says, thus keeping tissue cells healthier longer. Doses given to volunteers in the experiment: 600 units of vitamin E per day.

Earlier, the Minnesota Agricultural Experiment Station reported that when cattle appearing to be in perfect health were deprived of their vitamin E rations, they suddenly dropped dead of heart disease. When wheat germ with E was restored, the deaths from heart disease stopped.

TIGER'S MILK

Adelle Davis's recommendation for increasing your energy and alertness. Many Senior Citizens Clubs are using a glass of tiger's milk for breakfast and daytime pickups.

The basic recipe is:

1 quart regular milk
½ cup dried milk
½ cup brewer's yeast
small can frozen orange juice (unsweetened)

Blend in a blender or cocktail shaker. Keep in the refrigerator.

Some start with all orange juice, instead of milk. Or apricot, pineapple, or apple juice. Some add a raw egg.

Make up your own recipe from these possibilities:

BASES	FLAVORINGS	ADDITIONS
Milk	fruit pulp	brewer's yeast
Orange juice	apricot, pineapple,	powered skim
Apple juice	frozen orange	milk,
Tomato juice	juice, undiluted	lecithin
Pineapple juice	blackstrap molasses	desiccated liver
	lemon	apple cider vinegar
	honey	raw egg yolk

A commercial product called Tiger's Milk has been marketed which contains some of the ingredients mixed together in powdered form.

HOW TO APPLY PRINCIPLES OF THE HUNZA DIET TO YOUR NEEDS

The Hunzas are happy and serene, have no jails, no police, no divorces, and until lately had no doctors. They often live to be over 100 and are routinely sexually active at 90. Doctors who have visited and studied the Hunzas in their mountain environment attribute their excellent health to their diet. The facts of their diet: They eat nothing processed or refined, and until the last few years never ate sugar. They grow their food on fertile soil (all waste matter is returned to the soil). They eat raw vegetables, fresh and sun-dried fruit, espe-

cially apricots and apricot seeds which they eat almost every day, sprouted beans, freshly ground whole wheat flour, yogurt, a great deal of fowl and eggs, and only occasional meat.

Does it work? When rats were fed the food of the early Hunzas, a peaceful strain was developed with long lives and no disease. When other rats were fed a typical modern diet, they became irritable, tried to kill each other, and had many ailments.

The same good health, tranquility, and long life is found in Indians of the Yucatan, in Eskimos, and groups in Africa, South America, and the Pacific Islands. The one thing scientists say they have in common—eating their native natural diet without processed or refined foods.

MENTAL DISABILITY IS NOT INEVITABLE

Many mental disabilities, such as depression and forgetfulness, happen as we get older, we assume, but they are not inevitable and are often due to physical causes that are treatable.

Anyone who thinks he or she might be depressed more often and more severely than is normal, or has other mental problems, should take this test.

These are typical questions from the Renard Research Interview, developed by doctors at Washington University in St. Louis.

Circle the number 3 if the symptoms were severe enough so that you went to a doctor, if the symptoms were disabling, or necessitated your taking medication.

Circle the number 2 if the symptom was caused by a known physical condition.

Circle 1 if none of these apply.

Do you think you have always been
sickly the majority of your life?   1   2   3
Do you have shortness of breath on
exertion, or is it a recent change?   1   2   3
Do you have anxiety attacks?
(Spells of apprehension, fear,
uneasiness, plus shortness of breath
or palpitation; and one symptom
from the following list: chest pain,
weakness, sweating, dizziness,
numbness, visual blurring, trembling. Negative if the above symptoms have occurred only with medical or acute emotion-provoking
situations.)   1   2   3

Have you ever had amnesia?   1 2 3
Have you ever had sudden gains or
losses in weight? (In less than 2
weeks gained or lost more than 15
pounds, not related to medical dis-
ease.)   1 2 3
Do you have diminished sex drive?
(Positive if 50 percent or greater reduction in frequency of intercourse
not due to partner's refusal, etc.,
and lasting at least one month.)   1 2 3
Do you quit jobs without having an-
other one to go to? (Positive if occurred more than once. Negative if
only for legitimate reasons, such as
retirement.)   1 2 3
In your lifetime, have you ever had
any period of feeling depressed,
sad, blue, or down in the dumps
lasting two weeks or longer?   1 2 3
Has there ever been a time when
you were the opposite of
depressed—that is, too happy or too
enthusiastic for your own good?
This would be a time when you
were so high that others were concerned about it. (Must have lasted
at least one week.)   1 2 3
Have you ever taken any of the fol-
lowing drugs without a prescription,
or more than was prescribed: Marijuana? Uppers (amphetamines)?
Downers (barbiturates)? Narcotics?
Any other?   1 2 3
Did you ever think you drank too
much in general?   1 2 3

If you have more than a couple of 3's, show the
test and test results to your doctor and discuss
your possible problem with him.

CEREBRAL ARTERIOSCLEROSIS

This is the hardening of the arteries of the brain
that so devastatingly often robs the older person of
memory and other mental functions.
Some of the symptoms:

- Increased irritability over unexpected things
- Forgetting recent events, but remembering past
  events
- Inattentiveness, loss of interest
- Lessened capacity for work
- Periods of depression
- Occasional headaches and dizziness

- Occasional slurring of speech and groping for
  words
- Carelessness about personal appearance
- Personality changes
- Temper tantrums
- Obstinacy and stubbornness
- Regression to childish habits
- Crying spells

Sometimes there are weeks of complete nor-
malcy, followed by recurrence of symptoms.

MEDICATION CAN HELP

If the symptoms are caused by high blood pressure or by spasm of the blood vessels to the brain,
medicines for this condition will correct the mental
problem. If the general condition of the patient is
poor, vitamins and minerals and various medicines
can build him up again.

SOME OF THE OTHER MENTAL CHANGES

Changes in interpersonal relationships can
bring on mental decline. A person who has lost a
spouse or close friend or whose family has moved
away may show mental changes. If there is a
death, it is important that the children of aging parents encourage new interests and activities soon
after the mourning period has ended.

When an aging person feels unwanted or unloved, he may resign himself to old age and will
lose interest in things about him.

Physical disease, especially of a chronic nature,
can cause mental changes. And a severe illness can
trigger the onset of mental deterioration. It is not
uncommon to see people suddenly show marked
mental changes after having a serious illness. Encourage them to resume former participation in
family and community activities.

Symptoms can be precipitated by a temporary
emotional trauma. They often disappear completely when the problem is solved—a new love, a
new project, or recovery from a serious physical
illness.

MEMORY PILLS AND OTHER NEW WAYS
TO HELP AGING PERSONS HELP
THEMSELVES

As your parents become older, and less acute,
what can you do to help them?

First thing, doctors say, is to get them to the
doctor for a thorough medical examination. Many
times what seems to be hopeless mental deterioration is really caused by an undiagnosed medical

condition that can be treated, or even by poor eating habits.

Recent research shows that intelligence need not decrease with age. Nor does memory have to fade. Researchers at the University of Chicago found older people were so ingrained with the idea of losing their memory that they expected it. The real problem, the researchers found, was depression. Treat the depression, and memory usually returned to normal.

Another researcher says recent work indicates that the loss of intelligence often seen with aging is actually related to high blood pressure. In subjects with normal blood pressure, there was no intellectual drop.

The biggest breakthrough in research on aging may be the memory pills. One, called Cylert (made by Abbott Laboratories), has been shown to have excellent results in both animals and humans, tests reporting a 60 percent improvement in function. There have been no reported side effects. But at present the F.D.A. has approved the drug for use only in hyperactive children in the U.S. The drug is available in Europe (chemical name is magnesium pemoline).

Another new memory pill being tested is called Noctropyl. It even works in students to increase memory, according to studies being done in Wales. It is available in Great Britain, Belgium, and Sweden.

A third drug, called cyclandilate, has been shown to dilate blood vessels, treat artery disease, and halt mental deterioration in the elderly. It is being studied in England.

EDTA, a drug used to wash lead from your body in lead poisoning, is used by many doctors to remove calcium from hardened artery plaques of the elderly, improving circulation and mental functioning.

OXYGEN THERAPY

In New York, oxygen is being given to patients under pressure in a hyperbaric oxygen tank. Volunteers in the experiment go into the chamber for 90 minutes twice a day for 15 days. A number of reports suggest it may be of benefit for memory loss. Other studies are being done giving volunteers 100 percent oxygen without the hyperbaric tank to see if there is benefit, a practical at-home method if it can be done during sleeping hours.

Proponents of the memory therapy say the oxygen improves memory and other mental functioning, improves some cases of arthritis, increases energy and sex drive, improves chronic lung disease, and lowers blood pressure. However, some scientists believe the improvement is only temporary.

Some doctors say they can even see some improvement by having patients do a simple exercise designed to get more blood with oxygen to the brain cells. The exercise: Lie face down on the bed, with your head hanging over the edge to increase blood flow to the brain. Do for 5 minutes or so 2 or 3 times a day. Get up slowly so you don't get dizzy. Or use a slant board, with the feet 12 to 15 inches higher than the head.

A few of the places where the memory therapy is being done are: Florida Atlantic University, Boca Raton; Miami Heart Institute; V.A. Hospital, Gainesville, Fla.; Ocean Hyperbaric Oxygen Center, Lauderdale-by-the-Sea, Fla.; New York University; V.A. Hospital, Buffalo, N.Y.; University of Colorado Medical Center, Denver. Medicare and Medicaid usually will reimburse for the treatments, if they are prescribed by your doctor.

HOW TO PICK YOURSELF UP WHEN YOU'RE DOWN AND OUT

Lithium: This drug has for a long time been used to treat manic-depressive patients. Now it appears to also be effective for simple "unipolar" depression (without the mania phase).

Lithium's effect on alcoholism is also being studied, with some encouraging results so far.

Warning: Lithium has been reported to sometimes alter thyroid metabolism. Be sure your doctor regularly monitors you for goiter possibility if he puts you on it.

Tricyclic antidepressants: Since the 1950s several drugs have been prescribed successfully against depression. And they still work. However, many times doctors give too much. The response curve rises, reaches a peak, then falls again. At too high levels there can even be side effects such as seizures and measurable changes in the EKG. Pharmaceutical companies are now establishing optimum blood levels for each drug for the best effectiveness.

THE YOUTH DRUGS

For the past 20 years, thousands of patients have flocked to clinics in Europe to receive treatments with the controversial Rumanian "youth drug" called Gerovital. It is a mixture of procaine (novocaine) and several other substances that the developers of the drug claim are outstandingly effective in treating mental depression among the aged, as well as arthritis, heart conditions, memory loss, impotence, arteriosclerosis, high blood pressure, and Parkinsonism.

Actually there are two forms of the drug: KH-3, developed by Dr. Fritz Widemann of West Germany, which is one of the top 10 biggest over-the-counter sellers in West Germany; and Gerovital H-3, developed by Dr. Ana Aslan of Rumania, which is sold in Switzerland and in Rumania, and is given to patients through gerontology clinics set up on farms and in factories across the country. Both are sold in Great Britain. The best results reportedly come from the Rumanian kind, which is usually given in 3 injections a week, for 4 weeks, repeated in 2 weeks for patients past 60, in 2 months for those 35 to 60. Plain procaine without the various additions in H-3 seems to have no effect.

At first put down by U.S. doctors, the two drugs are now being tested by at least five research groups here. So far the tests look very promising. Rom-Amer Pharmaceuticals Ltd. of Las Vegas so far is the only company in the U.S. licensed by Rumania to distribute Gerovital. It is obtainable in Nevada to anyone.

DMAE (dimethylaminoethanol). This chemical, from which the vitamin choline is formed, has also been shown to have potential in slowing aging. It increased length of life by 30 percent in mice that received it in their drinking water. Clinical studies in people are underway.

Three new drugs. Meclofenoxate, kawain, and magnesium orotate all work against deposits of a chemical called lipofuscin found in the brain and heart during aging. They are available in several countries in Europe for the treatment of senile mental disorders.

Cell therapy. It is offered in England, Germany, Switzerland, and the Philippines. Probably the most well-known therapists are Dr. Peter Stephan at the Cell Therapy Center in London and doctors at the Clinique Générale La Prairie, where Dr. Paul Niehans first developed the technique in Clarens, Switzerland. The cell injections are made from fresh or frozen cells from sheep embryos. Those giving cell therapy do not claim that it extends life, but that it gives persons increased alertness and vigor with a renewed sense of well-being.

HELPS FOR MENOPAUSE

Menopause usually happens around age 50, but can occur later, or as early as age 35. Menstruation ceases, and progesterone and estrogen levels drop.

Calcium will help. The calcium level usually drops greatly when ovarian hormones decrease. Calcium is especially helpful if you have problems during the week in your cycle when you used to have premenstrual tension. Increase your calcium intake at those times. Some nutritionists claim that hot flashes, night sweats, leg cramps, and irritability can sometimes disappear in a single day if you take calcium plus a little vitamin D and either vegetable or fish oil (for vitamin E) to help assimilate the calcium.

Vitamin Bs can help. They will give you peace and tranquility to help overcome jangled nerves. Eat lots of liver, wheat germ, and brewer's yeast or take properly balanced vitamin B complex tablets. (Don't take just one of the vitamin Bs; they should be balanced with all the vitamin Bs.)

Lecithin can help. It will help the body use calcium and help maintain a hormone balance.

Vitamin E can help. Because of its benefits to circulation it is helpful for hot flashes.

The estrogen controversy. Estrogen therapy has been shown to bring relief from hot flashes and sweats, to counteract weakening of bones and low back pain, and to solve the problem of vaginal tissue that often becomes dry and tender. Some doctors think it should be continued indefinitely; others use it for a short time; some, not at all.

About half of postmenopausal American women have been taking estrogens, but the number is decreasing with the controversial report of studies that indicate women on estrogen have an increased rate of occurrence of cancer in the uterus (about 25 cases for every 100,000 users). Is it coincidence or has the estrogen caused the increase? Doctors don't know. Some say the statistical correlation doesn't even exist. But they urge women not to panic, since estrogen doesn't affect the incidence of uterine cancer nearly as much as obesity and other factors do. And obviously if you have had your uterus removed, you have no danger of cancer of the uterus.

They do recommend that before starting estrogen a woman see her doctor for a checkup and that women on estrogen should have a twice yearly checkup. You should join your doctor in deciding if your symptoms require estrogen, whether the benefits outweigh any risks. If you decide to take it, keep your dose levels as low as possible.

You should not take estrogen if you have had fibroid tumors, breast cysts, or a history of cancer, or if you are obese, smoke cigarettes, have high blood pressure, or high levels of cholesterol or tri-glycerides.

Caution: If your menstrual bleeding stops for many months, then starts again, if you have spotting between periods, or if bleeding becomes especially heavy, call your doctor.

If you decide to take estrogen, see Chapter 5 for the diet you should be on.

SEX AFTER SIXTY

Sex does not need to be missing from your life as you grow older, study after study shows. In fact, many women experience increased eroticism after menopause, just when they are expecting a decline. Nursing home administrators report that sex has become more popular in nursing homes than checkers. The biggest hazard for the oldsters is becoming overenthusiastic and falling out of the small beds.

Men and women can remain sexually active through their 70s, 80s, and 90s, doctors say, although frequency may decline. When impotence occurs, it is usually because the person expects it to, or has an unwarranted fear of a problem.

Being sexually active has bonus benefits, too. It has been reported to help persons with arthritis, perhaps by release of cortisone by the adrenal glands. Dr. George Ehruch, director of the rheumatology department at Albert Einstein Medical Center in Philadelphia, says many patients say they achieve six to eight hours of relief of pain after sexual activity.

Depression and suicide rates go down in the aged in groups where sex is prevalent, investigators say.

If you are not as active as you would like to be, read Chapter 11 for help with specific problems.

For drying of vaginal tissues that usually comes with aging: Increased intake of vitamin A and folic acid; use of vaginal hormone creams or K-Y jelly, inserted into the vagina every night just as a contraceptive cream would be, are helpful.

Warning: If you are in the midst of menopause, continue to use contraceptives for several months (check with your doctor for exact time) after your periods have apparently stopped. There is still a chance you can get pregnant.

SOME OF THE THINGS THAT TEND TO CAUSE WRINKLES THAT YOU CAN DO SOMETHING ABOUT IF YOU ACT EARLY ENOUGH

Drinking. It can cause tiny blood vessels to burst, causing small red lines. (Red lines can also be caused by high blood pressure or constant exposure to concentrated heat.) And drinking alcohol can rob the skin of moisture, making it drab and lifeless.

Smoking. It impairs circulation, causes skin to be yellow, sallow, and wrinkled. Dr. Harry Daniell reports in the *Annals of Internal Medicine* that the most heavily wrinkled people are almost always smokers, and that the amount of wrinkling is correlated to "an uncanny degree" to the amount and duration of smoking. "Smokers in the 40–49 age group were likely to be as prominently wrinkled as non-smokers 20 years older," he said.

Too much sun. It typically causes wrinkles and thick, leathery skin. Doctors call it the "Miami Beach Syndrome."

Frequent gaining and losing of weight. This can cause premature wrinkling and sagging because the skin becomes stretched, then relaxed.

Drugs. Tranquilizers, barbiturates, amphetamines, or other drugs can cause everything from premature aging to blisters, wrinkles, and sores.

REVITALIZING AGING SKIN

Moisturizers will not prevent wrinkling, but will help restore moisture to the outer layer of the skin.

Some doctors say keratin protein will help give you a smooth look. Another form of protein is collagen protein. You can get samples by sending 25¢ to Schmid Laboratories, Route 46 West, Little Falls, N.J. 07424.

Vitamin A acid (Rein A cream), available by prescription, reduces scaliness, makes skin smoother, diminishes mottling and blotchiness, and reduces hair plugs in follicles that often increase with age.

Wonderlift will temporarily help lift and smooth skin, but effects only last a few hours.

Some claim placenta and hormone creams will help smooth out wrinkles, but doctors recommended them only in strengths obtained by prescription. Some claim Eterna 27 enables underlying tissues to retain moisture and plumps out the skin.

EUROPEAN TECHNIQUES

Christine Valmy Shops have brought several European methods to the U.S., including electrocoagulation of skin albumin to lessen wrinkles (the de-wrinkling is said to last about four months), cleaning with various machines, light chemical peels, embryo cell treatments, paraffin masks.

AN AT-HOME TEMPORARY FACE LIFT

Apply egg white to the face, let dry while lying down and relaxing. After it has dried completely you can feel the tightening. Rinse it off with cold water.

THE BEST BEAUTIFIERS OF ALL

Sufficient sleep, keeping the face clean, regular exercises, fresh air, a *little* sunshine, proper diet, and a smile.

WHAT TO DO FOR ITCHY SKIN

1. Use Alpha-Keri, or other commercial bath oil, or a few tablespoons of peanut, olive, vegetable, or baby oil in the bath.
2. Cut down the heat in the house and humidify the air.
3. Avoid strong chemicals and strong drying soaps and detergents.
4. Include unsaturated fatty acids in the diet, especially cod-liver oil or lecithin.

If these simple measures don't work, then get three tests: a blood count, a blood sugar test, and a sedimentation test to determine if an underlying illness is causing the problem.

If you have frequent boils, athlete's foot, and other skin infections in addition to itching, it's a likely sign of diabetes. Older people are especially susceptible to skin changes from hidden diabetes. Itching skin with a yellow jaundiced look can mean liver disease, or if accompanied by a boggy feeling and bumpiness of the skin may mean insufficient thyroid hormones.

DO-IT-YOURSELF FACIAL SAUNA

Smooths and softens the skin and temporarily erases tiny lines. Bring a pot of water to a boil, remove from direct heat, hold your face about a foot away from it, and drape a towel over your head to catch the steam for 5 to 10 minutes.

DIET AND AGING SKIN

Make sure there is enough fat in your diet to provide oils and hormones for your skin and hair (but not greasy foods).

Stay away from sugar, chocolate, colas, and heavy spices.

Be sure your vitamins include vitamins A, B, C, D, and E every day—essentials for good skin.

IF YOU HAVE A VISIBLY RED NOSE

If there are visible capillaries close to the skin surface, beware of hot spicy foods such as chili, curry, hot peppers, and caffeine, and alcohol. They all cause dilation of the blood vessels. So can estrogen.

XANTHOMAS

These little white or yellow fatty papules can appear on the eyelids, tendons, hands, or joints. If you see them, go to your doctor to check for a lipid profile of your blood.

SHOULD YOUR SKIN BE ACID OR ALKALINE

Washing with alkaline soaps and detergents breaks down the skin's natural defense. When the skin is young, it only takes about 20 minutes to return to its natural acidic state, but when older it takes longer. Be sure to use soaps and shampoos that are neutral or slightly acid (a pH of 7 or under). Also see that shampoos contain protein (make sure the label says it's the hydrolyzed kind).

KEEPING HAIR HEALTHY

If you have dull hair (as well as dry scaly skin), you may not be getting enough unsaturated fatty acids (found in fish and vegetable oils) or vitamin A. Take cod-liver oil and wheat germ.

If you are losing your hair, it could be caused by (among other things) anemia, thyroid disease, or vitamin deficiency. Get a blood test and a thyroid test. Hair loss can also occur when estrogen level drops at menopause or if a person stops taking estrogen. It can also be due to pulling your hair back too tight or using too much heat on your hair. Hair loss can also occur in people taking heparin, coumadin, or certain other medicines, or while pregnant, or during a severe illness or severe stress.

Inositol has been helpful in treating baldness in many people. A commercial preparation of vitamins and minerals called Headstart has restored hair to many people who received no benefit from other treatment. Available from Cosmetic Labs., Box 18596, Atlanta, Ga. 30326.

WE'RE ALMOST AFRAID TO MENTION THIS . . .

Some scientists are reporting that three vitamins seem to restore color to graying hair—pantothenic acid, para-aminobenzoic acid (PABA), and folic acid. They have worked in humans and in animal experiments. Dr. Benjamin Sieve of Boston has claimed he has returned patients' gray hair back to normal with PABA. Dr. Carlton Fredericks has used a combination of PABA (100 mg), calcium pantothenate (30 mg), choline (2 grams), and B complex, plus a diet rich in B foods like liver, whole wheat, and brewer's yeast. He cautions it works in many people, but not all, and up to six months may be needed to restore the color.

Other people have found benefit from liver and iron injections, and from molybdenum.

Warning: If you dye your hair, be alert for lead poisoning. Many hair preparations contain lead, and doctors report many people with arthritis and even mental problems are actually suffering from lead poisoning from hair coloring. Their problems cleared up when they stopped using the coloring.

COSMETIC SURGERY—WHAT IT COULD DO FOR YOU

The techniques most often used to diminish signs of aging are these:

A face lift. Can tighten sagging skin of face and neck. Lifts and eliminates excess tissue. Can be used to remove double chins and turkey gobbler folds in the neck. Results usually last at least 5 years.

Blepharoplasty. Can remove wrinkles, bags, and bulges of the eyelids by removing fat and excess skin around the eyes.

Face peel and dermabrasion. Can reduce wrinkles, lines, tattoos, freckles, or acne scars.

Fibrin foam. Can be used to fill in depressions or deep lines.

Silicone injections. Can be used to fill in deep facial lines. Legal for use by only a few clinical investigators in major medical centers.

Hair transplants. Hair is taken from the back and sides of the head to the bald areas.

Electrolysis. Not expensive. Can be used to remove red lines from broken veins or remove warts and moles.

Body surgery. Can correct sagging breasts, droopy arm flesh, abdominal fat, and shape buttocks, hips, or thighs.

To check on a potential surgeon, write for his credentials to the American Board of Plastic Surgeons, 4647 Pershing Street, St. Louis, Mo. 62108.

FREE BOOKLETS
Plastic Surgery
American Academy of Facial Plastic and Reconstructive Surgery
2800 Lake Shore Drive, Suite 4008
Chicago, Ill. 60659

Aesthetic Surgery: What It Can and Cannot Do
American Medical Association
535 North Dearborn
Chicago, Ill. 60610

To see what a face lift would do for you, place your fingers high on your cheekbone in front of your ears. Pull lightly up and back on the skin to see how the excess skin is lifted around the cheek and jawline.

WHAT THOSE FABULOUS SPAS REALLY OFFER

Here's what it's really like inside the top glamour spas where the beautiful people go to relax and shape up.

THE GOLDEN DOOR

In the hills of Escondido, California, north of San Diego. $1250 per week.

Mostly for women, 10 weeks set aside for men. Limited to 24 guests at a time. Cuisine (800–1000 calories per day) prepared by a gourmet chef. You arrive in a gold limousine from the airport and walk through a Tunisian gold door to your room with marble birdbaths, crystal chandeliers, a dressing table full of free cosmetics, and a view of a courtyard garden. A maid unpacks your suitcase, brings you tea. The day begins at 6:45 A.M. with coffee, 500 milligrams of vitamin C, a pink sweatsuit, yellow terry-cloth robe and a two-mile walk. After breakfast: calisthenics, hot potassium broth, exercise on machines, a steambath, massage, exercise in a heated pool. After lunch: a finger and toe massage, manicure, pedicure, facial, hair treatment, a nap while wrapped in hot sheets and herbs. Then a dance class, lessons in makeup and skin care, water volleyball, yoga, and a walk to end the day. Alcohol is forbidden, and you can't smoke in public areas. The evening: a non-alcoholic cocktail time followed by a candlelight dinner.

LA COSTA

Also north of San Diego in southern California. $100 per day.

Co-ed. Accommodates 100 guests. Part of an 8,000-acre resort with a golf course, horseback riding, 25 tennis courts, several swimming pools, a movie theater, a gourmet restaurant. The program includes calisthenics, dancing, water exercises, yoga, facials, massages, a manicure and pedicure once a week, saunas, steambaths, herbal wraps, mineral whirlpool baths, medicinal waters, self-defense, isometrics, makeup, and hair styling. Evening entertainment includes movies, bridge, and cocktails. A physician gives diet lectures and makes up custom diets.

PALM-AIRE

At Pompano Beach, Florida. Midway between Palm Beach and Miami. $100 per day.

Twin facilities for men and women. Program includes water ballet, calisthenics, jogging, walking, deep breathing, belly dancing, gym, yoga, loofah scrub, body massage, facial massage, whirlpool, manicure, pedicure, and hair treatments. There are 5 golf courses, 19 tennis courts, 15 heated pools, arts and crafts, and an ocean beach for swimming. Evening entertainment includes dancing, films, lectures.

MURIETTA HOT SPRINGS

In Murietta, California. $240 for three days: $560 for one week.

Separate spas for men and women: children allowed in the summer. Tennis seminars in April and May. Golf, horseback riding, croquet, badminton, hot mineral baths, and mud baths available at all times. The program includes morning walks, exercise, gymnastics, tumbling, dance, gym equipment, facials, body massages, foot massages, salt wraps, yoga, whirlpool, water exercises. Evening includes dancing, bridge, a piano bar, and backgammon.

THE GREEN HOUSE

In Arlington, Texas, 12 miles east of Forth Worth. $1200 per week.

Accommodates 35 guests in Southern style luxury. Rooms have sunken tubs and canopy beds. You get breakfast in bed each morning with fresh rose, crystal, fine china and silver. The day's schedule: wake-up and breathing exercises, body control exercises with music, sauna, massage, spot reducing, manicure, whirlpool. Lunch is by the heated marble pool with a latticed ceiling under a glass dome with buckets of fern and other greenery. The afternoon includes water exercise class, face and skin analysis. Evening: a sumptuous low-calorie dinner, followed by astrology lecture, fashion show, jewelry display, diet discussion, a wine expert, or a yogi.

MAINE CHANCE

Nestled in Camelback Mountain in Phoenix, Arizona. From $850 to $1050 per week.

Elizabeth Arden's health and beauty resort with turquoise pools, plush greenery, bright flowers, palm trees, fine paintings, beautiful china and linens, antique furniture, and marble floors. A personal maid brings you breakfast in bed and afternoon tea and honey. The program includes exercises to music, steam cabinet, sauna, wax bath, whirlpool, massage, water exercises, face and scalp treatments, hand and foot massages, makeup class. In the evenings there are movies, trips to the theater, backgammon, bridge. On the last day you get a shampoo, set, manicure, and pedicure. Women only.

THE ASHRAM

In a secluded area in Calabasas, California, about 30 miles from downtown Los Angeles. $500 per week.

Only six guests at a time. Women and men, but no children. The full schedule includes a 7:30 A.M. meditation period, breakfast, a morning hike, a break for juice and rest, an outdoor exercise class, water exercises in the pool, water volleyball. After lunch is sunbathing or a massage, an afternoon walk, jogging, calisthenics, yoga, more meditation. Evening program includes dinner, discussion periods on raw foods, self-analysis, getting in touch with nature.

THE RENAISSANCE SPA

On Providence Island near Nassau in the Bahamas. $2000 for 10 days.

This is a health-oriented center, specializing in revitalization therapies. The spa directors say the center is concerned with helping the mature person counteract stress and to overcome sleeplessness, fatigue, loss of vigor, impotence, frigidity, poor muscle and skin tone, problems of weight, anxiety, and premature aging. The plush spa in the clean balmy airs of the Bahamas features succulent local fish and lobster caught fresh from the seas and fruits and vegetables from a local organic farm. Director of the center is Dr. Ivan Popov, former physician to the royal family of Yugoslavia, who has brought to the Bahamas many European techniques of nutrition therapy and revitalization. The program includes megavitamin therapy, massages, biostimulated fertile eggs, diet counseling (including tests to determine what vitamins and minerals are needed), seawater sprays, seaweed therapy, mud therapy, a natural cosmetic program, low-voltage electrotherapy for insomnia, and exercise.

SOME SPECIAL PROBLEMS OF AGING AND WHAT TO DO ABOUT THEM

All of the following disorders can occur at other ages, but are particularly prevalent as people mature. Many people suffer needlessly from them because they don't realize these disorders are not natural and can be treated. Here are some of the more important innovative treatments.

(Also see Common Ailments and the Most Up-to-Date Ways to Treat Them, Chapter 20.)

STOMACH BALLS

When the fibrous parts of fruits and vegetables don't pass properly from the stomach to the intestine (especially occurs in people who have had stomach surgery), they can form a ball, producing stomach distress and even vomiting.

Drink *raw* (not canned) pineapple juice, say Janice Feffer, R.D., and Dr. Richard A. Norton, of Tufts-New England Medical Center. Pineapple juice that has never been heated contains an enzyme that can break up the ball.

POLYPS OF THE LARGE BOWEL

Polyps are wart-like growths on the large intestine. The major symptom is rectal bleeding.

Polyps can be removed in the doctor's office or in a hospital. They could in the future become cancerous so they should be removed.

EXCESS SALIVA

The person may have to swallow constantly, or may even drool from the sides of the mouth or become nauseated. Your doctor can give you a belladonna-type medicine, to decrease salivation.

GAGGING AND CHOKING

Older people often have difficulty in swallowing so should chew foods thoroughly and avoid large bites.

They also tend to have too little gastric juice and stomach acid so should eat less at one time. Hydrochloric acid-digestive enzyme tablets are often helpful.

MORE FREQUENT URINATION

This may be caused by weakness of muscles and ligaments, or in men may be due to prostate enlargement.

Drink no fluids after dinner. Especially avoid alcohol, tea, and coffee in the evening.

Cut down on sharp, salty, and spicy foods.

If you need to take a diuretic medicine, take it in the morning and early afternoon, not in the evening.

If you need to take a belladonna medicine, take it in the evening since it will cut down the desire to urinate.

See your doctor to find the cause of your increased urination. It may be due to a kidney or bladder infection or other disorder.

PHLEBITIS

This is inflammation of a vein. It is dangerous because a piece of clotted blood can form, break off, and travel to the heart, brain, or lungs to cause heart attack, stroke, or lung embolism.

Prevent phlebitis by exercising regularly even if you are bedridden and have to do special in-bed exercises. (See Chapter 6).

If you have varicose veins, have them treated since they are particularly prone to phlebitis.

Don't wear constricting garters.

Seek early treatment for any infection of the legs or feet.

HEMORRHOIDS (PILES)

These are dilated varicose veins in the anus and rectum. They may be outside the anus or up inside. Symptoms of hemorrhoids are grape-size lumps on the outside of the rectum after a bowel movement, sometimes pain, bleeding, or a mixture of bleeding and mucus discharge.

Prevent hemorrhoids by trying to move the bowels regularly each day, by not spending more than 15 minutes in attempting to have a bowel movement, and by eating fresh fruits, vegetables, and whole bran products. (Remember, excessive straining can cause not only hemorrhoids, but also stroke and heart attack.)

See your doctor because they may sometimes be caused by something serious such as a tumor in the bowel, cirrhosis of the liver, or an infection.

Treatment may be by simple surgery, injections, or by banding with special rubber bands; or by keeping the stool soft, avoiding alcohol and spices, taking sitz baths, and applying ointments. Taking 50–150 mg of vitamin B_6 has been reported to clear up hemorrhoids in about a week.

TEARING

The lower eyelid may adhere less snugly than before, permitting tears to run out onto the cheeks. Or a tear duct may become clogged, causing tears to collect and spill over.

See an ophthalmologist. He can do simple surgery under local anesthesia to correct the eyelid, or probe the tear duct to open it up.

(Sometimes the edge of the eyelid turns inward, constantly scratching the eyeball with the eyelashes. This can also be corrected by simple surgery.)

EMPHYSEMA

A lung condition from loss of elasticity of lung tissue and overstretching; often follows years of bronchitis or asthma. Symptoms are shortness of breath, barrel chest, coughing, blue fingertips and lips. But sometimes there are no symptoms.

Prevent emphysema by eliminating early all the things that can cause development of bronchitis and asthma, and treat these respiratory ailments vigorously if you have them.

The chief treatment is avoiding respiratory infections.

NUMBNESS AND TINGLING IN HANDS AND FEET

Can be caused by diabetes, anemia, or an aftermath of a severe or prolonged illness, as a side effect from drugs, vitamin deficiency, alcoholism, or pressure on nerves from arthritis, a tumor, or other cause.

PROSTATE PROBLEMS

Symptoms of inflammation of the prostate are pain in the back or perineum, fever, blood or pus in the urine, frequent and sometimes burning urination.

Drink large quantities of fluids.

Avoid alcohol and highly seasoned foods.

See your doctor for antibiotics.

Take frequent hot baths.

If the prostate trouble advances to chronic inflammation and enlargement, there may also be a loss of sexual potency or premature ejaculation, decrease in the force and the amount of the urinary stream, dribbling of urine, difficulty in starting to pass urine, the need to get up several times during the night to urinate.

See your doctor. Because prostate enlargement interferes with the proper passage of urine and so can cause infections and kidney problems, it is essential that the problem be solved. (Stones can also form in the prostate and cause obstruction of urine.)

For an enlarged prostate, a physician should periodically massage the gland. It is not difficult to

do, and you can have him teach your wife to do it if you wish to cut down office visits.

Surgery may be necessary to remove the enlarged portion of the gland or the entire gland.

Every adult male, especially over age 60, should have a rectal examination at least once a year.

Note: There have been reports that vitamin F helps a high percentage of prostate cases. Vitamin F complex includes linoelic, linolenic, and arachidonic acids. You can also obtain these substances by taking lecithin. After three days, the dose was dropped to four tablets daily; after several weeks a maintenance dose of two tablets a day was established.

Several foreign studies have indicated that eating pumpkin seeds helps prevent prostate problems. The seeds have a beneficial hormone, the researchers believe. Others indicate that 15–150 mg of zinc per day is helpful.

SCIATICA

This severe pain courses along the sciatic nerve to the lower back and legs. Symptoms: pain is aggravated when you twist the body; is worse when sitting; is sometimes relieved by standing up or lying flat. Causes: pressure on the sciatic nerve by a tumor or from a herniated spinal disk, an injury such as spraining your sacroiliac, an infection.

The pain will often disappear by itself in a few weeks or months, but can be speeded up by bed rest (lie on your back with a pillow under lower back and under the knees; use a firm mattress). A hot bath or heating pad will occasionally give temporary relief.

See your doctor for pain-relieving drug and a muscle relaxant drug.

Injections of novocaine or other drug to block nerve may be given.

Vitamins may be given orally or by injection.

Traction may be necessary (stretching the leg by attaching weights).

POLYCYTHEMIA

In this progressive condition there are more and more red blood cells, so blood volume increases and blood thickens. Symptoms: Sometimes the skin is a reddish-purple; the person may have headache, dizziness, vague aches and pains. Cause is unknown.

Bloodletting will reduce blood volume and relieve symptoms.

Radioactive phosphorus and other chemical agents are helpful.

RECTAL ITCHING

Itching of the skin in the rectal and anal area is common in older people because their skin in this area tends to be thin, sensitive, and dry. The itching can also be caused by fungus infection, emotional disturbance, diabetes, allergy, excessive alcohol, highly seasoned foods, hemorrhoids, or excessive perspiration.

Avoid tight synthetic or heavy undergarments, and do not become overwarm while sleeping. Dust talcum powder on the area to reduce perspiration. Take warm baths and apply witch hazel. Try to stop scratching and do not use strong soaps.

Stop smoking. (Improves circulation.) Wash, rinse, dry and apply wheat germ oil several times a day.

See your doctor for helpful ointment or antihistamine tablets, and to determine the underlying cause.

WINNING THE FIGHT TO CONTROL PAIN

For local pain: Ice bags are helpful in relieving pain caused by injury and bruising. An ice cube held directly on a burn will stop the pain and usually prevent blistering.

For deep pain: Hot water bags, heating pads, and heat lamps are helpful. Be sure to guard against burning.

For bursitis: An injection of novocaine is often helpful, sometimes completely eliminating the pain with one shot.

For muscle pain: Muscle relaxant drugs often help.

In terminal cancer patients: Severe pain that will no longer respond to narcotics can sometimes be eliminated by a new technique of injecting alcohol or phenol into the spinal canal at the appropriate place. Sometimes surgery is used to cut nerve pathways and relieve pain. The controversial drug laetrile is also reported extensively to relieve cancer pain.

A NEW PAINKILLER

A new drug, nalbuphine, has been reported to be as effective as morphine, but not addictive. It should be available soon.

ELECTRONIC PAIN CONTROL

Dr. John E. Adams, neurosurgeon of San Francisco, and Dr. Donald E. Richardson, of New Orleans, are treating patients with severe chronic intractable pain by implanting electrostimulators in the brain that can act as a switching point to switch off pain impulses. Pain relief occurs in 50 to 75 percent of patients, depending on original cause of pain.

TWO NEW TREATMENTS FOR "INCURABLE" TIC DOULOUREUX

This severe facial pain is now being successfully treated by two different new surgical procedures. One technique is to use heat-controlled electrodes to delicately and precisely coagulate certain fibers of a particular cluster of nerve cells called the gasserian ganglion. The other technique, developed by Dr. Peter J. Jannetta, of the University of Pittsburgh, is to relieve vascular pressure causing irritation of the facial nerve cells by actually relocating the guilty blood vessels.

A NEW TECHNIQUE WITH ACUPUNCTURE

Dr. Ronald Dougherty of Syracuse, N.Y., has treated patients with standard acupuncture combined with a technique called transcutaneous nerve stimulation (TNS) produced by mild electrical stimulation of the skin at the traditional acupuncture sites. Of 100 patients (with bursitis, arthritis, migraine, low-back pain, or other chronic pain) 88 percent had relief of pain, Dr. Dougherty reports. Previously they had been severely addicted to drugs because of the severity of their pain. The acupuncture treatment was given on an outpatient basis once a week at Crouse-Irving Memorial Hospital in Syracuse. Patients were given TNS units to use at home for up to four hours a day.

SOME OF THE MAJOR PAIN CLINICS IN THE U.S.

If you have serious, long-lasting pain that cannot be helped by ordinary medical measures, there are a number of pain centers that have just recently been established in a number of medical centers to deal with this problem. Some techniques include neurosurgery, electrical stimulation, hypnosis, nerve blocks, biofeedback, muscle relaxation training, spinal injections, dietary instruction, acupuncture, psychotherapy, physical therapy, drug withdrawal.

Some treatments are done while you're in the hospital, others are given on an outpatient basis. Nearly all of the centers require that you be referred to them through your physician.

SOME PLACES TO GO:
Pain Center
     City of Hope National Medical Center
     1500 East Duarte Road.
     Duarte, Calif. 91010
Pain Treatment Center
     Hospital of Scripps Clinic
     La Jolla, Calif. 92037
UCLA Pain Management Clinic
     UCLA School of Medicine
     10833 Le Conte Avenue
     Los Angeles, Calif. 90024
Pain Center
     Mount Zion Hospital and Medical Center
     1600 Divisadero Street
     San Francisco, Calif. 94115
Portland Pain Rehabilitation Center
     Emanuel Hospital
     3001 North Gantenbein Avenue
     Portland, Ore. 97227
Pain Clinic
     University of Washington School of Medicine
     Seattle, Wash. 98195
Pain Center
     Rush Medical College
     Rush-Presbyterian-St. Luke's Medical Center
     1725 Harrison Street
     Chicago, Ill. 60612
Pain Clinic
     University of Illinois College of Medicine
     840 South Wood Street
     Chicago, Ill. 60612
Pain Clinic
     Mayo Clinic
     Rochester, Minn. 55901
Pain Management Center
     Mayo Clinic-St. Mary's Hospital of Rochester
     Rochester, Minn. 55901
Pain Unit
     Massachusetts Rehabilitation Hospital
     125 Nashua Street
     Boston, Mass. 02114
Pain Consultation Center
     Mount Sinai Medical Center
     4300 Alton Road
     Miami Beach, Fla. 33140
Pain Clinic
     Johns Hopkins University School of Medicine
     Baltimore, Md. 21205
Nerve Block and Pain Studies Clinic
     University of Virginia Medical Center
     Charlottesville, Va. 22903

Warning: If chordotomy is performed (cutting of certain nerve fibers in the spinal cord) to eliminate pain, almost 100 percent of patients are left with total or near-total sexual impotence.

IF YOU BECOME DISABLED

Whether the cause of disability is stroke, arthritis, multiple sclerosis, or another problem, there are people and institutions to help. Get help immediately. Your rehabilitation should start the minute your vital signs—pulse, respiration, and blood pressure—are normal.

SOME AIDS YOU MAY NOT HAVE HEARD ABOUT

An electric wheelchair.

A myoelectric arm. You attach it to the stump of an amputated arm, and you can move the fingers by contracting remaining muscles.

A still experimental device is a computer-typewriter you operate by sipping and puffing on a straw.

Check with a local rehabilitation center for these and other aids.

HELPFUL RESOURCES

Accent on Living
     Box 700
     Bloomington, Ill. 61701
     Magazine for people with disabilities
Free catalogues of patient-lifting devices
     Ted Hoyer & Co., Inc.
     2222 Minnesota Street
     Oshkosh, Wis. 54901
Free brochure on automobile hand-control devices
     Wells-Engberg Co.
     P. O. Box 6388
     Rockford, Ill. 61125
The Wheelchair Traveler
     Ball Hill Road
     Milford, N.H. 03055
     $3.55
     Lists hotels, motels, restaurants, and sightseeing attractions for the handicapped traveler
Free catalogue of wheelchairs, walkers, hospital beds
     Sears, Rocbuck & Co.
     Sears Tower
     Chicago, Ill. 60684
Free catalogue of patient aids, wheelchairs, walkers
     Everest & Jennings
     1803 Pontius Avenue
     Los Angeles, Calif. 90025
Free catalogue of aides, easy-on clothing
     Fashion Able
     Rocky Hill, N.J. 08553

WHERE TO OBTAIN NURSING CARE FOR A CHRONICALLY ILL OLDER PERSON

Check the following kinds of agencies:

- The local old-age-assistance bureau
- The social service department of a large nearby hospital

- The community visiting-nurse association
- Public-health nursing agencies
- Church, fraternal, and social organizations
- The department of welfare or department of social welfare
- Nurses' registries, either private or associated with nearby hospitals
- The county medical society

FINDING THE RIGHT NURSING HOME AT A PRICE YOU CAN AFFORD

LOOK AND COMPARE

The only way you can find a home that you like and can afford is to get out and look. Check local chapters of the American Nursing Home Association or the American Association of Homes for the Aging or write the American Nursing Home Association, 1025 Connecticut Avenue, N.W., Washington, D.C. 20036. Ask friends, doctors, nurses, medical society, church, and social agencies to recommend homes that they think are good. Call for literature and rates, and visit to compare facilities and costs. After you have narrowed your list to one or two, go back a second time *unannounced* and wander around to see how patients are treated. Check the kitchen, the grounds. How well kept up are things? How friendly is it?

CAN YOU AFFORD IT?

Many church, fraternity, and professional groups have nursing homes for their members at low cost. It may also keep a person from feeling like a complete stranger in new surroundings.

Some homes have lower fees for those who do not need constant care. For a bedridden patient, a flat rate may be most economical. For the ambulatory person, a home with varying fees for gradation of care could be better.

Many homes require the person to turn over a major part of his savings and Social Security. In return the home agrees to care for him for the rest of his days.

Sometimes costs will be paid by the public assistance program of the county or city welfare department.

FIND OUT WHAT YOU GET FOR WHAT YOU PAY

Some nursing homes add on fees for food, medicines, and doctors' visits. Get a written list of what specifically is covered.

LOOK FOR THE HOME'S LICENSE

Usually the state license will be posted in the office. If there is no license, ask the administrator why. If some standards are not met, you should know what they are and whether they are important to you. Government inspectors are supposed to check nursing homes for certain standards. Ask the administrator to show you a report.

CHECK YOUR MEDICARE OR OTHER INSURANCE

Not all insurance policies cover nursing homes. Check the fine print: sometimes the only way you can collect insurance payments is to spend several days in a hospital before you go to a nursing home. A veteran may have VA nursing home benefits.

MAKE SURE THE NURSING HOME IS CONVENIENT TO GET TO

Can you visit by public transportation or car? How much will it cost to travel back and forth? If convenient, more friends and relatives will visit.

EIGHTEEN QUESTIONS TO ASK WHEN YOU VISIT HOMES

The American Medical Association recommends that you ask the following questions:

1. What type of patient does the nursing home accept?
2. Is the home licensed by the state or local licensing agency?
3. Does the institution require a physical examination and a physician's summary of any needed treatment?
4. Is each patient's medical record kept on file so that prescribed treatments can be followed accurately?
5. Are there staff physicians who actually spend time in the nursing home with the patients and nursing home staff?
6. Does the nursing home report periodically on the patient's condition to his personal physician?
7. What level of nursing supervision is provided? What is the total number of nursing staff?
8. What provision does the home have for dental care of patients?
9. Are facilities and staff available for patient rehabilitation?
10. Are the facilities fireproof, in good repair, designed with fire escapes and adequate ramps for quick evacuation?
11. Are there rails in the hallways, grip bars in

bathtubs and next to toilets, and nonskid material on floors?

12. Are the kitchen and cooking area clean, with proper and adequate refrigeration, dishwashing, and garbage disposal facilities?

13. Does the nursing home prepare therapeutic diets when needed?

14. Is the general atmosphere home-like? Are floors clean? Landscaping attractive? Space sufficient for each patient?

15. What is the attitude of the staff and patients?

16. Are adequate recreational services available?

17. Can a patient bring his personal belongings and some of his furniture (a favorite rocker, for instance) to the nursing home?

18. Are there extra charges for drugs, special diets, extra nursing care, tray service, laundry, shampoos, haircuts, shaving, and the like?

DO YOU REALLY NEED A NURSING HOME?

A recent survey in one state showed that 80 percent of the patients in nursing homes were simply old patients with minor ailments who needed nothing more than pills and proper diet, not nursing care. If a member of your family is capable of independent living, then consider an apartment shared with someone the same age, or investigate communities designed for senior citizens. Consider having a parent live near you in a studio apartment so you can give help and companionship when needed, yet maintain privacy.

CONSIDER A VISITING NURSE

A need for occasional nursing may be filled by a visiting nurse on a daily or weekly basis. Contact a Visiting Nurse Association.

USE MEALS-ON-WHEELS AND OTHER FOOD SERVICES

Many older people do not eat well if they live alone. Meals-on-Wheels services deliver food to the home, or a senior citizens community center may have a dining hall where people can eat together.

PROPRIETARY HOME—RESIDENCE

These Senior Citizens' hotels or homes are for persons in their 70s, 80s, or 90s who are in good health but no longer wish to take on household responsibilities. The proprietary home or resident hotel offers food, shelter, cleaning services, and recreational facilities.

FOSTER HOME CARE

For the person who does not want an institutionlike setting, but no longer wants to manage his own household, being part of a foster family can be the answer. Private and public social service agencies supervise foster home placements with approved families and make the necessary financial arrangements.

CONVALESCENT HOMES

After a serious illness or surgery a period of recuperation can be had in a convalescent home. Operated by hospitals, religious institutions, or community agencies, the convalescent home is staffed by nurses and physicians who help the patient to recovery. Length of stay can vary from 2 to 6 weeks, depending on the patient's progress.

HEARTLINE

A service for senior citizens to answer questions and solve problems. Send your questions with a stamped self-addressed envelope to Heartline, 114 East Dayton Street, West Alexandria, Ohio 45381.

14

What You Should Know About Your Vision

Hold this at arm's length. Does it appear blurred? Even if you can read it clearly, don't jump to any conclusions. There's far more to good vision than reading the fine print. There's the big wide world around you. Only an optometrist or an ophthalmologist can make sure you're seeing it all as well as you should.

HOW TO MAKE YOUR EYEGLASSES LAST LONGER

Wash them with soap and warm water. Dry with tissue.

Have them adjusted periodically by your optician.

Never put them lens down. They can become scratched.

Keep them in a case when not in use, and put your name and phone number on the case.

ALWAYS LOSING CONTACT LENSES?

You can replace lost or damaged contact lenses by phone. Call prescription to Contact Lens Ser-

vice 1-800-848-7573. The cost is $40 per pair of hard lenses, $100 for Soflens.

VISION AND SPECIAL SITUATIONS

Golf. You can order special eyeglasses that have one correction for addressing the ball, another correction for watching where the ball goes.

Trap Shooting. You can order special glasses for seeing the gun sights and for seeing the target.

Contact Sports. Buy lenses and frames designed to take hard blows. Consider contact lenses.

Television. If children insist on sitting close to the set, it may mean they are nearsighted. Have their eyes examined. Have a soft light on in the room; avoid glare or reflection on the screen. Don't wear reading glasses for watching TV. If you are over 50 and have trouble seeing TV, you may want to get special glasses with a correction for the television distance. If you experience discomfort or your eyes water when you watch television, get a checkup.

Bifocals. Necessary when a single lens prescription is not satisfactory for seeing both far and near, generally after age 40. A bifocal lens has two parts—generally, the lower is for seeing near objects clearly, and the upper is for distance viewing.

Trifocals have an extra section for seeing at about arm's length, or a reading segment can be both at the top and bottom of a lens with the middle area focused for long distance.

Tips on wearing bifocals or trifocals: don't look down at feet when walking; hold reading material a little closer to body and lower your eyes (not your chin). Eyes must be aimed through the segment of the lens designed for your seeing job. Move the newspaper, instead of your head, until you can see the newspaper clearly.

IF YOU ARE EXPOSED TO UNUSUAL EYE HAZARDS

You should wear safety goggles or some kind of protective eye shield if you are exposed to flying metal objects, molten metal splash, welding arc, gases, vapors and fumes, dusts, and similar hazards. When maximum protection is needed, safety eyewear of industrial quality is a "must." It should fit properly and be inspected frequently.

NEW DEVELOPMENTS IN CONTACT LENSES

SOFT LENSES

These lenses are made of a very pliable substance for ease in wearing, and are almost impossible to dislodge; however, they are slightly more difficult to take care of and do not correct vision quite as well as the standard hard contact lens.

THE WET LENS

Old or new hard contact lenses can be treated with a special chemical that makes the lens attract water, thus floating it more freely on the tear layer of the eye, improving clarity and making lenses much easier to wear for longer times.

BIFOCALS

Bifocal contacts are ground for both far- and nearsightedness, with the part for close vision ground in the bottom of the lens, much as regular glasses are, but the line of division is not noticeable. Instead of being completely circular, one new bifocal design is straight on the bottom with the straight edge lightly resting on the lower lid of the eye.

NEW CONTACT LENS CLEANER

Bausch and Lomb has a new cleaner for Soflens made from an enzyme. It rids lenses of protein deposits that build up and cause cloudiness and discomfort. Use weekly or so to improve visual acuity and prolong life of lenses.

ORTHOKERATOLOGY—USING CONTACT LENSES TO GET YOUR EYES BACK TO NORMAL AGAIN

Contact lens specialists now are using contact lenses to actually change the shape of the cornea. Since it is the shape of the eye that usually causes poor vision, they use the contact lens to correct the shape to normal again.

The technique is to use a lens that is a little flat, which then flattens the eyeball a little. As the eye changes, the lenses are changed, little by little altering the eye back to its ideal shape. In many cases visual acuity can be brought back to 20/20. Or in some cases, people who are almost blind can be made to see again.

Doctors using Ortho-K say it's similar to orthodontics, which gradually moves teeth with braces.

On the average the treatment takes about two years and includes five changes of lenses. Some doctors have their patients wear "retainer" lenses a few hours a day to maintain the changed shape; others find the retainer lenses are not always necessary.

About 10,000 people have been treated this way so far.

For more information and the name of an optometrist in your area who practices the specialty, write the International Society of Orthokeratology, 6505 Alvarado Road, San Diego, Calif. 92120.

VISION PROBLEMS OF CHILDREN

It is estimated that 80 percent of learning during the first 12 years of life is through seeing. This is the critical period. Parents should watch carefully for these warning symptoms:

- Tilting the head to one side, frowning, squinting
- Placing the head close to a book or desk when reading or writing
- Difficulty in reading, or skipping words
- Excessive blinking or frequent rubbing of the eyes
- Frequent headaches or nausea
- Daydreaming

- Not being able to see what is on the blackboard
- Eyes inflamed, watery, or crossed
- Pupils of unequal size
- Eyelids red-rimmed, encrusted, or swollen

VISION OF BABIES

Warning of visual problems in a baby are inability to pick up small objects, missing toys when reaching for them, or bumping or stumbling over objects that should be seen easily.

As your child gets older, play visual games. Ask him if he can see something that you can see. Make sure one eye is not wandering from the other.

IS YOUR CHILD HAVING TROUBLE IN SCHOOL?

Perhaps a professional eye examination and hearing test might discover something you didn't know about your child. Watch for the signs that could indicate a vision problem.

Warning: Poor vision will not always make itself known. The child may show the signs we mentioned, but may not. He often compensates by using only the good eye. He functions normally, but the defective eye, through lack of use, gets progressively worse.

See test for amblyopia in Chapter 24.

Both teachers and parents should also be aware of the limitations of the famous Snellen eye chart. A child may score 20/20 on the school chart and still not have good vision for reading. Even the most comprehensive screening test will not detect all vision problems.

School eye examinations often come too late. All children should have professional eye examinations at birth and again between the ages of 3 and 4.

VISION PROBLEMS AS YOU GET OLDER

LOW VISION READING

If you have difficulty reading even with glasses, try special magnifying hand lenses or light-beam devices that can brighten the printed word. Also available are large-type printed materials and recorded literature.

SENIOR CITIZEN DRIVERS

The eyes' focusing ability is no longer as flexible as in youth and it becomes harder to switch from near to far objects. Side vision and sharpness of vision also tend to diminish with age. Traffic signals may appear less bright. Senior citizens with diminished vision should avoid driving at dusk or at night.

IF NIGHT VISION IS BELOW NORMAL

It can be improved by increasing intake of vitamin A. Check whether you can see the dividing white lines at night on the road when there is oncoming traffic.

FOR TIRED EYES

Try cotton pads dipped in witch hazel placed on your closed eyelids while you lie down.

THINGS THAT CAN GO WRONG WITH YOUR EYES

One out of every two people in the United States has refractive error in the eye. This means that the light rays entering the eye are bent too much or not enough, so that no clear image is formed on the retina of the eye. Three main types of refractive errors are:

1. Nearsightedness (Myopia). A person's eyeball is too long and the image in focus falls in front of the retina.

2. Farsightedness (Hyperopia). The eyeball is too short and the image falls behind it.

3. Distorted and Blurred Vision (Astigmatism). The cornea has an imperfect curvature.

AMBLYOPIA

Sometimes called "lazy eye." The vision is dim in one eye. The child tends to suppress the weaker eye and use only the stronger one, and the vision in the weaker eye is gradually lost. Correction of amblyopia traditionally consists of placing a patch on the good eye, forcing the child to use the amblyopic eye.

UVEITIS

Inflammation of the iris or other parts of the eye. Symptoms may range from a mildly red eye to severe pain and blurred vision. The condition can lead to cataract or glaucoma. It can usually be controlled by drugs.

CORNEAL DISEASE

The cornea, the transparent membrane at the front of the eye, can be affected by bacteria, fungus, and virus infections, injury, allergic reaction, nerve impairment, improper moistening and covering by the eyelids, and degenerative disorders.

Corneal infections or injuries must be treated promptly, or the cornea may become scarred or opaque, resulting in impaired vision or blindness. In such cases, corneal transplant may be able to restore sight.

RETINITIS PIGMENTOSA

Retinitis pigmentosa is an inherited disease that usually produces night blindness in children or adolescents, then later cuts down on the amount of side vision even in the light, resulting in "tunnel vision."

Sometimes the disease progresses to complete blindness. But many patients keep their reading vision throughout their lives, although it may be restricted to a small central part of the visual field. (The symptom of night blindness does *not* necessarily indicate retinitis pigmentosa.)

RETINAL DETACHMENT

Retinal detachment is a separation of the inner layer of the retina from its outer layer. The detachment can cause permanent impairment of vision. It occurs most often when a tear or hole develops in the retina from an infection, blood vessel disturbance, tumor, or injury. It has been described as a curtain being drawn across the eyes. You may also see soot-like spots or light flashes.

If retinal detachment is diagnosed in its early stages, it is often possible to re-attach the retina surgically and restore vision. If untreated, the detachment often becomes complete, and results in permanent blindness.

DIABETIC RETINOPATHY

Diabetic retinopathy is a disorder of the blood vessels in the retina stemming from diabetes. Visual impairment can result from swelling of the retina from leaky blood vessels, formation of scar tissue, and detachment of the retina. The occurrence of retinopathy is generally related to the duration and severity of the diabetes. Treatment is by laser beams to seal off the abnormal vessels or by vitrectomy (surgical removal of the vitreous).

MACULAR DEGENERATION

In many cases of degeneration of the retina only a small area of the retina called the macula is involved. The macula, in the center of the retina, is responsible for fine detail or reading vision. Damage to the macula usually results in a gradual loss of central vision. Persons 60 years of age and older are those most frequently affected by macular degeneration.

CROSS-EYES

An eye pointing in or out is caused by incorrect development of the eye muscles. It will not correct itself. A doctor should be seen for exercises or special glasses as early as age 9 months.

An operation to correct the muscular imbalance can be done at 3 to 4 years of age.

CATARACTS

A cataract is not a film that grows over the eye, but is a cloudiness of the lens itself that impairs vision. Some cataracts become progressively worse; some are stationary and never need treatment. Symptoms are: blurring of vision; or an object appears as though a chunk were missing; or there is a large black spot always in front of the eye; or lights appear double.

See a doctor. About 98 percent of cataracts can be cured by surgery.

An underground medicine: A compound called Orgotein has been successful in treating cataracts and other problems in animals, but is not approved for humans yet.

GLAUCOMA

In glaucoma, there is increased pressure within the eye that eventually may crush the optic nerve. Usually the pressure and the damage build gradually, but sometimes acute glaucoma occurs, and the person must have surgery within 48 hours to prevent blindness from strangled eye nerves.

Symptoms are: headaches or eye aches; fuzzy or blurred vision that comes and goes; watering of the eyes; poor vision in dim light; change in eye color; seeing rainbow halos around lights, and loss of side vision. If you have any of these symptoms, see a doctor to have a tonometer test (for eye pressure) and an eye examination.

In some people glaucoma can be controlled by medication to reduce pressure; others need surgery to improve the eye's drainage system and reduce pressure. Untreated, there will be loss of vision.

Pilocarpine, the usual drug used to reduce the dangerous pressure in the eye, can now be applied in a new way as a thin oval wafer that is placed inside the lower eyelid to give a steady week's supply without the four-times-a-day eyedrops that most glaucoma patients need.

Underground medicine: Marijuana has been shown capable of reducing eye pressure, but is seldom used.

CENTERS SPECIALIZING IN TREATMENT OF EYE PROBLEMS

Bascom Palmer Eye Institute
    University of Miami School of Medicine
    P.O. Box 875
    Biscayne Annex, Miami, Fla. 33152
Jules Stein Eye Institute
    Los Angeles, Calif. 90024
Lakeside Hospital
    2065 Adelbert Road
    Cleveland, Ohio 44106
Manhattan Eye & Ear Hospital
    210 East 64th Street
    New York, N.Y. 10021
Massachusetts Eye and Ear Infirmary
    243 Charles Street
    Boston, Mass. 02114

Scheie Eye Institute
    51 North 39th Street
    Philadelphia, Pa. 19104
University of Washington Hospital
    Seattle, Wash. 98195

FREE AT-HOME EYE TEST

The National Society for the Prevention of Blindness has prepared a free *Eye Test for Preschoolers* that you can use to test your child's eyesight at home. Write the National Society for the Prevention of Blindness, 79 Madison Avenue, New York, N.Y. 10016.

FREE BOOKLET
Sunglasses and Your Eyes
    Bausch and Lomb
    Rochester, N.Y. 14602

CHAPTER 15

The Things You Need to Know About Your Teeth

WHEN SHOULD TOOTH CARE BEGIN?

As soon as a baby cuts his first tooth. Pediatric dentists urge parents to wipe a baby's teeth daily with a soft cloth, tissue, or cotton until he is old enough to brush his own. Don't give him sweetened liquids or foods.

Let the child start trying to brush his own teeth whenever he wants to try, usually at about age 2.

A child should make his first trip to a dentist at age 3 or 4.

TOOTH CARE KIT

A dentist selected this collection of products for parents of babies and young children. The kit includes a small, soft-bristled brush, teething gauze, disclosing tablets, floss, a flossing device, toothpaste, and a brochure describing how to care for the teeth of babies and very young children.

Available from:
Babydontics P.O. Box 72
Fresh Meadows, N.Y. 11365
$2.00 + 25¢ postage.

HOW TO KEEP YOUR TEETH FOREVER

Choose a dentist who emphasizes preventive dentistry rather than just reparative dentistry. He should try to save teeth instead of proposing quick extractions.

Have regular dental checkups.

If you have a dental school in your area, go to their clinic. Many dental schools have free or low-cost clinics to give their students clinical practice; experts supervise.

Use disclosing dye. This dye stains plaque sticking to your teeth so you can see where to clean more vigorously.

Learn how to use dental floss. It is almost as important as brushing the teeth.

Stop eating sugar and refined carbohydrates, which encourage tooth decay.

If you notice bleeding of the gums, persistent bad breath, loose or flabby gums, or looseness or drifting of the teeth, consult your dentist immediately. These are signs of periodontal disease. If it continues, bony support may be lost and teeth become loose, and perhaps will have to be extracted.

Consider taking extra calcium. A deficiency of calcium in the diet is responsible for much periodontal disease. The dietary intake of calcium should be about 1100 mg per day minimum for the average adult. Most do not come near that. Take magnesium also.

THE MAJOR TOOTH KILLER—PERIODONTAL DISEASE

It starts as an inflammation of the gums (gingivitis); then bleeding and swelling occur; the gums pull away from the teeth, making pockets where germs and food particles collect; pus forms, the gums ulcerate; then the bone itself is attacked and destroyed. Without treatment, the teeth loosen and eventually come out.

THE SEVEN WARNING SIGNS OF GUM DISEASE

- Bleeding gums when you clean your teeth
- Bad breath
- Soft, swollen, or tender gums
- Pus from the gum line when you press
- Loose teeth
- Gums shrinking away from the teeth
- Any change in the way the teeth come together

WHAT TO DO TO PREVENT IT

- Brush your teeth properly and regularly
- Use dental floss
- Have your teeth cleaned professionally every 4 to 6 months
- Have periodic dental x-rays to detect damage
- If necessary, have surgery to eliminate pockets between teeth and gums

PERIODONTAL TOOLS

For special equipment for cleaning hard-to-get plaque near the gumline, see your druggist, or write to Mays Drugstore, 48 West 48th Street, New York, N.Y. 10036.

DENTAL NEWS THAT YOU CAN USE

IF YOUR CHILD HAS A TOOTH KNOCKED OUT

The tooth should not be cleaned, but should be wrapped in a wet cloth or placed in water. The child—and the tooth—should be taken to the dentist immediately. In many cases the dentist can replace the tooth in the child's jaw, and it will in time re-attach to the jaw and function normally. Also see your dentist if a tooth has been loosened.

If a tooth has been fractured and broken off a little, the original shape can often be restored by binding on a plastic.

If you have lost a filling or have broken a tooth, put candlewax, beeswax, or paraffin on the jagged edges until you get to the dentist.

DON'T CHEW ON ICE

Cold is bad for your teeth. So is switching from hot to cold food or drink. The rapid temperature change can cause microscopic cracks in the surface of the teeth and cause the enamel to break or chip. Fillings can pull away from the tooth, or loosen.

TAKE VITAMIN C

Vitamin C aids healing. Research shows if you use a vitamin C program before and after having dental surgery, tissue healing will occur in about half the time.

WHAT TO DO FOR TEETH STAINED BY TETRACYCLINE

Permanent teeth in children are frequently stained yellow or brown from earlier use of this antibiotic. Your dentist can bleach the stains clear with hydrogen peroxide applied warm for 30 minutes about once a week for eight weeks. This should be done by a dentist, not as a home treatment, since a rubber dam is needed to protect the gums from the hot bleach.

WHAT TO DO FOR SENSITIVE TEETH

Pain from hot, cold, or touch can be helped by a toothpaste containing strontium chloride. One brand is Sensodyne. Also try applying Chloraseptic, an anesthetic mouthwash.

HOW TO STOP TOOTH-GRINDING

This new method has been described by Drs. Marvin P. Levin and William Ayer of Walter Reed Army Medical Center, Washington, D.C.: clench teeth together as hard as possible for 5 seconds, then relax jaw for 5 seconds. Repeat 5 times. Continue 6 times a day for two weeks.

CANKER SORES

Taking tablets of *Lactobacillus acidophilus*, available from your druggist without prescription, will often restore the natural environment of the mouth and eliminate canker sore pain.

It has also been found that people who tend to get frequent canker sores can often prevent them by regularly taking folic acid tablets and vitamin C *with bioflavonoids*.

REFERRED PAIN FROM YOUR TEETH

Pains in the head, the ears, and even the neck, arms, and shoulders can be due to grinding of the teeth. If you have such pains and no one can find the cause, ask that your bite be tested.

Typical symptoms of faulty bite; a clicking sound accompanied by grating noises in the jaw or severe pain or wagging of the jaw from side to side when the mouth is opened or closed.

A NEW SUGAR THAT IS SUPPOSED TO REDUCE CAVITIES

Called Xylitol, studies in Finland indicate it not only reduces new tooth decay, but even reverses old cavities. Studies to confirm are now being conducted by the National Institute of Dental Research. Biggest problem: it's expensive. For free sample and more information, write Xylitol Information Bureau, P.O. Box 80, Cresskill, N.Y. 07626.

Fructose also is less carcinogenic than sucrose.

NEW KIND OF DENTAL X-RAY

A new method has just been developed in which x-rays of teeth can be taken by placing a pencil-shaped x-ray source *inside* the mouth and the film *outside*. It can't be used for all x-rays, but when it is used it will eliminate the discomfort of large bite-down films hitting the gums under present methods. The new method should also reduce the amount of radiation. It uses a high-speed system with special Polaroid film.

CAVITIES MAY BE CONTAGIOUS

Dentists have discovered that tooth decay can be catching. When hamsters with cavities were put in with hamsters who had no cavities, the ones with perfect teeth soon had as many holes as the first group.

A VACCINE AGAINST TOOTH DECAY?

Scientists are working on it. Dr. Martin Taubman of Boston, one of those trying to develop such a vaccine, says tests have been successful in rats, hamsters, and monkeys. After being vaccinated against the chief germs that cause decay, the animals were fed cookies and candy but did not get cavities. Animals not vaccinated and similarly fed got many cavities.

Another new approach: Dr. William Bowen, formerly of London, now at the National Institute of Dental Research in Bethesda, Md., is working on a pill or mouthwash that would have the same effect as the injection form.

A plastic adhesive is also being developed that can be sprayed or painted on teeth and bonded with ultraviolet light to protect teeth.

BOOKLETS
A Shopper's Guide to Dentistry
    Herbert Denenberg
    Consumer Insurance
    873 National Press Building
    Washington, D.C. 20004
Taking the Pain Out of Finding a Good Dentist
    Health Research Group
    2000 P Street, N.W.
    Washington, D.C. 20036
    Contains a directory of Washington, D.C., dentists.

CHAPTER 16

How to Get Psychiatric Help

HOW TO TELL IF YOU NEED PSYCHIATRIC HELP

Here are questions to ask yourself that could indicate you need help:

Do you have bouts of uncontrollable anger?

Are you becoming suspicious of everyone, especially those near and dear to you?

Are you performing activities that are weird?

Are you frequently too tired or too keyed up to sleep, or even to think or function properly?

Are you thinking seriously of suicide, or of murder or of sexual assaults?

Are you so nervous you need to use a pill when facing meetings or decisions, or to get you through the day?

Do you feel as if you want to run away?

Are you so depressed you have no interest in your family or friends?

Do you have an uncontrollable compulsion to perform certain acts or rituals without knowing why?

Do you sometimes seriously wonder if you are losing your mind?

Are you becoming or already are addicted to alcohol or other drugs?

Do you notice a decrease in your mental functioning, loss of memory, inability to think clearly?

Have you had a sudden or pronounced change in personality or behavior?

Do you hear voices from the air or see strange things?

If you answered yes to any of these questions, for yourself or a member of your family, don't put off getting professional help.

A GUIDE TO FINDING THE RIGHT THERAPIST

Talk to your family doctor about your problem and have him recommend someone appropriate.

Talk to a counselor or read about different approaches to therapy, decide which one suits you best, then find a therapist who uses that approach.

Ask if your therapist uses nutrition therapy, drugs, or other techniques, whether he thinks this is right for your case. Decide whether *you* think his approach is right for you.

In the first few sessions when the therapist is evaluating your problem, you evaluate him and determine if you are comfortable with him and confident.

Form an informal written contract with him in which the two of you decide specific goals you want to accomplish; also include details of time and cost.

RECOMMENDED:
Through the Mental Health Maze
    Sallie Adams and Michael Orgel
    Health Research Group
    2000 P Street, N.W.
    Washington, D.C. 20036
    $2.50

A Guide to Mental Health Services
    University of Pittsburgh Press
    Boston Children's Service Assoc.
    1 Walnut Street
    Boston, Mass. 02108
    $2.95
How to Judge a Mental Hospital
    F. H. Kahan
    American Schizophrenia Foundation
    610 South Forest Avenue
    Ann Arbor, Mich. 48104
    50¢
A Consumers' Guide to Psychiatrists
    Health Research Group
    2000 P Street, N.W.
    Washington, D.C. 20036
    $2.50

KEEPING DOWN COSTS FOR PSYCHIATRIC HELP

OBTAIN TREATMENT OUTSIDE A HOSPITAL WHENEVER POSSIBLE

With new forms of treatment, not as many patients need to be treated in the hospital. You may be able to obtain adequate help in an outpatient clinic, partial hospitalization facility, community mental health center, nursing home, halfway house, other "transitional" facility, and in the offices of psychiatrists and clinical psychologists in private practice.

You can find a nearby center by checking the yellow pages, asking your doctor, or contacting the psychiatry department of your closest hospital.

CONSIDER PARTIAL HOSPITALIZATION

Many hospitals allow patients to come in just for days or just for nights. Some even have programs treating patients in the evening or the weekend. There are about 90 federal (mostly Veterans Administration) and 600 nonfederal hospitals that have partial hospitalization services.

INVESTIGATE ALTERNATIVE THERAPISTS

A psychiatrist is an M.D. who specializes in the treatment of mental illnesses. As a physician, he can prescribe drugs or other forms of treatment needed for a serious mental problem. But if you feel you basically need psychoanalysis or counseling, you can work through a psychologist who, like a psychiatrist, is licensed by the state, but cannot prescribe drugs.

In addition to psychiatrists and psychologists, there are other persons who may be able to help: your family doctor, your clergyman, a social worker in a hospital or at a social agency. Most schools and colleges have psychiatric and psychological services, free or minimal in cost.

If you use a marriage counselor be sure the counselor is a member of the American Association of Marriage Counselors. If a problem is so serious as to endanger your safety or the safety of your family, you can ask the police or local courts for referral for psychiatric counseling at low cost.

In group therapy, you discuss problems with a group of people under the supervision of a professionally trained person rather than having an individual session.

USE TELEPHONE COUNSELING SERVICE

In many cities you can now dial a hot line for psychiatric help, either for emergencies or for general counseling with any emotional problem. There are often special numbers for alcoholics or drug addicts to call.

A National Directory of Hot Lines and Switchboards is available from Youth Emergency Services, 1423 Washington Avenue, Minneapolis, Minn. 55404.

TAKE ADVANTAGE OF FREE OR LOW-COST SERVICES OF SOCIAL AGENCIES

For example, the Jewish Board of Guardians in New York has a residential school for disturbed and delinquent boys and girls, a residence club for older adolescent boys who require a protected living environment, a child guidance institute, a child development center, a day treatment center for delinquent adolescent boys referred by the courts, and a camp for emotionally disturbed children.

Other typical agencies include the following:

Addicts Anonymous, Box 2000, Lexington, Ky. 40501.
Gamblers Anonymous, Box 17173, Foy Station, Los Angeles, Calif. 90017.
Neurotics Anonymous, 248 East 33rd Street, New York, N.Y. 10016.
Recovery Inc., 116 South Michigan Avenue, Chicago, Ill. 60603.

Also check your church, various government agencies in your area, and other organizations listed in the directory in the back of the *Whole Health Catalogue*.

OBTAIN INSURANCE THAT COVERS MENTAL ILLNESS

More and more insurance policies are offering coverage of mental illness. See that yours does.

HELP FOR THE HYPERACTIVE CHILD

The typical hyperactive child won't sit still, won't pay attention, can't concentrate, is cruel and mean to other children, and is a show-off.

The biggest help is coming from a drug called Ritalin, actually an *energizer*. But paradoxically—and no one really knows why—it calms overactive children, sometimes in minutes, and frequently makes them calm, happy, cooperative, and able to concentrate in school.

Other doctors report that Ritalin and Dexedrine are especially beneficial in children with learning, vision perception, and visual-motor coordination problems.

When Ritalin or Dexedrine do not work, some doctors find Benedryl or the tranquilizer chlorpromazine effective. Other investigators are using magnesium pemoline and the antidepressant imipramine, with varying reports of success.

Dr. Magda Campbell, at New York University Medical School, is treating schizophrenic, hyperactive, and extremely withdrawn children with cytomel, with a high improvement rate.

Other investigators have found success in working with the children using behavior management, giving special treats for good behavior and depriving play activities or television for unacceptable behavior. Some centers work with the children in special classrooms. Others use videotapes or parent groups to train parents to use the behavior modification treatments at home.

Simple classroom measures that help are placing the child close to the teacher and away from distractions, and giving him one-to-one attention through teachers' aides whenever possible.

Investigators stress that the hyperactive child should be helped to understand the nature of his difficulties and how treatment is intended to help the child help himself. The treatment then should make more sense to him and he will hopefully see it as one of his tools, not something forced on him by others.

DIET FOR BEHAVIOR DISORDERS

Dr. Bernard Rimland, of the Institute for Child Behavior Research in San Diego, has used vitamins on children at his institute with much success. Each child daily took vitamin B_3, B_6, pantothenic acid, vitamin C, and sometimes dilantin. There was definite improvement in 45 percent of the children, including those with autism.

THE ALLERGIC TENSION-FATIGUE SYNDROME

Many children have symptoms of tension and irritability, or its apparent opposite: lack of concentration, fatigue, listlessness, and drowsiness. They are often diagnosed as having behavior problems when they are really allergic to foods, pollen, or pets. Determining the offending allergen and eliminating it from the child's life will often cure the problem, allergists find.

HELP FOR ANXIETY

Too much caffeine may be your problem. Dr. John F. Greden, of the University of Michigan Medical School, warns that anyone drinking more than 600 mg of caffeine a day (7 cups of coffee or cola, or several headache tablets) is in danger of caffeinism.

Symptoms that can be caused are: shakiness, nervousness, irritability, palpitations of the heart, upsets in heart rhythms, low blood pressure, circulatory failure, nausea, vomiting, dizziness, stomach pain, diarrhea, frequent urination.

RECOGNIZING AND TREATING DEPRESSION

Many people suffer from depression without realizing it, and few of them will receive the treatment they should have or will even realize that they have a condition that *can* be treated. The person who feels no pleasure in life, the person who is always tired, and the underachiever are often really suffering from depression. Many older people who are diagnosed as being senile or having hardening of the arteries of the brain really have depression.

The symptoms of depression often begin so slowly that a person is not even sure when they started. He feels and looks tired and sad, perhaps with a smile to hide the melancholy. There may be tears or a lack of feeling, a progressive feeling of meaninglessness, a diminished interest and drive, apathy toward work, more and more effort required just getting through the day. There may be feelings of failure, of self-reproach, and of self-pity. There may be increased anxiety, increased irritability, heavy alcohol intake, neglected hair or clothes, difficulty in reaching a decision or in starting something new, sleep disturbances, or bad dreams. Sometimes the depression is steady and unrelenting. Sometimes it comes and goes.

YOU CAN MEASURE DEPRESSION ELECTRONICALLY

Doctors at Harvard University have discovered that tiny facial muscles mirror your mood. They ask a subject to imagine happy or sad situations while muscle activity is recorded by electrodes. Depressed subjects show low activity when asked to imagine a happy situation.

WHAT TO DO

See your doctor for anti-depression medication, such as lithium, and to check for diseases that can cause depression (hormone disturbances, anemia, viral infections, alcoholism, and other disorders).

Go on the Whole Health Diet.

Take vitamin and mineral supplements.

If blood sugar levels are low, try fructose (also called levelose) between meals.

Psychoanalysis or group therapy may be helpful.

Exercise. British doctors find brisk exercise doubles production of the hormone norepinephrine, which is an anti-depressant.

Warning: If someone you know becomes so depressed he threatens to commit suicide or shows other signs of planning to end his life, get professional help through a suicide prevention center, crisis intervention center, mental health clinic, family physician, hospital, or clergyman. Don't believe that people who talk about suicide don't commit it. They often do.

WELL-KNOWN PLACES TO GO TO FOR HELP

Some medical centers that specialize in the treatment of depression:

Columbia University College of Physicians & Surgeons
    Presbyterian Hospital
    722 West 168th Street
    New York, N.Y. 10032
Creighton University School of Medicine
    Department of Psychiatry
    10th and Castelar
    Omaha, Neb. 68108
Massachusetts Mental Health Center
    74 Fenwood Road
    Roxbury, Mass. 02119
Rush-Presbyterian Hospital-St. Luke's Medical Center
    1733 West Congress Parkway
    Chicago, Ill. 60612

SCHIZOPHRENIA

Schizophrenia can strike at any age, but is most prevalent in young people aged 16 to 30.

HOW TO RECOGNIZE IT

- Perceptual changes in seeing, hearing, touching, tasting, and smelling
- Alteration of the personality
- Insomnia
- Headache
- A change in skin color to a darker hue
- An offensive body odor
- Intense self-preoccupation
- Irrational crying fits
- Crippling fatigue
- Deep depression unrelated to external events
- Severe inner tension
- The feeling of being watched
- A sense of terror
- A fear of loss of self-control over one's thoughts and actions

WHAT IT'S LIKE TO BE SCHIZOPHRENIC

Colors may become brilliant or things may lose color. Objects may look different, flat, or with changed shape or size. You may have hallucinations, such as a snake on the floor, or voices speaking from the air, a person changing to something else. There may be feelings of needles sticking the skin, or worms crawling under the skin. Foods may taste strange. Smells may be different. Your mind may feel as if it is racing away from you or going to explode. You may feel someone is following you or trying to poison you, or that you are under the influence of outside divine or demon forces. There may be deep depression, crippling fatigue, withdrawal from the world.

WHAT TO DO

See your family physician or psychiatrist or go to a mental health clinic. Treatment methods include psychotherapy, electroshock, and drugs. Aftercare should include counseling and an aftercare clinic with guidance in readjustment.

MEGAVITAMIN TREATMENT FOR SCHIZOPHRENIA

Megavitamin therapy is the use of super-large doses of vitamins for treatment of certain diseases. One of the major uses is in treatment of schizophrenia and other mental disorders in a branch of psychiatry called orthomolecular psychiatry. Psychiatrists using the approach say it is able to save many patients who did not respond to other treatment.

The technique is still experimental and modifications are still being made as new information is learned, but here is the basis of the treatment at present:

Sugar is removed from the diet.

Refined starches are removed from the diet.

High amounts of protein are given.

The following supplements are given daily, usually for one year, with variations for different investigators in practice.

- A high-potency multiple vitamin-mineral capsule
- Liver tablets
- A general B-complex supplement
- Niacinamide (vitamin B_3), 3 to 30 grams per day
- Thiamine (vitamin B_1), 1 to 2 grams
- Pyridoxine (vitamin B_6), 100 to 500 mg
- Pantothenic acid, 200 to 300 mg
- Vitamin B_{12}, 1 mg by injection, 50 to 100 micrograms orally
- Vitamin C, 3 to 20 grams daily
- Vitamin E, 400 to 800 mg

- Zinc
- Magnesium

Sometimes folic acid is given (but some become worse on folic acid and do better on zinc and manganese).

This treatment must be given by a doctor. Specialists in the therapy claim 50 to 75 percent of patients can be helped.

A similar program has been used with some success in treating autistic children, children with learning disabilities, behavior disorders of aging, drug addiction, and several psychiatric disorders.

For more information about orthomolecular psychiatry write: The Huxley Institute for Biosocial Research, 1114 East End Avenue, New York N.Y. 10021.

Warning: Schizophrenic patients should never use marijuana in any from. Using marijuana in even small amounts can cause severe symptoms and an often violent relapse in an otherwise controlled patient, says Dr. Darold A. Treffert of Winnebago Mental Health Institute, Wisconsin. There is mounting evidence that alcohol also may be a hazardous substance for schizophrenics.

CHAPTER 17

What Every Consumer Needs to Know About Medicines

TWENTY WAYS TO SAVE MONEY ON MEDICINES

1. *Check mail order discount drugs.* A number of drug companies, and even Sears, Roebuck, sell drugs at a discount by mail. Good when speed of delivery is not important.

2. *Check special organizations.* A person with epilepsy can get medicine at reduced cost from the National Epilepsy League, 116 South Michigan Avenue, Chicago Ill. 60603. The Retired Teachers Association, the American Association of Retired Persons, and some insurance companies have reduced prices.

3. *Check your insurance policy.* About 35 percent of people have medical insurance that covers medicines, but many don't use it.

4. *Ask your doctor for free samples.* Doctors often have free samples left by detailmen from pharmaceutical companies. Many Planned Parenthood clinics have free birth control pills.

5. *Buy in large quantities where possible.* Check unit prices by size and brand, or ask the druggist whether a particular item is cheaper in quantity. However, check also on how long a medicine will last, whether you will use the larger quantity before it begins to deteriorate.

6. *Store drugs properly.* If directions say to keep a medicine in the refrigerator, keep it there. Keep caps on tightly to keep alcohol from evaporating and air from getting to medicines. Capsules of vitamins last longer than the tablet or liquid form.

7. *Always tell the pharmacist to "label as to content."* If a drug you stopped using is re-prescribed and your doctor knows the name of a medicine and how long you have had it, it may mean you can use the medicine again and save the expense of a new bottle. Don't use the leftovers on your own; always check with your doctor first.

8. *Use medicines properly.* The medicine may not work properly unless you take it exactly as directed. Don't stop taking a drug when you begin to feel better unless your physician says to. Often anything less than the full course of treatment may prevent the medicine from completely correcting the condition.

9. *Find the causes of your problems.* You may spend hundreds of dollars for sleeping pills for years and then find it's too much coffee before bed that is keeping you awake. Coughing? Don't buy lozenges, give up cigarettes. Constant colds? Maybe you really have an allergy.

10. *Make sure you really need the medicine.* According to an article in *Science,* many doctors write prescriptions simply as a way to end an office visit. Don't encourage your doctor to give you medicines you don't need.

11. *Do comparison shopping.* Stop in at local drugstores and ask their prices on some prescription medicines that you use frequently. (But keep

in mind that there are other things besides prices of drugs. Those who charge higher prices often offer extra services such as staying open late at night, delivering free, keeping records, preparing statements of purchases for income tax returns.)

12. *Keep checking prices.* Many pharmacists, when they realize a customer is comparison shopping, will give a low price on the first order and will raise the price on later prescriptions.

13. *Tell your pharmacist when you are able to have a prescription filled cheaper elsewhere.* It might get him to lower his prices.

14. *Count your pills.* It might be worthwhile *if* you have the time.

15. *Watch for tax chargers.* The general rule is that there is no sales tax on items that are a treatment. However, dental products, first aid products, and medical equipment *are* taxable.

16. *Discuss the price of medicine with your doctor.* Many doctors have already compared the costs of medicines in the drugstores near them.

17. *Use generic names when you can.* Sometiems a specific brand name is the best, and your doctor may definitely want it for you, but when all brands are basically alike, ordering the prescription by the generic name can save you money. Check with your doctor.

18. *Ask your doctor to use the new* Physician's Guide to Prescription Prices. It lists every prescription drug and its average cost. When there is a choice of equally satisfactory drugs or dosage forms, he can see which are most economical.

19. *Ask your pharmacist.* He can usually recommend the least expensive brand to do the job.

20. *Look up non-prescription medicines yourself.* Consult *Without Prescription* by Drs. Erwin DiCyan and Lawrence Hessman. It compares over-the-counter drugs by ingredients, action, side effects, and cost.

WHERE TO FIND MEDICINES YOUR DRUGSTORE DOESN'T HAVE

G. Strasswimmer, 1664 Second Avenue, New York, N.Y. 10021.
    Founded 1875. Has 500 different medicinal and herbal teas from camomile to uva ursi to zinnkraut. The staff speaks eight languages. Orders filled from overseas.

Kiehl Pharmacy, 109 Third Avenue, New York, N.Y.10003
    Founded 1851. Has many natural creams, lotions, and shampoos and many honeys including Scottish heather, Spanish orange blossom, Jamaican logwood, Tasmanian leatherwood, Hungarian acacia, and Greek hymettus.

Caswell-Massey Company, 518 Lexington Avenue, New York, N.Y. 10022
    Founded in 1752. Noted for its rare items such as boar bristle toothbrushes, bear grease, and snuff, including that used by George Washington and the Marquis de Lafayette. Free catalogue.

Corby Chemists, 988 First Avenue, New York, N. Y. 10022
    If your druggist doesn't carry vitamin C with bioflavonoids and vitamins without additives, you can get them from Corby Chemists, 988 First Avenue, New York, N.Y. 10022; Wilner Chemists 330 Lexington Avenue, New York, N.Y. 10016, or Freeda Foundation, 919 Third Avenue, New York, N.Y. 10022.

BE SURE YOUR MEDICINES ARE LABELED AS TO CONTENT

Know exactly what your medications are; do not accept an unknown remedy without explanation.

In emergency situations, immediate identification of a drug from the label may be lifesaving. It is difficult to know the right treatment when a person lies unconscious clutching an unlabeled bottle of little red pills.

The information can be invaluable when you change physicians or move to another locality.

If a warning is issued against the use of a particular drug, you would know if you are taking it.

QUESTIONS EVERY PATIENT SHOULD ASK HIS DOCTOR WHEN A DRUG IS PRESCRIBED

Write down the answers as your doctor gives them.

What is my diagnosis and how was it arrived at?

What is the name of the drug and what is it supposed to do?

What are the drug's possible side effects? What side effects should I be especially alert for and report?

Are there any conditions in which the drug is unsafe?

How often should the drug be taken, before or after meals, for how many days?

Should the prescription be refilled and under what circumstances?

What precautions should be observed while taking the medicine? Should certain foods or activities or other medications be avoided?

How long should I wait before reporting to the doctor if there are no changes in symptoms?

Do I need another appointment?

WARNING: MEDICINES MAY BE DANGEROUS TO YOUR HEALTH

It is estimated that each year 100,000 Americans die and 300,000 are hospitalized from adverse drug reactions. With any drug there is always the chance that adverse reactions will occur. Protect yourself.

Never insist the doctor give you a prescription if he is not sure it's necessary.

Make sure you understand all directions thoroughly.

Always tell a new physician of past drug reactions, even if they were mild. The next one may be more severe.

Any time a label is missing, a medicine turns color, is congealed or more concentrated, has started to crumble, or smells like vinegar, throw it out immediately. Always discard medicines on their expiration date.

Always tell your doctor of any other medicine you are taking in addition to the one he prescribed for you, even if it is something as simple as aspirin or sleeping pills. And tell him if you are not responding to a medicine.

SOME UNLUCKY SIDE EFFECTS OF COMMONLY USED DRUGS

Call your doctor if you are taking medicine and any of the following signs of a reaction occur:

- Nausea and vomiting
- Wheezing or shortness of breath
- Inflammation of the eyelids and reddening of the eyes
- A skin rash, itching, or hives
- Blood in the urine
- An agitated or upset emotional state
- Diarrhea

Note: Guard against your child's being given tetracycline. It can cause permanent mottling of the teeth.

EVEN ASPIRIN

It's a great medicine—it relieves pain, reduces fever, reduces inflammation, and it's cheap. But it can cause side effects, too, particularly acting as an anti-clotting agent, thus often causing stomach bleeding or aggravation of ulcers.

Here are the rules doctors recommend concerning aspirin: Don't take them for stomach distress (including products like Alka-Seltzer that contain aspirin). Don't take during pregnancy, especially last three months. Don't take if they give you stomach upset or if you have an ulcer. Don't mix with beer, wine, or liquor; the mixing increases stomach irritation. Don't take if you are taking other medicine for arthritis, for thinning the blood, for diabetes. Always take with a full glass of water. Keep away from children; an overdose can kill.

Note: If you chew up aspirin before swallowing or crush it to a powder and mix it with a juice, it will cause fewer problems to your stomach.

BEWARE OF MIXING

Milk or antacids or anything with calcium will interfere with the action of tetracycline. Unfortunately tetracycline sometimes upsets the stomach so you tend to reach for a Tums. Don't do it. Tetracycline and penicillin should never be given together. They counteract each other.

Insulin can be neutralized by certain antibiotics or by aspirin. Sedatives can counteract antidepressants. Aspirin can counteract gout pills. Some of the new arthritis drugs can potentiate blood thinning by anticoagulants. Nose drops can counteract blood pressure pills. Antacids or Kaopectate can counteract digitalis.

Some foods can be deadly combined with medicines. If you are taking tranquilizers, do not eat chicken livers, bananas, avocados, canned figs, broad beans, soy sauce, yogurt, Camembert, Gruyère, cheddar or American cheese, sour cream, or Chianti, unless you check with your doctor. They could kill you in combination with certain tranquilizers.

Certain herb teas can change the rate of absorption of certain medicines, making them ineffective. Some herbs contain caffeine which can cause problems.

Nicotine from cigarettes can interfere with some medicines, and some mint cigarettes contain atropine and scopolamine that affect the nervous system.

Note: Whenever you are given a prescription, your doctor should ask if you are taking any other medication in case there is a conflict. If he doesn't ask, volunteer the information on other medicines you are taking.

DRUGS AND DRINKING

Don't drink alcohol when you are taking drugs. The mixture, if it involves a barbiturate, for example, can kill you.

THE ONE THING YOU SHOULD ALWAYS DO WHEN YOU TAKE AN ANTIBIOTIC

Get a supply of Bacid or Lactinex (or any preparation of *Lactobacillus acidophilus*) and take one each time you take the antibiotic. It will keep your body resupplied with good germs that have been killed off by the antibiotic when it killed the bad germs. Bacid or Lactinex puts good germs back into your system and so helps prevent diarrhea, vaginal yeast infections, fungus infections, and irritability. Eating a cup of yogurt each day will do the same thing. Use for children (½ cup) as well as adults. Always finish the full amount when an antibiotic is given to you. Otherwise hidden lingering infection can start up again.

IF YOUR DOCTOR GIVES YOU A PRESCRIPTION FOR CORTISONE

Be sure to tell him if you have a history of tuberculosis or ulcers. Cortisone should then not be given.

UNDERGROUND MEDICINES

There are many medicines used in other countries that are not approved by the F.D.A. in the United States, but are nevertheless used secretly by many U.S. doctors because they feel they and their patients should have freedom of choice in the treatments they use and because they feel the drugs are so beneficial to their patients it is worth the risk involved to use them. We list some of the "underground medicines" in other sections with the conditions they are used to treat.

CHAPTER 18

If You Must Be Hospitalized

HOW TO JUDGE A SURGEON

Look him up in the *Directory of Medical Specialists* (it's in most libraries) to learn his background and to determine if he is a fellow of the American College of Surgeons.

Make sure he is "board certified" in his specialty. This means he has taken several years of specialty training after medical school, has at least two years' experience, and has passed an examination.

Check his reputation with other doctors and nurses that you know.

Find out how frequently he does the particular operation you need done. You do not want a surgeon who does the operation only occasionally.

Make sure he is on the staff at a good hospital, one that is accredited by the Joint Commission on Accreditation of Hospitals, preferably one that is a research or teaching institution or is affiliated with a medical school.

WAYS TO SAVE MONEY WHEN YOU HAVE TO GO TO THE HOSPITAL

MAKE SURE TIME IN THE HOSPITAL IS NOT WASTED

Frequently days are wasted in the hospital because of improper scheduling. If you are lying around with no work being done, you might as well be at home. Discuss with your doctor what's going to happen and when.

Avoid entering the hospital on weekends if possible since services may be reduced and you may have to wait for tests to be done on Monday. Most admitting is done on Sunday, with heavy testing on Monday; so Tuesday, Wednesday, and Thursdays are best days for admission to avoid delays.

HAVE TESTS DONE BEFORE HOSPITAL ADMISSION

Many tests can be done just as well *outside* the hospital before you go in. Check with your doctor. Check your insurance to see if it will cover.

INSIST ON A WARD OR SEMI-PRIVATE ROOM

Many hospitals now have only semi-private rooms, but some hospitals still give people a higher-priced private room without asking preference. It will make a considerable difference in your bill.

PASS UP AIR-CONDITIONING

If you have a choice, choose a non-air conditioned room. It is less expensive, and actually better than an air-conditioned room for recovery:

BRING YOUR OWN PILLS WHENEVER YOU CAN

Medicines always cost more in the hospital. One aspirin may cost 50 cents, a sleeping pill $2. But some hospitals will not allow you to bring in your own medication. Check with your doctor. Naturally, you will not under any circumstances take anything without your doctor knowing about it.

DON'T TAKE MORE DRUGS IN THE HOSPITAL THAN YOU HAVE TO

Don't ask for a pill if you don't really need it. Not only are drugs expensive, but the more you take, the more side effects and interactions you are apt to have, which can cause complications and a longer hospital stay.

Unfortunately patients often are not told the names of the medications they are taking, why they are taking them, and what side effects to be alert for. ASK!

TRY TO CUT DOWN LABORATORY COSTS

Most laboratory tests, of course, are really necessary; but sometimes tests are done to satisfy supervising physicians, for research data, or simply because certain routines of testing have been set. Ask your doctor to go easy on ordering tests and not burden you with anything that isn't really necessary.

AVOID DUPLICATION OF TESTS

Speak out if the hospital wants to repeat tests done earlier in the doctor's office.

AVOID UNNECESSARY SURGERY

If there is any doubt in your mind about whether you really need surgery, get a second opinion from another doctor.

GET UP AND MOVE AROUND AS SOON AS POSSIBLE

Start doing as much as possible for yourself as soon as possible. Early moving around means faster recovery and fewer complications.

USE NO-FRILLS FACILITIES WHENEVER YOU CAN

More and more hospitals are offering no-frills care for patients who are well enough to help themselves. The patients make their own beds, take meals in the cafeteria, are free to play cards or visit with others, but are still on hand for follow-up care. The room bill is about 40 percent less.

DON'T STAY IN THE HOSPITAL ANY LONGER THAN YOU HAVE TO

Sometimes a whole day can be lost waiting for discharge. Make sure you know what the hours of discharge are at your hospital and how far ahead of time the proper papers have to be signed.

DONATE BLOOD

Most hospitals give you a choice of paying for blood or having a friend or relative donate an equivalent amount. You can also donate blood now to the American Red Cross and the American Association of Blood Banks, so in the future you or your family can have blood transfusions free.

FOR A CHILD, CHOOSE A HOSPITAL WITH ROOMING-IN

You can do many of the things for your child that might require expensive special nursing services.

IF YOU ARE A VETERAN, TAKE ADVANTAGE OF BENEFITS

If you have a service-connected injury or illness, you can go to a VA hospital. Even if your problem is not service-connected, if beds are available, you can sometimes be treated in a veterans' hospital free. And sometimes the VA authorizes care in non-federal hospitals for service-connected disabilities. Check with your local VA office.

BE AN OUT-PATIENT

Many people go to the hospital as an in-patient, staying all night, when they could have the same services performed as an out-patient, coming in for tests or treatment, then going home, eliminating the cost of the hospital room. More and more minor surgical procedures are being done this way if your doctor requests them.

Sometimes, of course, hospitalization is vital. But don't get hospitalized for convenience—either yours or the doctor's—if you are trying to save money.

BE TREATED AT HOME

Hiring a registered or practical nurse for at-home care can make it easier on the family, offer good care, and still be cheaper than staying in the hospital. Or you can have a visiting nurse come every day to give medicines and check on your condition; or you can use homemaker services with someone to come in to shop, cook, clean, and care for children.

CHECK YOUR HOSPITAL BILL

If the hospital does not automatically itemize your bill, ask them to do it. Check each item. Do not pay any item you think incorrect without discussion.

DELIVERING?

If it's late at night and labor pains are still slow, it may pay to sit outside the hospital and wait for a while. Many hospitals begin their billing day at midnight, so you could save an entire day's billing by checking in a few minutes after midnight instead of before.

HOW TO HEAL FASTER IF YOU HAVE SURGERY

TAKE ZINC TABLETS

Studies show that zinc as an amino acid complex makes wounds heal better and faster and with fewer complications. Many surgeons now give zinc and amino acid for a week before as well as after surgery and say healing occurs about twice as fast.

TAKE VITAMINS

Several vitamins, such as A, C, and E, also speed healing, so many surgeons give high doses of vitamins and minerals before surgery and during the recovery period. In Japan surgeons say large doses of vitamin C (2 grams per day) have prevented patients from ever getting serum hepatitis from blood transfusions.

MOVE AROUND AND EXERCISE

Even in bed you can contract your feet and leg muscles. Sit up and walk as soon as your doctor says you can. This will not only help you heal faster, but also help prevent dangerous blood clots from forming in the leg veins. (See Chapter 6 for in-bed exercises.)

YAWN

Yawning helps inflate the lungs postoperatively, helping to clear bronchial secretions and prevent pulmonary complications that often occur after surgery. Yawn five deep yawns every hour for the first postoperative days.

NEW TREATMENT FOR BROKEN BONES THAT AREN'T HEALING

Several investigators have reported that fractures will heal faster when small amounts of electricity are applied to them. The mild electrical current stimulates bone growth and even induces healing in fractures that have refused to heal for years.

Another aid: take bone meal or other forms of calcium to encourage union.

TO REDUCE GAS PAINS

Drink from a glass, not from a straw, to reduce amount of air swallowed.

Move around as much as possible; at the very least turn from one side to the other frequently.

Don't eat beans, peas, or Chinese noodles.

If you're able, kneel in bed with head and arms touching, resting on the bed, rear end in the air to let gases rise.

WHAT TO DO BEFORE YOU GO TO THE HOSPITAL TO REDUCE COMPLICATIONS LATER

If you are a smoker, stop smoking several days before surgery.

If you usually drink large amounts of alcohol, cut down before entering the hospital.

If you have had a recent cold or other respiratory infection, postpone elective surgery.

If you take medication to reduce high blood pressure, work with your doctor to discontinue it a few weeks before surgery.

If you have been taking cortisone, ACTH, or similar drugs prior to surgery or if you have sickle cell anemia, inform the anesthesiologist and surgeon about this.

Loose or infected teeth should be removed if there is time.

Have plenty of rest and nourishing foods for the weeks preceding an operation.

Take your vitamin and mineral supplements.

The night before surgery, wash your hair and take a shower. Recent reports show this simple step cuts wound infection rate in half.

CHECK YOUR BIORHYTHM

Many surgeons are beginning to schedule their surgical patients (when there is a choice) for the days when their biorhythm charts show that their body cycles are up. Biorhythms are the ups and downs everyone has in their physical, emotional, and intellectual cycles. They are chartable, and many researchers believe they can enable you to determine the days that are most dangerous to your body, when your defenses are lowest and you are most vulnerable to stress. The technique has been used extensively in industrial plants, especially in Japan, to reduce industrial accidents, and now is being used by many surgeons there, in Switzerland, and by a few in the U.S. and Canada. Mortality and complication rates have gone down significantly.

To order your Biorhythm Chart worked out for a year, send your birthdate and $3.95 to Biorhythm Research Institute, 401 Market Avenue, N. Canton, Ohio 44750, or watch for ads in newspapers and magazines.

HOW TO GET THE TRUTH FROM THE HOSPITAL WHEN YOU ARE A PATIENT

Call on the outside line of your phone, pretend you are a relative, and ask about your condition.

Prepare a list of questions to ask your doctor when he stops by your room each day.

Ask to see your chart. (Patients are now allowed to; in fact the U.S. Department of Commerce now recommends that patients have absolute right of access to all their medical records.)

THE PATIENTS' BILL OF RIGHTS

A set of Patients' Bill of Rights was recently formulated by the American Hospital Association. A book explaining the rights has been given to all hospitals, clearly spelling out the requirements for patient care and the following rights:

1. The patient has the right to considerate and respectful care.

2. The patient has the right to obtain from his physician complete current information concerning his diagnosis, treatment, and prognosis in terms the patient can be reasonably expected to understand. When it is not medically advisable to give such information to the patient, the information should be made available to an appropriate person in his behalf. He has the right to know by name the physician responsible for coordinating his care.

3. The patient has the right to receive from his physician information necessary to give informed consent prior to the start of any procedure and/or treatment. Except in emergencies, such information for informed consent should include but not necessarily be limited to the specific procedure and/or treatment, the medically significant risks involved, and the probable duration of incapacita-

tion. Where medically significant alternatives for care or treatment exist, or when the patient requests information concerning medical alternatives, the patient has the right to such information. The patient also has the right to know the name of the person responsible for the procedures and/or treatment.

4. The patient has the right to refuse treatment to the extent permitted by law, and to be informed of the medical consequences of his action.

5. The patient has the right to every consideration of his privacy concerning his own medical care program. Case discussion, consultation, examination, and treatment are confidential and should be conducted discreetly. Those *not directly* involved in his care must have the permission of the patient to be present.

6. The patient has the right to expect that all communications and records pertaining to his care should be treated as confidential.

7. The patient has the right to expect that within its capacity a hospital must make reasonable response to the request of a patient for services. The hospital must provide evaluation, service, and/or referral as indicated by the urgency of the case. When medically permissible a patient may be transferred to another facility only after he has received complete information and explanation concerning the needs for and alternatives to such a transfer. The institution to which the patient is to be transferred must first have accepted the patient for transfer.

8. The patient has the right to obtain information as to any relationship of his hospital to other health care and educational institutions insofar as his care is concerned. The patient has the right to obtain information as to the existence of any professional relationships among individuals, by name, who are treating him.

9. The patient has the right to be advised if the hospital proposes to engage in or perform human experimentation affecting his care or treatment. The patient has the right to refuse to participate in such research projects.

10. The patient has the right to expect reasonable continuity of care. He has the right to know in advance what appointment times and physicians are available and where. The patient has the right to expect that the hospital will provide a mechanism whereby he is informed by his physician or a delegate of the physician of the patient's continuing health care requirements following discharge.

11. The patient has the right to examine and re-

ceive an explanation of his bill regardless of source of payment.

12. The patient has the right to know what hospital rules and regulations apply to his conduct as a patient.

If at any time you feel these rights have been transgressed, ask to see the social service representative or a person found in some hospitals called an ombudsman.

IF YOU ARE HOSPITALIZED IN A MENTAL HOSPITAL

The following is a list of the Mental Patients' Bill of Rights as formulated by the Mental Patients' Liberation Project of New York City.

1. You are a human being and are entitled to be treated as such with as much decency and respect as is accorded to any other human being.

2. You are an American citizen and are entitled to every right established by the Declaration of Independence and guaranteed by the Constitution of the United States of America.

3. You have the right to the integrity of your own mind and the integrity of your body.

4. Treatment and medication can be administered only with your consent; you have the right to demand to know all relevant information regarding said treatment and/or medication.

5. You have the right to have access to your own legal and medical counsel.

6. You have the right to refuse to work in a mental hospital and/or to choose what work you shall do and you have the right to receive the minimum wage for such work as is set by the state labor laws.

7. You have the right to decent medical attention when you feel you need it, just as any other human being has the right.

8. You have the right to uncensored communication by phone, letter, and in person with whomever you wish and at any time you wish.

9. You have the right not to be treated like a criminal; not to be locked up against your will; not to be committed involuntarily; not to be fingerprinted or "mugged" (photographed).

10. You have the right to decent living conditions. You're paying for it and the taxpayers are paying for it.

11. You have the right to retain your own personal property. No one has the right to confiscate what is legally yours, no matter what reason is given. That is commonly known as theft.

12. You have the right to bring grievance against those who have mistreated you and the right to counsel and a court hearing. You are entitled to protection by law against retaliation.

13. You have the right to refuse to be a guinea pig for experimental drugs and treatments and to refuse to be used as learning material for students. You have the right to demand reimbursement if you are so used.

14. You have the right not to have your character questioned or defamed.

15. You have the right to request an alternative to legal commitment or incarceration in a mental hospital.

WHAT TO DO TO AVOID UNNECESSARY SURGERY

Don't go directly to a surgeon for medical treatment. A surgeon is more likely to suggest surgery than some other form of treatment. Your first visit should be to an internist or family practitioner who will refer you to a surgeon if he thinks an operation may be needed.

When surgery is recommended, obtain an independent opinion from another qualified surgeon. *Always* do this if you have been told you need one of the operations often done unnecessarily, such as hysterectomy, gallbladder or hemorrhoid surgery, or removal of tonsils.

Have your family doctor *and* your surgeon explain the alternatives to surgery, and both benefits and possible complications of the alternatives and of the surgery.

Don't push a doctor into performing surgery if he does not think it is needed.

ANNOUNCEMENT

Blue Cross and other health plans in several states have announced that they will offer subscribers the opportunity to obtain a second professional opinion before undergoing non-emergency surgery. All charges related to the second opinion—the doctor's fee and the costs of any x-rays or laboratory tests needed—will be paid for by the insurance plan.

FREE BOOKLET
A Shopper's Guide to Surgery
    Herbert D. Denenberg
    National Liberty Corporation
    Valley Forge, Pa. 19481

IF YOUR CHILD FACES SURGERY

Tell your child the truth about what will happen at the hospital, explain the reason for the operation, that people in the operating room will be wearing masks, that he will be fast asleep during the operation so he won't feel pain, that when he wakes up the operation will be over. Be as relaxed and casual and reassuring as you can when you talk about it.

Buy him reading books and coloring books about going to the hospital.

Let him visit the hospital if it's possible. (At Children's Hospital of the East Bay in Oakland, Calif., nursery school children are taken on tours of the hospital so that they know what a hospital is like before hurrying there in an emergency. Some hospitals send personally addressed postcards to children before they come.)

Parents should be prepared properly, too. They need to be told how to treat their child, what they should or should not do in the hospital.

When the child gets to the hospital, introduce him by name to the nurse who will see him most. Tell the nurses the child's nickname, what foods disagree with him, what words he uses for going to the bathroom. Leave them a list noting all this.

Children should be allowed to wear their own pajamas if they want, and to wear regular clothes during the day when possible.

Allow your child to bring a nice soft blanket or favorite cuddly toy.

Remember to tell your child many times that you will be back, that he or she will soon be going back home.

Say good-bye at the end of visiting, do not slip out unnoticed.

Visit often, stay as long as you can, bring along little presents.

At the earliest date, take your child home.

NEW VISITATION POLICIES

In some hospitals parents are limited to only a few hours of visiting a day. Other hospitals are even worse, not allowing parents to visit more than a few times a week, with the children feeling abandoned at what seems their moment of greatest need. Try to get unlimited visiting, and even to stay all night if permitted.

At present some two-thirds of British hospitals allow unrestricted visiting. In the United States, only about 15 percent do.

Dr. Robert S. Mendelsohn of Michael Reese Hospital in Chicago says, "We should drop the term visiting 'privileges' . . . Visiting is not a privilege, but a right of every patient and family."

The American Academy of Pediatrics has proposed not only liberalization of visiting hours, but also increased facilities for parents staying overnight and changes in rules so children can visit parents in the hospital.

At the Yale Child Center in New Haven, Conn., when mothers worked with children, children after surgery had lower blood pressure, took fluids more easily, had less fever, less vomiting, cried less, needed the doctor less often, and recovered more quickly.

Le Bonheur Children's Hospital at the University of Tennessee reports "the majority of these mothers are useful and helpful. Their children have fewer falls out of bed, and other accidents. Acute anxiety in mother and child is reduced. Time of floor nurses is saved, and nursing cost is cut."

Several organizations have been formed to crusade for liberalization of visiting hours. A newsletter, *Mother Care for Children in Hospital*, 16 Berwyn Road, Richmore, Surrey, England, is available for persons who want to work for such facilities in their local areas.

RECOMMENDED:
Johnny Goes to the Hospital
    Jospehine Sever
    Houghton Mifflin
    1 Beacon Street
    Boston, Mass. 02107
The Hospital
    Mabel Pin
    Houghton Mifflin
    1 Beacon Street
    Boston, Mass. 02107
Linda Goes to the Hospital
    Nancy Dudley
    Coward, McCann and Geoghegan
    200 Madison Avenue
    New York, N.Y. 10016
Your Child Goes to the Hospital
    Ross Laboratories
    Division Abbott Laboratories
    Columbus, Ohio 43216

CHAPTER 19

What You Need to Know About Health Insurance

Four out of five Americans have health insurance of some kind. Yet most don't know that their insurance usually covers much less than they thought, or perhaps doesn't cover their problem at all. When they find it out, it's too late.

THE BEST BUYS IN HEALTH INSURANCE— HOW TO KNOW WHAT YOU SHOULD HAVE

Read your policy to see which one of these you have.

Hospital Expense Insurance. This pays all or part of the cost of hospital room, board, x-rays, medicines, and other expenses. Some plans reimburse the patient. Others pay the hospital directly.

Surgical Expense Insurance. This pays part or all of the cost of an operation. The amount paid depends on the nature of the operation.

Medical Expense Insurance. Under this plan, visits to a doctor's office or his house calls are reimbursed, according to a limit set in the policy.

Major Medical Expense Insurance. This insurance helps to pay the cost of extended sickness or injury. The policies generally have a deductible clause: typically, the patient pays the first $100 or $200 himself, then the plan pays 80 percent of the balance, up to some limit, perhaps $25,000.

Loss-of-Income Insurance. This insurance, also called Disability Income Insurance, pays benefits when the insured person is unable to work because of illness or injury.

Prepaid Group Health Plans. In these plans, like Kaiser-Permanente, you pay a yearly fee to a group of health specialists for regular checkups and treatment, and sometimes stays in a hospital.

Dental Insurance. Some plans are offered by state dental societies. Other plans are offered by companies through group insurance for their employees.

Cooperatives. A cooperative is operated by a Board of Directors, chosen from its own membership, which contracts with a medical staff for provision of services on a salary rather than on a fee-for-service basis.

Health Maintenance Organizations. This is comprehensive medical care, with emphasis on preventive and maintenance medicine to try to keep the patient healthy and *out* of the hospital. The idea is to collect fees to keep people well instead of to cure them after they're sick.

HOW TO GET THE MOST OUT OF YOUR HEALTH INSURANCE DOLLAR

KNOW WHAT YOUR BENEFITS ARE

A lot of people don't use the insurance they have, and actually pay medical bills themselves when they are covered by insurance.

On the other hand, you may not be covered for something for which you think you are insured. Read the fine print.

DON'T LIE WHEN YOU APPLY FOR INSURANCE

If you hide the fact you have or had some injury or illness, no matter how minor or how long ago, you may find an insurance company using this as an excuse not to pay.

BE SURE YOUR CHILDREN OBTAIN THEIR OWN COVERAGE AS THEY GET OLDER

Most policies don't cover children after age 19, or if they are self-supporting.

DON'T HAVE ELECTIVE SURGERY UNTIL YOU READ YOUR POLICY

Many policies have a waiting period before they pay for routine surgery, such as removal of tonsils or treatment of a hernia. Before you schedule surgery, check to see if your policy will be in effect. There also may be a waiting period for benefits to be paid for treatment for a pre-existing condition.

BUY INSURANCE AT WORK IF YOU CAN

Group contracts are much less expensive than individual contracts. If you can't get insurance through an employer, perhaps you belong to a professional, social, fraternal, or farm workers organization that offers an insurance plan.

If you leave a job, be sure to check what provisions there are for members when they change jobs. You may choose to convert all or part of your coverage to an individual contract.

CHECK YOUR HOSPITAL BILL

Insist on knowing what charges are for. You may legitimately owe them or you may not.

COMPARE POLICIES

There may be a huge difference in what different policies offer. Shopping around can pay.

MAKE SURE YOU HAVE ENOUGH BENEFITS

Try to get a policy that has these features:

- Guaranteed renewable to age 65, or even better, for life
- Applies to all family members' medical expenses, rather than just one person's
- Has no exclusions that could leave you uncovered (many policies cover psychiatric expenses inside a general hospital, but not in a psychiatric hospital)
- Is in line with medical costs as you know them in your area
- Covers any pre-existing illness so long as you didn't know you had the illness
- Covers as many extra costs as possible, such as x-rays, medicines, lab tests, private nurses

AVOID DUPLICATIONS OF INSURANCE

Provisions of your car insurance often overlap provisions of your health insurance. You may not need medicine insurance for auto accidents except to cover other people.

Also if both husband and wife work, there may be duplicate insurance coverage. Ask your insurance agent if some adjustment can be made to reduce coverage and reduce premiums.

If you do have overlapping policies and one pays you directly instead of the hospital, it is sometimes possible to collect from both policies.

CHECK INTO YOUR POLICY AT YOUR JOB

Find out whether the insurance at work is best for you or is adequate. Even though much less expensive, it may not offer sufficient protection.

BUY THE INSURANCE THAT FITS YOUR OWN SPECIAL NEEDS

A young couple usually needs insurance that pays right from the beginning without any deductibles for you to pay, and they need protection for pregnancy and delivery and the accidents and operations their children are likely to have. They are less likely to come down with an expensive illness.

A young unmarried person who is healthy might be best off with a comprehensive major medical rather than Blue Cross or Blue Shield. One trouble with Blue Cross and Blue Shield is that a young healthy person pays the same premium as a 60-year-old. A comprehensive major medical takes into consideration the policyholder's age, occupation, and state of health.

A middle-aged or older couple mostly needs major medical, since they are more likely to develop long-term expensive diseases, and their children are most likely to get hurt in costly auto accidents.

WATCH OUT FOR THESE TRICKY TERMS

Some insurance policies do not cover bills for very long. Some cover a hospital stay of 365 days, others for only three weeks. If you're hospitalized for a long time, the latter can be disastrous.

When insurance plans have a deductible (an amount you pay yourself before you get any benefits), the deductible amount can run from $100 to $1000.

Some plans pay only 75 percent of the expenses for any illness. So if you have an expensive $100,000 illness and you have one of these plans, you'll have to pay $25,000.

Many policies cover you for only a fixed amount for a hospital room, no matter what the actual room rate is, and it will cover your surgical expenses only up to a fixed limit, no matter what the actual cost. If your policy has a limit of $50 a day in a hospital and you're in a $150-a-day hospital, you pay the difference.

Sometimes hospital care is not covered for the first six or eight days. The average hospital stay is about eight days!

By using the "pre-existing conditions" clause, many policies don't pay costs of cancer, heart disease, tuberculosis, and mental disorders. If a policyholder of six months developed cancer, for example, the company might claim that the condition existed before he took out the policy.

GET AN INSURANCE POLICY THAT COVERS OUT-PATIENT TESTS

Many insurance companies will pay for tests only if they are done in a hospital, a ridiculous waste of money and time, since many of the tests can be done in a few hours, and the patient dismissed.

BE SURE YOU ARE COLLECTING WHAT YOU CAN FROM MEDICARE

Things keep changing under Medicare, so you may have different benefits now from when it first began.

IF YOU ARE RELATED TO THE MILITARY

The Civilian Health and Medical Program for the Uniformed Services (CHAMPUS) is available to dependents of serviceman, retired servicemen, and dependents of deceased servicemen. The benefits also apply to the National Oceanic and Atmospheric Association and the Commissioned Corps of the Public Health Service. Millions are eligible to get treatment at civilian medical facilities if it isn't conveniently available from the military, and have most of their bills paid. Only about one-tenth the people eligible are taking advantage of it. If you think you are eligible, contact your County Veteran Service Officer or CHAMPUS, Denver, Colo. 80240.

SEVEN QUESTIONS TO ASK ABOUT YOUR MEDICAL INSURANCE

1. Who can renew or cancel the policy?
2. What are the daily benefits?
3. What expenses are not covered?
4. Will pre-existing conditions be covered?
5. What are the exclusions and how long is the waiting period, if any?
6. What are the premium rates and can the rates be raised at a later date?
7. Is the company licensed?

Warning: If you are married less than nine months, sometimes ten, most policies will not make any maternity payments.

GOOD PLACES TO FIND OUT MORE ABOUT HEALTH INSURANCE

National Association of Blue Shield Plans
    211 East Chicago Avenue
    Chicago, Ill. 60611
Health Insurance Institute
    277 Park Avenue
    New York, N.Y. 10017
National Council of Senior Citizens
    1627 K Street, N.W.
    Washington, D.C. 20006
Delta Dental Plans Association
    211 East Chicago Avenue
    Chicago, Ill. 60011

HOW TO GET THE MOST FROM MEDICARE

Medicare is a program of health insurance under Social Security that helps millions of Americans 65 and older pay for health care.

Most people 65 and older are automatically eligible for the *hospital insurance*, which pays for care in a hospital.

You can also sign up for *medical insurance*, which helps pay doctor bills and other medical items and services not covered under hospital insurance. The medical program is voluntary: no one is covered automatically.

If you are not certain whether you are eligible for either program, call any Social Security office for information.

BE SURE TO SIGN UP EARLY

To make sure you get the full protection of Medicare, starting with the month you reach 65, you must sign up with your social security office at least a month before your birthday.

You may sign up for medical insurance only during specified periods. The first period begins three months before the month you reach 65 and ends three months after. If you miss your first chance to sign up, you will have other opportunities during the first three months of each year. If you wait more than a year to sign up, your premium will be higher. After three years, you can no longer sign up at all.

THE BENEFITS COVERED

Your *hospital insurance* will pay the cost of room and meals in semi-private accommodations (2 to 4 beds), regular nursing services, drugs, supplies, and appliances. It will not pay for doctor bills, private duty nurses, telephone, or television.

The *medical insurance* part of Medicare helps pay for physicians' services given in the doctor's office, the hospital, or your home, as well as for out-patient hospital services in an emergency room or out-patient clinic. It does not cover routine physical checkups, eyeglasses, hearing aids, immunizations, dental care, orthopedic shoes, and services provided outside the United States.

Benefits are occasionally changed. You can call any Social Security office for more detailed information about latest regulations.

RECOMMENDED:
Your Medicare Handbook
    U.S. Printing Office
    Washington, D.C. 20402
    35¢
    A booklet explaining all phases of Medicare.
Heartline's Guide to Medicare
    114 East Dayton Street
    West Alexandria, Ohio 45381
    $1.50
    Questions and answers, large print, sample claim form with instructions.
A Shopper's Guide to Health Insurance
    Herbert Denenberg
    Blue Cross Association
    Box 4389
    Chicago, Ill. 60680
    Free

20

Common Ailments and the Most Up-to-Date Ways to Treat Them

ALLERGIES

HOW TO RECOGNIZE THEM

If you have some illness that simply won't go away despite treatment, it may be due to an allergy. Suspect an allergy if you have: frequent sneezing, a snuffy runny nose, watery eyes, sinus trouble, asthma, unexpected skin rashes, hives, headaches, earaches, coughing, dizziness, diarrhea, constipation, stomachache, gas pains or even when you have frequent unexplained fatigue, depression, or mental problems. In an infant or young child there may be colic or diarrhea, he may spit up large amounts of formula, he may have extreme likes and dislikes in foods, he may be cranky or irritable, he may have a persistent night cough, he may constantly push his nose up or sideways to get more air.

WHAT TO DO

Determine the Cause

Is it something (dust, chemical vapors, animal danders, feathers, pollen, molds, cosmetics) you are breathing?

Is it something (foods, drinks, medicines) you are eating or drinking?

Is it something (fabrics, poison, plants, metals, woods, plastics, medicines, cosmetics, soaps) you are touching?

Could your pets be causing the trouble? Cats, dogs, hamsters, birds, all can cause allergy. Put your pet with friends for several weeks, clean the house thoroughly; if your symptoms stop, you can be almost sure it was the pet.

Could it be additives in foods and medicines? Red and yellow dyes especially have been incriminated in many allergy attacks, even causing crying spells, mental confusion, depression, delusions, and other psychiatric symptoms.

ALLERGY-PROOF YOUR HOUSE AND LIFE

If you are allergic to dust, keep furnishings simple, avoiding overstuffed furniture, shag, chenille, feathers, or down. Use two pillow cases on each pillow, sealing both ends. Use only washable toys. Bathe pets in Dust Seal. Have house cleaned frequently, including closets, furniture, drapes, mattresses, and box springs. Electric heat or hot water is preferable to forced air heat, which circulates dust. In homes heated by a forced air system, install a good two-stage electronic air cleaner or put several layers of cheesecloth under registers to filter out dust. Use air conditioning, central if possible. Replace filters frequently. Don't set temperatures more than 12 degrees lower than outdoors. Keep away from tobacco smoke, kerosene, oil, paint, and insect sprays. No matter how much you love a pet, if you are allergic to it, you must get rid of it. If you have pollen allergy, keep the windows and doors closed during the season. Have an air conditioner in the car. Avoid garden work where pollen gets stirred up from the weeds and dirt.

If you are allergic to any foods, especially avoid them during hay fever season, because they will add to your respiratory symptoms.

Use eyedrops for itching and burning eyes.

See your doctor for antihistamine drugs to lessen dripping, congestion, and itching. Ask him also whether you should have a series of injections, starting out with very small doses and gradually increasing, to build up your immunity.

WHAT'S NEW

Recent research shows respiratory allergies can be caused by bacteria and molds growing in humidifiers, air conditioners, and drip pans of refrigerators. Clean equipment frequently and use a germicide.

Office workers are being plagued by a new type of allergy—to the chemicals in no-carbon copies. The substances can cause inflammation of the skin, eye and other irritations.

If you are allergic to insects: an insect sting first aid kit is available from Center Laboratories, 35 Channel Drive, Port Washington, N.Y. 11050.

RECOMMENDED:
The Complete Allergy Guide
  Simon and Schuster
  1230 Avenue of the Americas
  New York, N.Y. 10020
  $9.95
Hayfever Holiday
  Public Affairs Division
  Abbott Laboratories
  North Chicago, Ill. 60064
  Free
  A state-by-state listing of ragweed counts.

ANEMIA

HOW TO RECOGNIZE

Symptoms are fatigue, low energy, and pale skin and mucous membranes. More severe anemia: pounding of the heart, shortness of breath on exertion, rapid pulse, headache, loss of appetite, dizziness, and ringing in the ears.

WHAT TO DO

For iron deficiency: eat foods rich in iron, such as liver, lean meat, molasses, egg yolk, nuts. Take daily supplements of iron tablets.

FOR PERNICIOUS ANEMIA

Injections of liver extract or vitamin B_{12} continued throughout life.

Note: There are many causes of anemia, including diet deficiencies, inability of the body to process vitamins properly, chronic blood loss from an ulcer, hemorrhoids, excessive menstrual flow, worms, or even cancer. You must see a doctor for proper diagnosis and treatment.

ARTHRITIS

HOW TO RECOGNIZE

Joint pain and swelling and loss of mobility in joints, also fever and weight loss in rheumatoid arthritis.

Arthritis occurs in children as well as in adults.

WHAT TO DO

Stay slim to reduce burden on joints.

Get plenty of rest, especially when there is inflammation or fever; locally rest a joint when it is inflamed.

Exercise, work with hands, move about when there is no inflammation. Maintain good posture and breathing habits.

Get heat treatments, take hot tub baths, use hot moist towels, heat lamps, use heating pad, paraffin baths. (Although some doctors claim ice packs work better. Test for yourself.)

Use massage.

Live in a hot, dry climate.

Take drugs, such as aspirin (especially as magnesium and copper salicylate), injections of gold salts, cortisone, hormones, phenylbutazone, antimalarial drugs, and indomethacin. (Watch for the many side effects of these drugs. With cortisone take vitamin D and calcium to keep bones strong.)

WHAT'S NEW

Taking folic acid vitamin pills.

Sleeping in a sleeping bag. To increase heat on joints.

A new drug called Orgotein. Being tested for humans, and is already in use by veterinarians.

A new copper-aspirin combination called copper aspirinate. In clinical tests appears to be some 20 times more effective than aspirin.

Zinc sulfate. At the University of Washington patients with chronic rheumatoid arthritis were given zinc sulfate tablets three times daily and had less joint tenderness, swelling, and stiffness.

Pills containing gold. These new pills are faster and more effective than ordinary injections of gold, say developers at Smith, Kline and French Laboratories. The pills, called Auranofin, are being further tested now in Argentina, Sweden, and South Africa. The pills are reported to take effect in about five weeks (injections take about three months to take effect) with dramatic reduction of joint pain, swelling, and stiffness.

A new drug to stop aspirin damage. A hormone called prostaglandin E₂ has been shown to prevent the damage to the digestive system often caused by aspirin and indomethacin. Dr. Max M. Cohen said at a meeting of the American College of Surgeons that the prostaglandin worked by increasing the protection of the digestive system against acid.

Three new experimental drugs. Sulindac has been shown effective in the treatment of rheumatoid arthritis, osteoarthritis, and especially ankylosing spondylitis. At present available for investigational use only in the U.S., but may be released soon. It is long-lasting (two pills a day needed) and non-irritating to the stomach.

Penicillamine, reported at a recent meeting of the Arthritis Foundation, is approved in the U.S. only for investigational use at present. It appears comparable to gold in providing slow but long-term benefits in some patients, who can be identified only by trial and error. The drug is currently making international history because it is being simultaneously tested in the U.S.A. and U.S.S.R. on a cooperative basis. In the past it has been used successfully to treat Wilson's disease, a rare illness of the liver and the nervous system.

Cloprednol, a hormone product, is helpful in controlling the symptoms of rheumatoid arthritis, with fewer side effects than other steroids now in use. It is still in the investigational stage in the U.S., but is available in Mexico.

A new five-finger exerciser for hand mobility. This small, plastic "Hand Gym" has been shown to prevent or slow down development of hand disabilities caused by rheumatoid arthritis and osteoarthritis. Five minutes of daily use improved muscle strength, range of motion, and useful hand function in a majority of rheumatoid and osteoarthritis patients after two months, studies show. Available from Krewer Research Laboratories, Point Lookout, N.Y. 11569.

Acupuncture. It's helping many, especially those with osteoarthritis. For referral to a qualified acupuncturist in your area, contact Acupuncture Information Center, 127 E. 69th Street, New York,

N.Y. 10021, or National Acupuncture Research Society, Suite 1508, 505 Park Avenue, New York, N.Y. 10022.

Swedish clinic methods. A number of clinics in Sweden and other European countries treat arthritis with a partial fast for several days in which the patient eats no solid foods, has only vegetable and fruit juices, vegetable broths, and herb teas. After this the diet consists of raw fruits, vegetable salads, yogurt, wheat germ, brewer's yeast, seeds, nuts, vegetable soup, potatoes, prunes, raisins, cottage cheese, kelp. Treatment also includes alternating hot and cold showers (15 minutes very hot, about 3 minutes cold), massage, heat treatments, therapeutic baths, exercises, daily naps, and large amounts of the B vitamins and vitamins C and E.

Spare parts. When joints are badly destroyed by arthritis, sometimes replacement with an artificial joint is the most satisfactory answer. The major artificial joints now being used are hip (widely used, dramatically effective), feet (gives pain relief and increased walking ability), knee (still experimental), shoulder (early results are encouraging), and wrist (gives limited motion). Contact local chapter of the Arthritis Foundation for recommended surgeons nearest you who do the operation you might need.

SOME LEADING ARTHRITIS CENTERS

Hospital for Special Surgery
    Rheumatology Department
    535 East 70th Street
    New York, N.Y. 10021
Robert B. Brigham Hospital
    125 Parker Hill Avenue
    Boston, Mass. 02120
UCLA Hospital
    Division of Rheumatology
    10833 Le Conte Avenue
    Los Angeles, Calif. 90024
Joe and Betty Alpert Arthritis Treatment Center
    1050 Clermont Street
    Denver, Colo. 80220
Massachusetts General Hospital
    Arthritis Unit
    32 Fruit Street
    Boston, Mass. 02115
Mayo Clinic
    Rochester, Minn. 55901

HAMMER AND BROOM EXERCISES

1. Hold a hammer near its head with your elbow bent. Turn your wrist from left to right and back. Let the weight of the hammer swing your hand over as far as possible each time. Repeat 3 to

6 times with each hand. As you improve, shift your grip farther toward the end of the handle so that the weight of the hammer makes you work harder.

2. Stand with your back against a wall with your heels, buttocks, shoulder blades, and head touching it. Grasp a broomstick or cane in both hands and raise it as high above your head as possible, keeping your elbows as straight as you can. Then lower your arms. Repeat.

3. Grab a broom and push it up as if you were shoveling snow over your right shoulder. Change your grip and repeat the motion over your left shoulder. Repeat.

From "Home Care Programs in Arthritis," courtesy: Arthritis Foundation.

Also see Chapter 7 for hand-strengthening exercises.

TWO UNDERGROUND MEDICINES

DMSO, short for dimethyl sulfoxide, has been shown to reduce pain and increase joint mobility in many persons with osteoarthritis and gout. It has the unique property of being absorbed almost instantly through the skin to the blood stream, thus going quickly to all parts of the body. Research reports indicate DMSO is also effective for: reducing pain and swelling in bursitis, tendonitis, sprains, and strains; reviving hands and feet damaged by frostbite, saving amputation; stimulating healing of open wounds and burns, even when infection is present; reducing pain after surgery; clearing up the ulcers and stiff tissues of scleroderma; relieving pain of shingles, phlebitis, and bedsores.

In the U.S. it can be used legally only on horses, dogs, plants, and in patients in a few medical centers on a limited experimental basis. You can buy DMSO freely in Canada, Japan, Mexico, and many European countries, where it is used frequently. Some people order an industrial grade of the chemical from a farmers' mail order catalogue or chemical or industrial supply house, but this can be dangerous because of unknown impurities. Since the medicine is approved for use in dogs and horses, many veterinarians order it and bootleg it to doctors and friends.

Orgotein, a new anti-inflammatory drug, is being studied in 11 major medical centers in the U.S. and in other countries. It has an outstanding safety record in the trials of its use for arthritis, cataracts, and inflammations of the genito-urinary tract. Investigators are very enthusiastic over its benefits. Orgotein is already available to practicing physicians in Austria, and in the U.S. is available from Diagnostic Data Company in California to veterinarians to treat dogs and horses.

HELPFUL BOOKS AND BOOKLETS

Rheumatoid Arthritis; Osteoarthritis; Gout
The Arthritis Foundation
1212 Avenue of the Americas
New York, N.Y. 10036
Free

How to Cope With Arthritis
National Institutes of Health
Dept. 42
Pueblo, Colo. 81009
60 cents

Flexible Fashions, Publication 1814
Superintendent of Documents
U.S. Government Printing Office
Washington, D.C. 20402.
20 cents
Clothing ideas for women with arthritis.

Your Garden and Your Rheumatism
Canadian Arthritis and Rheumatism Society
900 Yonge Street
Toronto 5, Canada
25 cents
Aids to gardening.

Self-Help Devices
Institute of Rehabilitation Medicine
New York University Medical Center
400 East 34th Street
New York, N.Y. 10016
$4.00
Descriptions, sources, and prices of hundreds of devices.
193 pages.

Toomey J. Gazette
Box 147
Chagrin Falls, Ohio 44022
Suggestions for dealing with disabilities.

ASTHMA

HOW TO RECOGNIZE
Symptoms are wheezing; difficulty in breathing.

WHAT TO DO
Determine what is bringing on the attacks, whether a respiratory infection, cigarette smoke, paint fumes, dust, mold, a cat, dog, bird, or horse, feather pillows, ragweed, or other pollen or food.

Keep in good physical condition, avoiding colds and getting chilled.

Keep windows in the bedroom closed at night. Keep your home at a relative humidity of 45 to 50 percent.

Treat colds, sore throats, and infections promptly.

Keep your diet well balanced and nutritious, eliminating food you are allergic to.

Keep away from paint fumes, dust, and tobacco smoke that may irritate the bronchial tubes.

Give up cigarette smoking completely and irrevocably.

Try to avoid anything that makes you cough.

Get enough exercise.

Get plenty of rest.

FOR THE ACUTE ATTACK

At the first sign of an attack, take a medication for bronchodilation.

To keep mucus loose, drink lots of fluid. Coffee is particularly good because caffeine dilates bronchial tubes and makes breathing easier.

Iodine salts in tablets or in solution are good expectorants.

Use a vaporizer to liquefy mucus.

Other things that sometimes help: daily doses of potassium iodide; drugs such as fenspiride, disodium cromoglycate, and if necessary, corticosteroids; lung lavage with salt water; postural drainage of bronchi; vitamin C.

WHAT'S NEW

Researchers warn that excessive use of aerosol sprays that are designed to relieve asthmatic attacks can actually trigger attacks in some patients. The side reactions have become so prevalent that some allergists urge that they not be used in asthma at all, nor in emphysema or bronchitis. Others feel that they can still be used, but in moderation. They say if you use a device more than three times a day, you are using it too much.

Latest research shows viral infections can trigger asthma attacks, often being related to a person's first attack, as well as later attacks.

Evidence has been found that many asthma sufferers are allergic to cockroaches and tiny pieces of insects often found in house dust. Patients found sensitive can be given desensitization shots.

A new anti-asthmatic steroid spray with no serious side effects, known as beclomethasone, has become available in prescription in England, Scandinavian countries, West Germany, Australia, New Zealand, and Canada. It is under test in the U.S.

PURSED-LIP BREATHING

Place a candle on a table and adjust the height of the wick to the level of your mouth, about 6 inches from your lips. Place both hands on the upper abdomen. Inhale deeply, pressing your hands inward and upward and blow against the flame so as to bend it without extinguishing the candle. Do this exercise for five minutes once or twice daily. Increase the candle distance 2 to 4 inches each day until you are able to bend the flame at 36 inches.

BACK TROUBLE

HOW TO RECOGNIZE

Pain may be in the back or may be referred to the leg. It can be due to stress from heavy lifting, bad posture, muscle imbalance, or may be caused by infection, strain, injury, kidney disorder, a tumor, or even to one leg being a tiny bit longer than the other.

WHAT TO DO

Lose weight if you are overweight. If your weight is normal, stay there.

Treat flat feet (see test for flat feet, Chapter 24).

Use heat.

Sleep on a flat, hard mattress, with a board between mattress and springs.

When you stand, keep lower back flat. When you work in a standing position, put one foot up on a footrest.

For driving, use a hard backrest; sit close enough to steering wheel so knees are bent to work the pedals.

If you work at a desk all day, get up and move around periodically.

Wear properly fitted shoes. See an orthopedic specialist about the possibility of lifts in one shoe.

For acute pain, try aspirin or muscle relaxants, bed rest, and warm baths.

Lift heavy weights properly, bending your knees rather than bending over, and using your leg muscles, not your back, to push up.

Sleep on your side curled up, not on your stomach. You want your back to be curled forward, not arched. If you have trouble maintaining this position, bend your knees toward your chest and put a pillow between them to keep your upper leg from falling down and putting stress on your back muscles. If you must sleep on your back, put a pillow or two under your knees so your back lies flat on the bed.

Do sit-ups and leg raises in the morning to loosen your spine, which may have stiffened overnight.

Keep in shape with regular swimming, brisk walking, or other exercise.

Sit erect; cross your legs to stretch muscles. Don't sit uninterrupted for long periods; get up frequently and stretch. Stop and stretch every hour or so when driving a car.

Avoid bucket seats in a car.

Avoid lifting heavy things or shoveling snow.

Heating pads, whirlpool baths, and bed rest sometimes help relieve pain temporarily.

See your doctor for definitive diagnosis (back pain can be caused by many things from slipped disc to kidney disease or cancer) and for medication or nerve blocks to relieve pain.

Osteopathic manipulation to realign joints and muscles helps many.

Surgery is necessary for about 5 percent of patients.

WHAT'S NEW

Acupuncture is relieving many cases. Be sure the person doing it has been trained in China.

An enzyme called chymopapain, made from papaya, when injected into a ruptured disc chemically digests the protruding tissue. It has given relief in about 80 percent of patients tested.

An implanted electronic device has been developed that when activated by the patient blocks pain impulses to the brain. Available to patients with severe pain who have found no relief by other means. The surgery is done at the Sister Kenny Institute in Minneapolis.

For an acute attack, see Chapter 7 for exercises to relieve low back pain.

RECOMMENDED:
Orthotherapy by Dr. Arthur Michele
    M. Evans & Co.
    216 East 49th Street
    New York, N.Y.
    $6.95
The Bad Back Booklet
    Simmon's Company
    1 Park Avenue
    New York, N.Y. 10016
    Free

BLADDER AND KIDNEY INFECTIONS

HOW TO RECOGNIZE

Painful and frequent urination. Urine sometimes is cloudy or bloody.

WHAT TO DO

Take showers instead of baths.

Wear cotton panties or cotton-crotch pantyhose instead of nylon; nylon holds in heat, increasing chance of infection.

Don't put off urinating when you have to go.

Drink lots of fluids.

If you drink huge amounts of citrus juices, cut down. They sometimes make people prone to urinary tract infections.

Eliminate sugar from the diet.

See doctor immediately for sulfa or antibiotic treatment, which should be continued for six to eight weeks and until two cultures free from infection are obtained.

WHAT'S NEW

If you keep urine acid, it retards bacteria growth. Use cranberry juice, plum juice, or a product called IsoPh.

For chronic bladder infections in women after sexual intercourse, known as honeymoon cystitis, the new treatment is an antibiotic taken immediately after intercourse. It is usually given for about one year, then discontinued.

Canadian doctors have found that daily use of a new low-dose antibiotic (trimethoprim sulfamethozazole) cuts recurrences of urinary tract infections to virtually zero.

Blacks should not take sulfa, which is often used to treat urinary tract infections, unless they have a test to make sure they do not have a blood enzyme deficiency called glucose-6-phosphate-dehydrogenase. If they do have this problem, taking sulfa can cause a serious sudden anemia and even death.

A newly reported simple treatment to prevent further recurrences of infection: Drink lots of fluids and urinate every two hours during the day, and once or twice at night.

A newly discovered old-fashioned remedy for cleansing the bladder: Cut up a watermelon into small cube-sized pieces (use pear if watermelon is not available) and eat a piece about every five minutes throughout the day. Do not eat or drink anything else that day. For the next three days, eat all the melons and fruits of any kind that you want for meals. On the fourth day resume your normal diet.

BRONCHITIS

HOW TO RECOGNIZE

A tight chest and deep coughing.

WHAT TO DO

If your coughing gets mucus and pus up, then do not use a cough suppressant, but ask your druggist for a decongestant expectorant to open up your chest.

If your cough is not getting anything up, ask for a cough suppressant.

If there is wheezing, use a bronchodilator expectorant.

Abstain from alcohol, which makes bronchitis worse.

If there is evidence of bacterial infection with thick yellow or green sputum, some doctors recommend antibiotics.

Use a vaporizer or steam.

Do not smoke; avoid air pollutants of all kinds.

If you frequently have bronchitis, you should have an influenza vaccine for protection each fall.

WHAT'S NEW

Highly spiced chicken soup and other hot spices can help unclog mucus of lungs and nose in bronchitis and other respiratory infections, according to Dr. Irwin Zement, a respiratory disease specialist at UCLA School of Medicine. In the *Journal of the American Medical Association* he recommends lots of garlic, pepper, curry powder, hot chili, and other spices.

Most helpful of all, researchers say, is to drink a gallon of fluid each day.

BUNIONS

WHAT TO DO

Go to a doctor or a podiatrist for injections to draw off fluids to reduce size, or for surgery to straighten toe.

WHAT'S NEW

A treatment called osteotripsy, which requires a small incision on the side of the toe through which a drill is inserted to cut down calcium deposits and bony bumps.

CARPAL TUNNEL SYNDROME

This is a weakness caused by compression of a nerve going through the wrist.

HOW TO RECOGNIZE

A tingling sensation plus decreased feeling in the hands, increasing weakness of the wrist and hand, sometimes shooting pains.

WHAT TO DO

See your doctor. Surgery is frequently necessary.

WHAT'S NEW

Many cases are being treated successfully with vitamin B_6, avoiding the need for surgery. See *Vita-*

min B_6: The Doctor's Report, by Dr. John M. Ellis and James Presley, Harper and Row, 10 East 53rd Street, New York, N.Y. 10022, $7.95.

DIVERTICULOSIS

Diverticula are tiny pockets in weakened sections of the wall of the large intestine. If they fill with fecal material and become infected, it is known as diverticulitis. Surgery is sometimes necessary to prevent rupture and peritonitis.

WHAT TO DO

Avoid alcohol. Eat a high-fiber diet, with whole grain bread, whole grain cereal, fruit, and vegetables. Take bran tablets (one study at the Royal Infirmary in England showed that bran tablets were even better than bulk laxative plus a high fiber diet).

EPILEPSY

Epilepsy is due to an abnormal nerve discharge in an injured portion of the brain. The injury can be produced by a blow, an infection, a stopped-up blood vessel, lack of oxygen, impaired circulation, or by injury before birth.

HOW TO RECOGNIZE

Symptoms can be so mild that the victim doesn't even notice them. They might only be a spell of dizziness, a momentary loss of consciousness, a rhythmic jerking of the arm or eyes, a staring off into space; or there can be a full-blown seizure with violent jerking of the entire body.

WHAT TO DO

Seizures usually can be prevented with medication; sometimes they clear up spontaneously, sometimes brain surgery is necessary.

Write to the National Epilepsy League for a list of physicians especially skilled in diagnosing and treating epilepsy. (For proper diagnosis a doctor should take a detailed history, obtain an awake and sleep EEG, blood count, urinalysis, x-rays, and do a neurologic examination. In addition, psychological testing, serum calcium, glucose tolerance, and pneumoencephalography may be advisable.)

With your doctor, try different medications for several months to find the best one. (What is good for one type of epilepsy may aggravate another type, so that medication must be carefully selected.)

WHAT'S NEW

A new drug. Sodium valproate is proving exceptionally effective in treating certain types of epilepsy. The drug is awaiting final F.D.A. approval, but is now available from Abbott Laboratories to neurologists or family physicians with specialty training in neurology. (Patients with focal, temporal lobe, or traumatic epilepsy do better on carbamazepine, specialists say.)

Epilepsy Diet. A number of research studies have shown that a special diet will help the person with epilepsy, reducing the number of seizures in most, sometimes eliminating them completely.

The diet: high protein with plenty of eggs, liver, nuts; whole grains, low carbohydrate (only 10 to 30 grams per day); increased fat with equal amounts of saturated and unsaturated fats; supplements of calcium, magnesium, and manganese; vitamin supplements, especially A, C, D, E, and the B vitamins (including folic acid). The dieter avoids: sugar, breads, cereals, pastries, fluorides, additives, butter substitutes. Have your doctor contact Miller Pharmacal in West Chicago for further details.

Epileptic persons can obtain life insurance and low-cost medications from the National Epilepsy League, 116 South Michigan, Chicago, Ill. 60603.

RECOMMENDED:
Total Rehabilitation of Epileptics
U.S. Government Printing Office
Washington, D.C. 20402
$1.25

FATIGUE

HOW TO RECOGNIZE
The fatigue that doesn't have an obvious cause is the fatigue to be concerned about.

WHAT TO DO
Change your diet so you have egg, meat, or other protein for breakfast; eliminate sugar and heavy alcohol intake. Take vitamin and mineral supplements, including iron and brewer's yeast.

See your doctor for possible vitamin B$_{12}$ shots and for a general work-up. Fatigue can be caused by iron deficiency, folic acid deficiency, several kinds of anemia, hormone upsets, underactive thyroid, hyperventilation, hypoglycemia, liver disease, early heart or lung failure, an infection such as mononucleosis, depression, or cancer.

GALLSTONES
Stones may form in the gallbladder and be present for years before causing trouble. The major trouble occurs if they move from the gallbladder to the bile duct and get lodged there, in which case they produce excruciating pain.

HOW TO RECOGNIZE
Vague discomfort and pain in the upper abdomen, indigestion, nausea, intolerance to fatty foods, possible slight jaundice.

The stones will show up on x-ray.

WHAT TO DO
Usual treatment is removal by surgery.

WHAT'S NEW
A new drug called chenic acid that is already used in Europe. It dissolves the gallstones and usually makes surgery unnecessary.

Dr. Sergey A. Tuzhilin, of the First Moscow Medical Institute in Moscow, reports that lecithin tablets taken daily will change bile acid composition and help dissolve the gallstones.

Stay off fat-free diets. Your gallbladder does not empty properly without some fat; in experimental animals fed little or no fat, gallstones will form.

Some doctors claim a quart of tomato juice a day will help.

GOUT

HOW TO RECOGNIZE
Because uric acid crystallizes and collects in joints, there is inflammation and pain in a joint such as the big toe.

WHAT TO DO
Eliminate high uric acid foods: sweetbreads, brains, liver, sardines, anchovies, gravies, beer, and other alcohol.

Drink a great deal of water.

See your doctor for prescription medicines to counteract excessive accumulation of uric acid.

WHAT'S NEW
There is evidence that a low-carbohydrate diet, eliminating all sugar and refined starches, will help.

HEADACHE
Sinus trouble, tension, colds, allergies, hunger, smoking, high blood pressure, hypoglycemia, ill-fitting dentures or imperfect bite, an illness coming on, or even a brain tumor can cause headaches; some headaches can be life-saving warning signals to you.

WHAT TO TRY

Fresh air and exercise.

A hot cup of coffee or tea.

A drink (unless it's a migraine headache, which alcohol makes worse).

An aspirin (or aspirin substitute).

A protein snack.

A neck and scalp massage, a heating pad, or a soak in a hot bath.

Meditation or relaxation exercises; biofeedback exercises.

An antihistamine (and if you think your headaches are caused by an allergy, try to avoid the offending food or substance).

Lying down in a dark, quiet room, with a cold wet towel on the forehead.

For a sinus headache: a hot shower to open up passages.

In children who often become dehydrated from hard playing, a large glass of water will help!

If headaches occur often, are severe, seem to be increasing in intensity, are accompanied by other symptoms, or if a severe headache comes on suddenly in a youngster or teenager, it can be serious; call your doctor.

WHAT'S NEW

For migraine headaches, ergotamine preparations, Sansert, Diazepam, propanolol, and methysergide often help. (Doctor's advice and prescription needed.) Some migraine sufferers can stop an attack by breathing oxygen from a tank stored at home.

There is new evidence that headaches can be caused by birth control pills and even by getting too much sleep.

Acupuncture. It sometimes works for chronic migraines.

A NEW HELP FOR HEADACHE THAT REALLY WORKS

The new technique of biofeedback is helping even the worst cases of migraine headache as well as tension, cluster, and other headaches. Subjects learn to produce a relaxed state and reduce blood flow to the scalp. Dr. Joseph Sargent at the Menninger Foundation reports that three out of four migraine sufferers were significantly helped, many of them freed from disabling headaches for the first time in decades. The foundation is looking for participants in their studies of migraine, sinus, tension, and cluster headaches and Raynaud's disease. For further information call or write:

Headache Research and Treatment Project
The Menninger Foundation
P.O. Box 829
Topeka, Kans. 66601

Do-it-yourself acupressure. Dr. Howard Kurtland, neurologist of San Francisco, says he has stopped giving medicines for headache pain and uses this method instead: Press thumbnail into the triangle of flesh between the thumb and index finger for 15 to 30 seconds. Repeat as necessary.

A yoga exercise for headache. This alternate breathing exercise will help relieve tension headaches and also open up sinus passages.

Sit comfortably; keep your spine straight but not rigid. Place the right thumb on the right nostril, inhale deeply through the left nostril (expanding the abdomen) to the count of 5. Close the left nostril, release the right nostril and exhale (pulling in the abdomen) to the count of 10. Without stopping, inhale again through the right nostril to the count of 5 and exhale through the left nostril. As your lungs expand, increase your breathing times to 8 seconds for inhalation and 16 for exhalation.

Ice cream headache. Ever eat something cold and get an immediate head pain? Decrease the pain by curling your tongue back and pressing it against the roof of your mouth, says the *New England Journal of Medicine*.

HEARING LOSS

Can be caused by ear wax, enlarged or infected adenoids or tonsils, colds, allergies, sinus infections, cigarette smoking, or nerve damage.

WHAT TO DO

See your doctor.

WHAT'S NEW

An electrode implanted in the inner ear is helping some deaf people hear some sounds; but the surgery is still experimental. It can help only patients who suffered hearing loss after they had learned to speak normally. It gives them a one-tone signal that does not sound like normal speech or music, but helps the patients read lips and talk more intelligibly.

Hearing-ear dog. Just becoming available. Dogs trained by the American Humane Association in Dallas to signal deaf people when the baby cries, the doorbell or phone rings.

FREE BOOKLET
Migraine—Information for Patients
   Dr. Donald Dalesio
   Organon Pharmaceuticals
   West Orange, N.J.

HEPATITIS

Caused by a virus that attacks the liver, it can be transmitted from person to person, by polluted water, or by a contaminated needle used for injections.

HOW TO RECOGNIZE

Symptoms are: fever, nausea, loss of appetite, weakness, headache, muscle pain, yellow color to skin or whites of eyes, urine may be dark, stools may be pale.

There may be pain under the ribs.

Symptoms can be so mild that a person doesn't know that he has the disease, or they can be serious enough to cause debilitating effects for months or even death by liver failure.

WHAT TO DO

See your doctor.

WHAT'S NEW

Hepatitis has been found to be astoundingly prevalent among hospital personnel and unwittingly spread by them. One public health survey showed 58 percent of physicians and dentists in one state showed evidence of having had hepatitis at some time. Among general surgeons it is estimated that about 50 percent *have* the clinical disease.

New experimental treatment: Most people recover from hepatitis naturally after a few weeks of rest and general treatment. But about 10 percent carry the virus in their blood indefinitely and become carriers of the disease. Doctors are finding that using interferon, a natural body substance that protects against illness, seems to wipe out the remaining virus.

New vaccine. Hepatitis B, also known as serum hepatitis, is frequently transmitted sexually. New research shows that when one spouse gets the disease, the other can be injected with a special gamma globulin shot called HBIG for protection.

Vitamin C. Giving it intravenously often clears hepatitis in 48 hours, new studies show.

HERNIA

Another name for hernia is a rupture, which actually is a weak spot in the muscle wall through which a part of your intestine or other organ can protrude, making a lump in the skin.

HOW TO RECOGNIZE

Inguinal hernia: The intestine begins to bulge out in the groin, forming a soft lump that can be felt through the skin. It sometimes becomes bad enough to extend down into the scrotum where the testicles are contained.

Femoral hernia. Most common in women. The bulging-out is in the upper thigh.

Umbilical hernia. The navel protrudes. Usually occurs in children.

Postoperative hernia. Bulging can occur if the incision does not heal properly after an operation.

Hernias may be aggravated by lifting, straining, coughing, sneezing, or in straining for a bowel movement when constipated.

WHAT TO DO

See a doctor immediately. Strangulation can develop, in which a loop of intestine gets caught and its blood supply cut off, causing gangrene of the intestine, a very dangerous condition.

Treatment: a simple operation to repair the weakness in the muscle.

HIATAL HERNIA

Because of weakness in the diaphragm muscle, a small part of the stomach protrudes up through the diaphragm opening and sometimes spills gastric juice up onto the delicate linings of the esophagus.

HOW TO RECOGNIZE

Symptoms are: heartburn, indigestion, chest pain, belching, and flatulence.

WHAT TO DO

Take antacids.

Eliminate sugar and refined carbohydrates from the diet.

Lose weight if obese.

Stop smoking.

Do not wear girdles or other tight things around abdomen.

Cut down fats, citrus juices, chocolate, alcohol or other foods that seem to bring on heartburn.

Elevate the head of the bed, or use several pillows when sleeping.

If symptoms still do not clear, surgery may be necessary.

WHAT'S NEW

Old-fashioneds with angostura bitters do not seem to produce the same problems other alcoholic drinks do.

HYPERVENTILATION

This is "overbreathing," usually caused by anxiety or by habit.

HOW TO RECOGNIZE

The patient first becomes lightheaded, tired, and may develop a sensation of suffocation. This may be followed by numbness and tingling of the arms and legs, along with dizziness and blurred vision. This often frightens the person so that he breathes even more deeply and faster, causing chest pain, muscle spasm, and even fainting.

WHAT TO DO

Breathe in and out of a paper bag to build up carbon dioxide.

Try to discover the anxiety triggering the episodes, and work with your doctor to combat it.

KIDNEY DISEASE

Kidney disease can occur in anyone, even children. Those most susceptible are people whose families have a history of kidney disease and those with high blood pressure. It often follows a streptococcal infection of the throat, tonsils, or sinuses.

HOW TO RECOGNIZE

Burning or difficulty during urination, more frequent urination, particularly at night, passage of bloody-appearing urine, puffiness around eyes, swelling of hands and feet, especially in children, pain in the small of the back, just below the ribs, high blood pressure.

WHAT TO DO

See your doctor and increase your water intake. (Animal experiments show that some kidney disease can often be prevented and cured by extra water intake for 7 to 14 days. In humans, the equivalent would be several quarts of water a day.)

KIDNEY STONES

Stones can occur in the kidneys, bladder, or anywhere in the urinary tract.

HOW TO RECOGNIZE

Acute attack of pain in the pelvic region, possible nausea, vomiting, chills, and fever.

WHAT TO DO

Take large amounts of vitamin C and Bs, eliminate sugar and refined starches from the diet, reduce calcium intake; increase magnesium.

Stop drinking milk and eating milk products such as ice cream because of the large amount of calcium.

Sometimes the stones can be dissolved by medicines.

Sometimes they must be crushed or removed by surgery.

WHAT'S NEW

Drink cranberry juice; or the juice pressed from raw beets (not cooked), sipped by the teaspoonful all day. (Do not drink beet juice in large amounts, it can make you sick.) Some patients say after drinking the beet juice, which stimulates the kidneys to eliminate gravel and stones, they can often hear the stones hit the toilet bowl as they urinate.

MENSTRUAL CRAMPS

WHAT TO DO

Curl up with a heating pad. Take aspirin. Massage back, abdomen, and legs to stimulate circulation. Sometimes using a birth control pill with estrogen will help.

WHAT'S NEW

Orgasm often relieves menstrual cramps.

Dr. John C. Jennings of the University of Tennessee is finding that indomethacin will relieve pain and cramps when taken three times a day with meals. But it is a prescription drug, and will not be approved for this use until further tests are done, he says.

Vitamin B_6 is often helpful.

MONONUCLEOSIS

Usually affects young adults, particularly those living in groups, such as college students, soldiers, nurses.

HOW TO RECOGNIZE

Fever, sore throat, swelling of glands of neck, weakness and fatigue, sometimes skin rash.

A blood test gives definite diagnosis.

WHAT TO DO

See your doctor. Since liver damage and other serious complications can occur, bed rest and medical care are essential.

Early reports are coming in on benefits from vitamin C treatment.

PARKINSONISM (PARKINSON'S DISEASE, SHAKING PALSY)

All tremors are not Parkinsonism. There are also tremors caused by alcoholism, lithium poisoning, multiple sclerosis, dilantin intoxication, brain tumors, acute infectious states, and even arthritis. Parkinsonism usually begins at about age 55.

HOW TO RECOGNIZE

Short jerky steps and scuffing of the feet when walking. Sense of heaviness in an arm or leg, followed by gentle tremor in one hand.

Handwriting small, difficult to read, speech blurred, chewing difficult, movement an effort.

Body often stooped, with hands and arms out in front.

Face muscles masklike and motionless.

Gum muscles shrink, so dentures may be loose. Many muscles rigid.

The intellect is not damaged, but the person is often depressed.

WHAT TO DO

See your doctor for L-dopa and other medications. It is also helpful for the patient to have speech therapy, to do stretch and pull exercises, to have neck traction to reduce neck rigidity, to have electrical stimulation of muscles, to have whirlpool baths, and to have hot and cold packs.

WHAT'S NEW

Surgery, including cryosurgery (surgery with a freezing cold probe into the brain that has been producing 93 percent success in abolishing tremor).

Other new treatments include electrical stimulation of the brain and oxygen treatment in hyperbaric chambers.

PNEUMONIA

Pneumonia can be caused by bacteria or by viruses. The most dangerous pneumonia is caused by the influenza virus, which can cause death.

If pneumonia affects one or more lobes of the lung, it is called *lobar pneumonia*. If both lungs are affected, it is sometimes called *double pneumonia*. If it is mostly around the bronchial tubes, it is called *bronchopneumonia*.

HOW TO RECOGNIZE

Cough, sharp chest pains, blood-streaked sputum, high fever, often starting with a shaking chill.

Viral pneumonia usually has a gradual onset; the patient is chilly but doesn't have shaking chills. His cough produces only a little sputum. Breathing is rapid, but he has no respiratory distress. Bacterial pneumonia starts very abruptly, with shaking chills and fever; there is heavy sputum production and shortness of breath. This type of pneumonia often follows an upper respiratory infection.

WHAT TO DO

A doctor should always be called. Usually home treatment is possible, but often hospitalization is required. Patients with viral pneumonia can usually be treated at home with aspirin for the aches and fever. Patients with bacterial pneumonia usually need erythromycin or other antibiotics.

PREMENSTRUAL TENSION

HOW TO RECOGNIZE

Tension, fatigue, moodiness, and irritability occurring for several days before the menstrual period.

Bloating and puffiness of tissue.

WHAT TO DO

Limit the amount of fluid you drink in the days before your period.

Eliminate salt, sugar, and carbohydrates from your diet; this will produce water loss for several days.

Ask your doctor about diuretic pills to rid the body of excess fluid.

Have tests done to see if you are secreting too much aldosterone hormone from the adrenal glands before your period. If so, medicine can counteract.

Hormones sometimes help, and many women on birth control pills say they no longer have premenstrual problems.

SHINGLES (HERPES ZOSTER)

HOW TO RECOGNIZE

Mild discomfort of the trunk, abdomen, neck, arms, or legs which develops into a severe burning pain.

Blisters form over reddened skin; they later dry up and leave little pink scars.

WHAT TO DO

See your doctor.

WHAT'S NEW

Injection of a local anesthetic like procaine or lidocaine has been found to stop pain and cause blisters to scale and fall away in 7 to 10 days.

Good results are being reported with a combination treatment that includes a corticosteroid drug to reduce inflammation and help prevent scarring, gamma globulin to help control the virus, tetracycline to prevent secondary bacterial infection. The treatment has proved very effective in patients tested, with relief of pain, shorter duration of blisters, and lessened pain.

SICKLE CELL ANEMIA

Sickle cell anemia is an inherited blood disorder. It is *not* contagious. The red cells are long, pointed, and often curved like a sickle. They sometimes stick together, clogging small arteries and veins, which causes many of the symptoms.

HOW TO RECOGNIZE

Paleness of fingernails, toenails, mucous membranes of the gums and inside the eyelid.

Yellow color of the whites of the eyes.

Shortness of breath, especially after exercising.

Frequent headaches.

Episodes of severe abdominal pain.

Pain and swelling of joints, especially hands and feet.

Frequent loss of appetite.

Excessive thirst.

Swelling of lymph glands in neck and under armpits.

Difficulty in fighting infections, with frequent colds or flu.

Leg ulcers, especially around ankles.

Dark urine.

Repeated fatigue.

Crisis attacks that may resemble ulcer, appendicitis, gallbladder attack, rheumatic fever, or heart disease.

WHAT TO DO

Go to a sickle cell clinic or your doctor to have proper lab tests done.

Drink four or five glasses of water, juice, or other beverage daily. Loss of fluids can cause a crisis attack.

Take folic acid tablets along with other vitamins each day.

Stay away from alcohol. It is notorious for making blood cells sickle and bringing on a crisis.

Avoid drugs that contract the blood vessels or produce an acid condition. Check with your doctor on *all* medicines you take.

Avoid low-oxygen areas, they can cause cells to sickle.

Avoid getting chilled and avoid infections; they cause crisis attacks.

Avoid general anesthesia for surgery or dental procedures whenever possible; have a local anesthesia instead.

TREATING A CRISIS

Take a hot bath, or apply local heat. Have someone massage the painful area. Drink a lot of fluids. Keep warm. Wear loose clothing to prevent constriction of the blood supply. If the attack is severe, go to the hospital *immediately*.

IF YOU HAVE SICKLE CELL TRAIT

You have *one* of the sickle cell genes, but *not* both. You can pass the gene on to your children, but you yourself will probably have no symptoms. You can live a full, normal life. Sickle cell trait can *never* turn into sickle cell anemia.

WHAT'S NEW

University of Michigan researchers report successful results using zinc tablets in sickle cell anemia patients (six pills a day). The treatment, still experimental, decreased the number of sickle cells in the blood and relieved symptoms.

At Florida Institute of Technology, encouraging results were found in a small number of patients using buffered aspirin and daily inhalation of oxygen.

At the University of California, San Francisco, a new drug called dimethyladipimidate (DMA) has been shown to have an anti-sickling effect in the laboratory. Clinical studies in people have not been done yet.

RECOMMENDED:
Sickle Cell: A Complete Guide
    Pavilion Publishing Company
    Box 668
    Riverhead, N.Y. 11901
    $2.00

SYSTEMIC LUPUS ERYTHEMATOSUS (SLE)

HOW TO RECOGNIZE

Pain, similar to arthritis, and rash. SLE mimics many other diseases, so often is misdiagnosed.

Symptoms usually become much worse with exposure to sun.

WHAT TO DO

See your doctor for determination of the type and severity. Some of the medical treatments used include liquid nitrogen, a malaria drug called Plaquenil, and cortisone.

ULCER

HOW TO RECOGNIZE

Burning pain in the stomach relieved by taking food, milk, or antacid.

Three factors that raise your risk of getting an ulcer are: *smoking cigarettes, overusing aspirin,* and *drinking too much caffeine*.

And if you already have an ulcer, these same factors will aggravate it.

WHAT TO DO

Eat six small meals a day instead of three large ones (studies at the University of South Florida show six meals produce half as much acid in a day as three meals do).

Use antacid medicines to counteract stomach acids causing the trouble.

Don't smoke.

Don't use aspirin.

Cut down on coffee, colas, greasy or highly spiced foods.

Reduce tensions.

See your doctor for medicines.

WHAT'S NEW

A new drug, cimetidine, which blocks acid secretion, promotes healing and apparently has no side effects. It is said it produces complete healing in a few weeks. Has proved very effective in England; has just been approved by the F.D.A. in the U.S.

Diet concepts are changing: for example, doctors now believe milk can aggravate an ulcer, first giving temporary relief, but then causing higher acid secretions. Low-carbohydrate diets are also proving beneficial.

ULCERATIVE COLITIS

Similar to a stomach ulcer, but it occurs in the intestine. The lesions look like burns—red, inflamed, sometimes oozing blood or pus.

HOW TO RECOGNIZE

Severe diarrhea, sometimes loss of weight, sometimes blood in the stools, weakness.

In advanced cases, there may be arthritis, joint pains, or skin disorders.

WHAT TO DO

Treatment at the moment is filled with controversy. Some doctors prefer bland, low-residue diets without fruits and vegetables; others stress a high-fiber diet, eliminating all sugar and refined starches.

Both groups recommend rest, relaxation, decrease of tension, and plenty of vitamins and minerals.

VAGINAL INFECTION

Many things can make a vaginal infection get started: too much sugar in the diet; antibiotics that kill the good germs as well as the bad germs and so change the normal bacterial picture of the vagina; a change in hormones from pregnancy or birth control pills; a generally run-down condition; or even the beginning stages of diabetes.

HOW TO RECOGNIZE

Vaginal discharge, odor, itching.

WHAT TO DO

Take sitz baths in salt water, washing the salt water into your vagina and cleansing the area with your fingers; or use a mild salt water douche once or twice a day until discharge clears.

If antibiotics are causing a discharge, keep it under control by taking lactobacillus. Some doctors are even having women insert the lactobacillus capsule Do Fus directly into the vagina to counteract infecting yeast or fungus organisms.

Eliminate sugar (which provides the nutrients the infection needs) from your diet.

Do not have intercourse when you have a discharge since your husband can become infected and then reinfect you later.

If discharge becomes green or yellow, becomes heavy, has a very bad odor, or itches or burns you, then see your doctor for medication.

Under no circumstances should you ignore medical treatment because you are too embarrassed or shy to discuss this with your doctor. The condition commonly occurs in all women.

WHAT'S NEW

Many women using vaginal deodorant sprays are complaining of itching, burning, vaginal discharge, rashes, and other problems from sprays.

Colored and perfumed toilet tissue, bubble baths, and some detergents can also cause such irritation.

Douching has also been implicated as a factor in inflammation of the fallopian tubes (salpingitis) and pelvic inflammatory disease. Drs. Hans Neumann and Alan De Cherney of the Yale New Haven Hospital in Connecticut studied more than 800 women and found that of the women with the gynecologic problems, almost 90 percent were frequent douchers—a three times higher rate than the non-diseased women. The two physicians speculate that overdouching may contribute to ascending infections by whatever organism happens to be in the vagina.

Latest research indicates that, of drugs used to fight vaginal fungus infections, the ointment form applied locally is more effective than pills.

Note: Do not douche before going in for a gynecological exam. It makes the Pap test less accurate, and also makes it impossible for the gynecologist to determine what your troublesome discharge is or how bad it is.

If you have repeated vaginal infections without apparent cause, you should have a test for diabetes.

VARICOSE VEINS

HOW TO RECOGNIZE

Varicose veins tend to develop in persons who stand or sit a great deal. Venous blood accumulates in the legs, making the legs feel heavy and full, tired and painful, and actually stretching the veins. The enlarged veins usually appear between ages 20 and 30. If you don't have them by age 40, you won't get them at all.

WHAT TO DO

Make sure your heels aren't too high, shoes too small, or clothing too tight.

For temporary relief use elastic stockings, elevate the legs, and massage.

For permanent relief have surgery to remove the overstretched veins. (Circulation is not disturbed since there are many other veins to supply the legs and feet.)

WHAT'S NEW

A new procedure that may eliminate need for surgery has been described by Dr. Eli Perchuk of Queens Hospital Medical Center in New York. He says excellent results were obtained using a syringe to remove blood from the varicose vein and injecting a chemical solution (sodium tetradecyl sulfate) with another syringe to close off and collapse the vein.

VENEREAL DISEASES

You can get VD from intercourse, from anal or oral sex, even from mutual caressing and petting.

HOW TO RECOGNIZE GONORRHEA

Discharge from the penis, swelling, pain, or redness of the tip of the penis or of genitals in women.

Pain and burning during urination.

Cloudy urine, sometimes a bit of blood.

Mushroomlike odor in women. (In the woman, symptoms may be absent or so mild that in 80 percent of women they go unnoticed.)

After a week or two these symptoms may disappear, but the person is still infected, and can pass the infection to a partner. The bacteria are now invading higher in the body. There may now be: heat, pain, swelling or feeling of heaviness in the genitals, the lower pelvis, or around the anus; pain with bowel movement, or release of pus; enlarged prostate; difficulty in urinating; pain during or after intercourse or during a vaginal examination; low fever, nausea, headache; irregular, painful menstruation.

HOW TO RECOGNIZE SYPHILIS

A painless sore called a chancre on the penis, vagina, lips, tongue, tonsils, or other site of contact.

Tender and swollen glands in the groin.

If treatment is not begun, the second stage appears four to eight weeks later, with infection throughout the body. Symptoms now may include: skin rashes, bumps or sores anywhere on body, eye inflammation, painful bones, swollen glands, hair falling out.

If the symptoms are still not recognized and treated, a third stage may occur anywhere from 3 to 30 years later with lesions in many organs, and the victim may develop syphilitic heart disease, or become crippled, blind, or insane. A pregnant women with the disease can infect her newborn child, or even kill it from the infection.

WHAT TO DO IF YOU SUSPECT GONORRHEA OR SYPHILIS

Go to your doctor or a clinic immediately for firm diagnosis.

SUMMARY OF THE MOST COMMON
SEXUALLY TRANSMITTED DISEASES

All of these diseases can be passed on without sexual contact as well.

DISEASE	INCUBATION	USUAL SYMPTOMS	TREATMENT	POSSIBLE COMPLICATIONS
GONORRHEA Cause: bacterial	1-30 days	Local, genital discharge, pain; often no symptoms in men; usually no symptoms in women	Penicillin, other antibiotics for patient and all sex contacts	Pelvic inflammatory disease, sterility, arthritis, blindness, eye infection in newborns
SYPHILIS Cause: spirochete	10-90 days	First stage: painless pimple on genitals, fingers, lips, breast; second stage: rash, sores, swollen joints, flu-like illness; latent stage: none	Antibiotics for patient, all sex contacts	Brain damage, insanity, paralysis, heart disease, death; damage to skin, bones, eyes, liver, teeth of newborns
HERPES PROGENITALIS Cause: viral	30 hours -6 days	Swollen, tender, painful sores on genitals	None considered completely effective	Severe central nervous system damage or death in infants infected during birth
NON-GONOCOCCAL URETHRITIS Cause: bacterial	5-28 days	Local discharge, frequent urination; often no symptoms	Antibiotics for patient and regular sexual partners	None
TRICHOMONAS VAGINALIS Cause: protozoan	4-28 days	Copious discharge, intense itching, burning and redness of genitals and thighs; painful intercourse; often no symptoms in men	Flagyl tablets for patient and regular sexual partners	Causes nausea in alcohol users
MONILIAL VAGINITIS Cause: fungal	Unknown	Thick, cheesy, offensive discharge; intolerable itching, skin irritation	Nystatin vaginal tablets and/or creams for patient and sexual partners; also antifungal creams or suppositories	Secondary infections by bacteria; mouth and throat infections of newborn
VENEREAL WARTS Cause: viral	30 or more days	Local irritation, itching	Podophylin tincture or surgical removal	Can spread enough to block vaginal opening
LICE, CRABS Cause: 6-legged louse	4 weeks	Intense itching, pin-head blood spots on underwear; small eggs or nits on pubic hair	Kwell cream, lotion or shampoo; cleansing of bed linen and clothing	None
SCABIES Cause: itch mite	4-6 weeks	Severe nighttime itching, raised gray lines in skin where mite burrows	Same	May infest elbows, hands, breasts, and buttocks as well as genitals

Adapted from chart of U.S. Public Health Service Center for Disease Control.

Take the entire course of penicillin or other antibiotic prescribed for you.

Tell all sexual partners immediately so they can have an examination to see if they are infected.

Go back for your follow-up tests to see that the disease is completely cured.

Do not have sexual intercourse for one month after receiving treatment.

WHAT'S NEW

The Sweden story. The number of cases of gonorrhea has tripled in the last 10 years in the U.S.; the number of cases in Sweden has dropped to one half. The reason, experts believe, is the promotion of condoms by the government.

HERPES VIRUS

Genital infection with herpes virus, sweeping the country, is similar to the herpes virus that causes cold sores and fever blisters, may be spread sexually, or through cuts and scrapes. Symptoms: clusters of small blisters, pain, fever, or fatigue for up to 12 days. Once infected, a victim can expect recurrent outbreaks for awhile even though he or she has not been reinfected. The virus apparently remains in the body, reactivated by such diverse things as menstruation, intercourse, overheating, fever, sunburn, overexertion, neurosurgery, acupuncture, tight underwear, or severe stress.

Hot moist packs applied to the genital area four times a day for 10 minutes has been claimed to bring about rapid healing *if it is begun early when the attack first begins*.

Abstain from sex when lesions are evident or recurrence is suspected.

Several drugs being used in Europe look promising for treatment, but have not been sufficiently tested yet. Some ointments will help relieve pain, but not cure.

HOW TO HELP PROTECT YOURSELF FROM GETTING VD

Apply Vaseline or other protective ointment before intercourse.

Use a condom in sexual intercourse, and/or a contraceptive foam or jelly.

Underground Medicine: An iodine compound called Proganasyl, designed to treat nasal infections, was tested in prostitutes and seemed to protect them from gonorrhea for 24 hours when inserted into the vagina before intercourse. The use has not been approved by the F.D.A.

Note: All 50 states now permit children to be treated for venereal disease in public health clinics without the consent or knowledge of parent or guardian. In addition, nearly all states permit the sale of condoms to those under 16.

VD HOTLINE

Operation Venus is a free national VD hotline. Volunteers will provide the name of the nearest public VD clinic or private physician who treats patients free or for minimal fees, and will provide information over the telephone on all sexually transmitted diseases. Will send printed materials to individuals and schools. The toll-free telephone number: (800) 523-1885.

RECOMMENDED:
VD Handbook
> P.O. Box 1000 Station G
> Montreal, Canada H2W 2N1
> Free

The Straight Story on VD
> Hans H. Neumann with Sylvia Simmons
> Warner Paperback
> 75 Rockefeller Plaza
> New York, N.Y. 10020
> $1.25

Various pamphlets are also available from the U.S. Public Health Service Center of Disease Control, 1600 Clifton Road, N.E. Atlanta, Ga. 30333, and the Massachusetts Public Health Department, VD Division, Government Center, 600 Washington Street, Boston, Mass. 02203. Free.

CHAPTER 21

Do-It-Yourself Emergency Techniques for Saving a Life When There Is No Doctor Around

FIRST AID KIT—WHAT SHOULD BE IN IT

Make sure your first aid kit—the one in the house, the one in the car, and the one in the boat—include all of the following:

- A first aid manual
- A bandage scissors or other blunt-pointed scissors
- Tweezers or forceps
- A fever thermometer
- One or more disposable enema packages
- A roll of 1-inch finger bandage
- A roll of 2-inch roller bandage
- A tin of Band-Aids
- A package of double-ended cotton applicators
- Cotton
- Sterilized gauze squares in envelopes
- A roll of adhesive tape
- A plastic bottle of eye-drops
- A plastic bottle of isopropyl alcohol or 70 percent grain alcohol
- Triangular bandage for sling or dressing
- Small package of salt
- Baking soda
- Safety pins

SIX VITAL RULES IN EMERGENCIES WHEN A LIFE MAY BE AT STAKE

1. Keep calm, and keep victim calm.
2. Maintain breathing using artificial respiration when necessary.
3. Stop serious bleeding.
4. Do not move victim unless necessary for safety.
5. Prevent shock by covering victim and raising legs or lowering head slightly.
6. Give nothing by mouth if unconscious or semi-conscious.

HELP!

1. Dial the police 911, or 0 for operator, or look under Ambulance in the yellow pages.
2. State your specific need and the nature of the injuries.
3. Tell the location where help is needed.
4. Give the number of the telephone you are calling from.

Always carry identification, so in case of an accident, your family can be contacted. If you are taken to a hospital, ask that your family doctor be contacted.

IF YOUR DOCTOR DOESN'T ANSWER

To get a doctor in an emergency, go to the nearest large hospital's emergency ward, or call the county medical society number for doctors on call.

DISASTERS

For emergency housing, food, clothing: contact the American Red Cross or the Emergency Division of the local Department of Welfare.

BLEEDING

Wash wound and surrounding area with soap and water. Hold sterile pad or clean cloth over wound until bleeding stops. If necessary apply pressure at pressure points.

Apply gauze dressing. If blood comes through first dressing, do not remove it, but cover with another layer.

Elevate the limb.

DEEP WOUNDS

Stop bleeding with any cloth, do not worry about sterility. Most important is to stop the bleeding.

Get medical help immediately.

Do not put antiseptic or ointment on deep wounds.

GO AT ONCE TO A DOCTOR OR EMERGENCY ROOM IF . . .

- There is spurting bleeding (seconds may count)
- Bleeding continues beyond 4 to 10 minutes
- There is foreign material in the wound that does not wash out easily
- The wound is a deep puncture wound
- The wound is long or wide or may require stitches
- A nerve or tendon may be cut (particularly in hand wounds)
- The wound is on the face or wherever a noticeable scar would be undesirable
- The wound has been in contact with unclean soil or manure
- The wound is from a bite (animal or human)
- Signs of infection appear (pain, reddened area around wound, swelling)

WHERE TO FIND AND USE PRESSURE POINTS

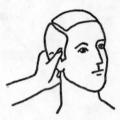

Bleeding from head, above level of eye: Press against head with finger just in front of ear.

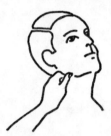

Bleeding below level of eye, above jawbone: Press against hollow spot in jawbone (about an inch in front of angle of the jaw).

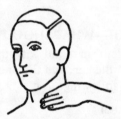

Bleeding from neck, mouth, throat: Hold thumb against back of neck, fingers at side of neck a little below Adam's apple (in hollow just before windpipe, not over windpipe). Press finger toward thumb.

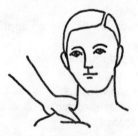

Bleeding armpit, shoulder, upper arm: Finger or thumb goes in hollow behind victim's collarbone; press against first rib.

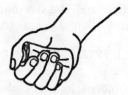

Bleeding from palm: Place thick sterile pad (rolled) in palm, close fingers over it; bandage into closed fist.

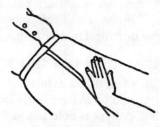

Bleeding from leg: Place heel of hand in middle of depression on inner side of thigh (just below line of groin). Press down against bone.

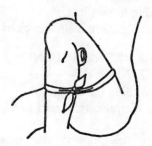

Bleeding below knee: Place pressure pad behind knee, lock lower leg against pad. Tie in place.

If direct pressure, pressure dressing, pressure points, and raising the limb have failed—use a tourniquet.

Use any cloth, belt, stocking, scarf, torn clothing twisted tight with a stick; do not use wire, rope, or anything that will cut into flesh.

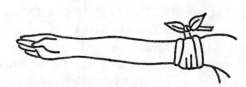

Place tourniquet between wound and heart, but not on or near edge of wound.

Tourniquet must be loosened every 15 minutes or gangrene may set in and cause eventual loss of limb.

Leave tourniquet in full view, do not hide or cover.

IF SOMEONE STOPS BREATHING—HOW BREATHING CAN BE STARTED UP AGAIN

RECOMMENDED RESCUE BREATHING TECHNIQUE

Clear the throat—wipe out any fluid, vomitus, mucus, or foreign body with fingers. For drowning victims, turn head sideways a moment to drain water from mouth.

Place victim on his back.

Tilt the head straight back—extend the neck as far as possible. (This will automatically keep the tongue out of airway.)

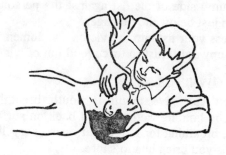

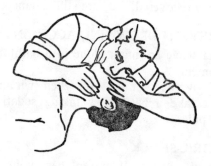

Blow—with victim's lips closed, breathe into nose with a smooth steady action until the chest is seen to rise. (Or breathe into mouth, holding nose closed.)

Remove mouth—allow lungs to empty.

Repeat—continue with relatively shallow breaths, at rate of about 20 per minute. For infants only shallow puffs should be used.

Note: If you are not getting air exchange, quickly recheck position of head, turn victim on his side and give several sharp blows between the shoulder blades to jar foreign matter free. Sweep fingers through victim's mouth to remove foreign matter. DO NOT SLOW UP. If you can see the chest rise and fall, all within reason is being done.

CHOKING

If person can breathe, leave him alone.

If a choking child cannot breathe, turn him head down over your knees and hit him between the shoulder blades.

If something is high in the throat: use a handkerchief to grab the tongue and pull outward; reach in throat and pull out object.

THE HEIMLICH MANEUVER

Stand behind the victim and wrap your arms around his waist.

Grasp your right fist with your left hand with the thumb side of the fist against the person's abdomen just below the rib cage.

Press your fist into the victim's abdomen with a quick upward thrust to force food out of windpipe.

IN DROWNINGS

You can give mouth-to-mouth breathing in water by holding victim's head back on surface of water, breathing for him about once every 10 seconds as you bring him to shore.

Recovered victims must be hospitalized for blood chemistry studies. Even if they appear to be completely recovered, they are still in danger.

PREVENT DROWNING ACCIDENTS

Never leave an infant alone in a bathtub even for a moment.

Don't overexert or show off when swimming.

Don't take a bath after taking sedatives or sleeping pills.

IN ELECTRIC SHOCK

Turn off current. If current cannot be turned off, push victim from live wire with board or pull off with rope. Do not touch or you may be electrocuted yourself.

Begin mouth-to-mouth breathing. Don't give up. It may take as long as 8 hours of mouth-to-mouth breathing before electric shock victim recovers. Keep up rescue breathing until doctor arrives.

The victim has been struck by lightning, you may touch victim and begin mouth-to-mouth breathing right away without danger to yourself.

SIGNS OF SHOCK FROM SERIOUS BLEEDING OR INJURY

Limpness, or unconsciousness, shallow breathing, weak pulse, dilated pupils.

SIGNS OF IMPENDING SHOCK

Weakness, fast weak pulse, pale face, skin cold and damp, forehead and palms sweaty, chills, nausea, shallow or irregular breathing.

TREATMENT FOR SHOCK

Raise victim's feet or lower head.

Protect from cold or wet ground. Cover lightly.

Give fluids if patient is able to swallow. Do not force fluids. Do not give alcohol.

FAINTING

Stretch person out in flat position.

Loosen clothing.

Give nothing to swallow.

Call doctor if person is unconscious very long.

IF YOU COME UPON SOMEONE WHO IS UNCONSCIOUS

Try to determine the cause.

Check for identification card or tag for any illness.

If breathing has stopped, start mouth-to-mouth breathing.

Do not give fluids.

Call doctor.

(If a person is unconscious or is confused and faltering, he may be a diabetic in need of sugar. Check for an identification card, and give him some sugar, or candy, a mint, or a soft drink.

IF A HEART ATTACK OCCURS

CARDIAC RESUSCITATION (EXTERNAL HEART MASSAGE)

This procedure should be used by a doctor or other trained person such as a Red Cross trainee (the Red Cross offers free courses in emergency first aid techniques) because it can be dangerous if done improperly, injuring internal organs and perhaps damaging the heart further. So use it *only* on an unconscious person whose breathing has stopped and whose heart has stopped beating. Use it *only* if mouth-to-mouth breathing fails, you feel no pulse, you fear the person is near death, and you cannot get immediate help.

Place victim on back.

Find pressure area on lower half of breastbone (sternum). (It is one or two inches above the soft spot in the lower chest where the breastbone ends.)

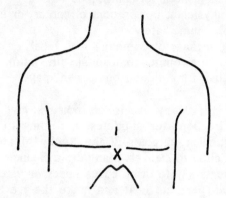

Kneel at victim's side. Press down firmly with heel of your hand on pressure area.

The rhythm is to press down 1 to 2 inches, once every second.

Have another person give mouth-to-mouth resuscitation. (If you are alone, press down on breastbone 15 times, then give 2 mouth-to-mouth inflations.)

Continue until doctor arrives, or person begins breathing for himself.

FOR SMALL CHILDREN

Press with two fingers on the *middle* of the breastbone.

Rhythm is to press down 1 inch per second.

SIGNS OF STROKE

Face is red or pale gray, pupil of one eye may be larger than other.

Part of body may be weak or cannot be used, one corner of mouth may droop.

Speech may be difficult or slurred.

Patient may be unconscious.

WHAT TO DO

Keep patient quiet. If breathing has stopped, begin rescue breathing.

Call doctor immediately.

HEAD INJURIES

Have victim lie down on his side so air passage does not become blocked.

Control bleeding, but do not press upon possible skull fracture.

Do not move head if there is bleeding or clear fluid coming from nose, mouth, or ears.

Call physician immediately.

HOW TO RECOGNIZE A BRAIN CONCUSSION

There may be headache, vomiting, a stiff neck; pupils of the eye may be unequal.

HOW TO TELL IF A BONE IS BROKEN

Part looks deformed. Arm or leg is swollen in one place; finger pressure causes severe pain. You cannot move part without severe pain. The skin may be broken (compound fracture) or may not be broken (simple fracture).

TREATMENT

The purpose of treatment is to keep the part from moving.

Have the patient lie down.

Stop any serious bleeding by pressure and bandaging.

Cut clothing away gently so injured part is not moved.

If skin is broken, apply clean dressing, but no antiseptic.

If skin is not broken, cover with cool compresses.

Put something soft around injured area to protect it, then make splint out of boards, broomstick, tightly rolled newspapers, anything rigid. Splint on *both* sides of injury and continue the splint far enough to include adjacent joints and so prevent motion. Fasten splint with cloth or bandages in at least three places.

Call an ambulance or take patient to hospital.

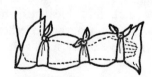

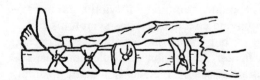

FOR POSSIBLE NECK OR SPINE INJURY

If a victim cannot move his fingers or toes or has a tingling or numb feeling in any part of his body, he may have a broken neck or spine.

Do not bend or twist him in any way. Do not put a pillow under his head. Don't pull him out of a wrecked car unless there is danger of fire. Don't lift him or move him.

Don't rush him to the hospital. Wait for an ambulance or physician to come. (If you absolutely must move him, keep his back and neck straight by making an emergency stretcher from a door, a ladder, planks of wood, or a coat fastened around two poles.)

POISON!

Speed is essential. Act before the body has time to absorb the poison. If possible, one person should begin treatment while another calls a physician or an ambulance.

WHEN TO SUSPECT POISONING

There is a strange odor on the breath, discoloration of lips or mouth, pain or burning sensation in the throat, empty bottles or opened packages near children, evidence in mouth of eating wild berries or leaves, unconsciousness, confusion, or sudden illness when access to poisons is possible.

FOR INHALED POISONS

Get victim to fresh air immediately. Apply rescue breathing if breathing has stopped.

Keep victim quiet and warm.

Do not give alcohol.

Do not become a victim yourself by breathing the same fumes.

Call a physician.

Warning: Do not mix bleaches, household cleaners, ammonia, or vinegar together. Some such home mixtures give off harmful gases.

FOR SWALLOWED POISONS

Give water or milk immediately to dilute poison.

Do not induce vomiting if victim is unconscious, is having convulsions, has symptoms of severe pain or burning or has swallowed kerosene, gasoline, lighter fluid, toilet bowl cleaner, rust remover, drain cleaner, lye, acid, iodine, washing soda, ammonia, insecticide, paint thinner, or any strong corrosive or bleach.

Do induce vomiting for any poison that is *not* corrosive. Stick your finger or spoon at back of victim's throat, or give 2 teaspoons of salt in glass of warm water, or give one ounce of syrup of ipecac (one tablespoon for child), plus water.

Call physician, poison control center, or nearest hospital immediately.

Bring package or container with label, or sample of victim's vomitus to hospital with victim.

See chart for antidotes on opposite page.

Warning: Many labels on poisons give the wrong directions for antidotes, according to Dr. Barry Rumack, director of the Rocky Mountain Poison Center in Denver. Many drain cleaners and lye products say to drink citrus juices or vinegar, which can generate heat and make the lye burn more severe.

WHAT TO DO NOW TO GUARD AGAINST THE FUTURE

Buy a universal antidote for poisoning called Unidote from your pharmacist and keep it in your medicine chest *at all times*. Also keep on hand syrup of ipecac (to induce vomiting) and activated charcoal (to carry toxins from the system).

In Foster City, Calif., the police department provides residents with strips of miniature stop signs. Children can easily be taught the meaning of the stop sign. Parents can place them on pill bottles, insect sprays, or any poison. If you want stickers or your local police department wants to know how to begin such a program, write to Chief of Police, 1040 Hillsdale Boulevard, Foster City, Calif. 94404.

THESE PLANTS CAN BE DANGEROUS

They can cause severe symptoms, and even death, if eaten.

- Azalea leaves, stems, berries
- Bleeding heart, any part
- Boxwood
- Buttercup
- Castor bean
- Cherry leaves, twigs
- Daffodil bulb, narcissus bulb, hyacinth bulb, crocus bulb

- Dieffenbachia, elephant ear
- Foxglove
- Ground cherry
- Hemlock
- Holly
- Horse chestnut
- Hydrangea
- Iris, any part
- Jimson weed (stinkweed) flowers, leaves, seeds
- Larkspur, any part
- Lily of the valley, any part
- Mayapple
- Mistletoe
- Mushroom (80 kinds)
- Nightshade

- Oleander, any part
- Peach leaves, twigs
- Poinsettia
- Pokeweed
- Privet berries
- Rhododendron leaves, stems, berries
- Rhubarb leaves
- Sweet pea, any part
- Tomato leaves and potato leaves
- Wisteria pods, leaves, stems, berries
- Yew, berries, foliage

The Sinister Garden. Describes 56 common poisonous plants with identifying drawings. Available free from Wyeth Laboratories, P.O. Box 8299, Philadelphia, Pa. 19101.

SPECIFIC ANTIDOTES FOR SPECIFIC POISONS

If you know exactly what the poison is, give these specific antidotes before taking the person to the hospital.

IF THE PERSON TOOK THIS POISON:	DO THIS:
Alkalis, lye, ammonia, drainpipe cleaners, washing soda	Give salad oil, cooking oil, melted butter, or a glass or two of milk.
Acids	Do not force vomiting. Give a cup of milk of magnesia, or 2 tablespoons of baking soda in pint of water, then raw egg whites in water. Or a glass or two of milk. Or about ¼ glass of any salad or vegetable oil.
Petroleum distillates, kerosene, gasoline, benzine, naphtha, lighter fluid, inflammable cleaning fluids.	Do not force vomiting. Give ½ cup of mineral oil. Give strong coffee or tea. Keep warm to combat shock. Give artificial respiration if necessary.
Sleeping pills, barbiturates, sedatives, opiates, codeine, morphine, paregoric	Induce vomiting. Give strong black coffee. Keep patient awake, walk him about. Give artificial respiration if necessary.

IF THE PERSON TOOK THIS POISON:	DO THIS:
Salicylate overdose, aspirin, headache and cold pills, oil of wintergreen	Induce vomiting. Give syrup of ipecac. Or 1 teaspoon baking soda in one pint of water. Give strong coffee.
Carbolic acid, phenol, creosote, creosol disinfectants	Do not force vomiting. Give soapsuds immediately. Or give Epsom salts (2 tablespoons per pint of water). Then large amounts of lukewarm water. Also give flour or cornstarch diluted in water. Or raw egg whites in water. Do not give alcoholic drinks.
Iodine	Give flour or cornstarch in water; bread; large amounts of starchy substances. Induce vomiting. Repeat starch and vomiting until vomited material has no blue color.
Wood alcohol, rubbing alcohol, denatured alcohol, methanol	Induce vomiting. Give tablespoon of baking soda in quart of warm water. Repeat vomiting, then soda solution. Follow with glass of milk containing teaspoon of baking soda.

POISON CONTROL CENTER NUMBERS

ALABAMA
  Montgomery .... (205) 265-2341

ALASKA
  Juneau .... (907) 588-6311

ARIZONA
  Tucson .... (602) 884-0111

ARKANSAS
  Little Rock .... (501) 661-2242

CALIFORNIA
  Berkeley .... (415) 843-7900

COLORADO
  Denver .... (303) 388-6111

CONNECTICUT
  Hartford .... (203) 566-3456

DISTRICT OF COLUMBIA
  Washington .... (202) 835-4080

FLORIDA
  Jacksonville .... (904) 354-3961

GEORGIA
  Atlanta .... (404) 656-4839

HAWAII
  Honolulu .... (808) 531-7776

ILLINOIS
  Springfield .... (217) 525-7747

IDAHO
  Boise .... (208) 384-2494

INDIANA
  Indianapolis .... (317) 633-5490

IOWA
  Des Moines .... (515) 281-5785

KANSAS
  Topeka .... (913) 296-3708

KENTUCKY
  Frankfort .... (502) 564-4830

LOUISIANA
  New Orleans .... (504) 527-5822

MAINE
  Augusta .... (207) 623-1511

MARYLAND
  Baltimore .... (301) 382-2668

MASSACHUSETTS
  Boston .... (617) 727-2700

MICHIGAN
  Lansing .... (517) 373-1320

MINNESOTA
  Minneapolis .... (612) 378-1150

MISSISSIPPI
  Jackson .... (601) 354-6650

MISSOURI
  Jefferson City .... (314) 635-4111

MONTANA
  Helena .... (406) 449-2544

NEBRASKA
  Lincoln .... (402) 477-5211

NEVADA
  Carson City .... (702) 882-7458

NEW HAMPSHIRE
  Concord .... (603) 225-6611

NEW JERSEY
  Trenton .... (609) 292-5616

NEW MEXICO
  Santa Fe .... (505) 827-2663

NEW YORK
  Albany .... (518) 744-2121

NORTH CAROLINA
  Raleigh .... (919) 829-3446

NORTH DAKOTA
  Bismark .... (701) 224-2348

OHIO
  Columbus .... (614) 469-2544

OKLAHOMA
  Oklahoma City .... (405) 427-6232

OREGON
  Portland .... (503) 228-9181

PENNSYLVANIA
  Harrisburg .... (717) 787-6436

RHODE ISLAND
  Providence .... (401) 521-7100

SOUTH CAROLINA
  Columbia .... (803) 758-5664

SOUTH DAKOTA
  Pierre .... (605) 224-5911

TENNESSEE
  Nashville .... (615) 741-3644

TEXAS
  Austin .... (512) 453-6631

UTAH
  Salt Lake City .... (801) 328-6191

VIRGINIA
  Richmond .... (804) 644-4111

WASHINGTON
  Olympia .... (206) 753-5871

WEST VIRGINIA
  Charleston .... (304) 348-2971

WISCONSIN
  Madison .... (608) 266-1511

WYOMING
  Cheyenne .... (307) 777-7275

If your state or local poison control center or your doctor is unavailable, a poison control center in Nebraska will answer all long distance calls night or day. Call (402) 553-5400.

For suspected food poisoning, doctors can call a 24-hour hot line in Atlanta, (404) 633-3311.

SNAKE BITE

Severe swelling or instant sharp pain usually means the snake is poisonous. Also bite marks from poisonous snakes usually show the puncture holes from the fangs at the front of the bite mark (see drawing below). Poisonous snakes in the U.S. are rattlesnakes, copperheads, moccasins, and coral snake.

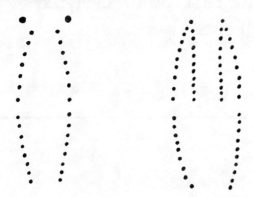

Poisonous bite   *Non-Poisonous bite*

Place a tourniquet between the bite and the heart (loosen every 15 minutes, move up further if swelling spreads).

Sterilize a sharp knife or razor blade with alcohol or by holding in flame; pinch the skin together and make ¼ to ½ inch light (*not* deep) cuts across the puncture marks.

Suck out venom for 30 minutes with suction cup or by mouth (unless you have sores in your mouth), and spit out.

Keep victim still as possible.

Contact a doctor or hospital immediately for an antivenom injection.

Do not give coffee, whiskey, or other stimulant; it will make poison spread faster.

Precautions: Wear high leather boots to protect your ankles in snake country. Look before you step or put your hands somewhere. Carry a snake bite kit in snake country.

SPIDER BITES

Watch out for the Black Widow Spider and the Brown Recluse Spider. Both are poisonous and prevalent everywhere. The Black Widow is shiny black, ½ inch long, has an hourglass red or orange spot. The Brown Recluse lives in dark corners indoors and out and has a dark violin-shaped mark on its back extending from its head.

Symptoms: pain at bite, pain in abdomen and back and chest, spreading to legs. May also have chills, dizziness, convulsions, paralysis, nausea, weakness. Rash may appear later, or severe ulcer of skin.

Save spider to show doctor.

Wash with soap and water.

Apply ice pack.

Put on paste of baking soda and water.

If any severe abdominal pain occurs, put patient in tub of really hot water and call doctor immediately.

SCORPION STING

Scorpions are prevalent in the South and West.

Apply ice immediately.

Place tourniquet above site of sting.

Place entire arm or leg in ice water.

Remove tourniquet after 5 minutes, but keep limb immersed in ice water for 2 hours.

Call doctor for antivenom.

Do not use Demerol for pain; it potentiates effect of venom.

Note: In life-threatening situations from venom poisoning, vitamin C given intravenously has proven beneficial.

The illustrations in this section were drawn with permission from *Emergency Family First Aid Guide,* Cooper Publishing and Simon & Schuster, Inc., 1230 Avenue of the Americas, New York, N.Y. 10020, $1.95.

CHAPTER 22

Help-Yourself Health Tips and Minor First Aid for Everyday Problems

RECOMMENDED SCHEDULE FOR IMMUNIZATION

AGE	IMMUNIZATION
2 Mo.	Diphtheria, tetanus, whooping cough, trivalent oral polio vaccine
4 Mo.	Diphtheria, tetanus, whooping cough, trivalent oral polio vaccine
6 Mo.	Diphtheria, tetanus, whooping cough, trivalent oral polio vaccine
1 Yr.	Measles, rubella, mumps, tuberculin test
1½ Yrs.	Diphtheria, tetanus, whooping cough, trivalent oral polio vaccine
4–6 Yrs.	Diphtheria, tetanus, whooping cough, trivalent oral polio vaccine
14–16 Yrs.	Tetanus, diphtheria; and thereafter every 10 years
Adults	Diphtheria-tetanus every 10 years (for contaminated wounds a tetanus booster is needed if it has run more than five years since last vaccination). Rubella—in women who have not had German measles and who are not pregnant and will not be for 3 months. Mumps—in men who have not had it. Influenza—each fall for persons subject to risk or with debilitating or chronic diseases.

Note: Children immunized against measles before the age of 13 months may be inadequately protected and should be reimmunized, says a research report in the *Journal of the American Medical Association.*

Experts in the field now recommend that measles immunization be deferred until about age 15 months, except during measles outbreaks when vaccinations should be given any time after 6 months. These children should then be revaccinated after 15 months.

WHAT HAPPENS TO VACCINATIONS WHEN YOU GROW UP?

Some give you life-long immunity. Others do not, and must be renewed. Pediatricians are very thorough in keeping up with children's immunizations, but adults' doctors tend to ignore their patients' immunization needs. Study the recommended immunization schedule and make sure you and your family are keeping up with the proper shots.

PETS CAN BE HAZARDOUS TO YOUR HEALTH

Because of the contagious bacteria and viruses they carry, animals can give you many diseases.

BRUCELLOSIS
(UNDULANT FEVER)

Resembles flu with headache, fatigue, chills, sweating, loss of weight. May last for days or months with repeated attacks. Carried by: *unpasteurized milk, cattle, pigs,* or *goats.*

LEPTOSPIROSIS
(SWINE HERDER'S DISEASE, INFECTIOUS JAUNDICE)

From mild flu-like symptoms to a severe, fatal form. Carried by: *cattle, pigs, dogs, cats, rats, sheep, goats, skunk, foxes, mice,* other animal life, or you can get from *swimming in farm ponds or streams* contaminated by urine from farm animals.

VIRAL ENCEPHALITIS
(SLEEPING SICKNESS)

Fever, confusion, delirium, or coma. Carried by: *birds, mosquitoes.*

Destroy mosquitoes and larva where possible; eliminate stagnant pools of water; use screens.

PSITTACOSIS
(PARROT FEVER)

Resembles pneumonia with fever and headache. Carried by: wild or pet birds, especially *parrots, parakeets, pigeons, turkeys, chicken.*

Buy birds only from reputable dealers. Don't feed pet birds from your lips. When cleaning cages, do not inhale droppings, wash hands afterward.

Q-FEVER

Vague symptoms with fever. Carried by: *cattle, sheep, goats,* or you can get by inhaling their dust or drinking their raw milk.

RINGWORM

Skin infection. Carried by: *dogs, cats,* other animals, or their bedding.

TULAREMIA
(RABBIT FEVER, DEER FLY FEVER)

Small sore occurs at site of infection, followed by fever and symptoms similar to flu. Carried by: *rodents, rabbits, flies, ticks.*

Avoid drinking raw stream water, use rubber gloves when dressing wild game, cook wild game thoroughly.

ROUND WORMS

They can attack vital organs and cause pneumonia, anemia, blindness, retardation, brain damage, impairment of heart, lungs, and liver. Carried by: *dogs, cats.*

Remove dog and cat droppings in areas where children play. Cover children's sandboxes when not in use. Discourage children from eating dirt, always have them wash hands after playing in dirt.

Have a veterinarian test a stool specimen from pet dogs or cats every six months for possible infection.

CAT SCRATCH DISEASE

A virus transmitted by cat scratch or bite. In 10 to 30 days there is fatigue, headache, low-grade fever, swelling of lymph node near scratch. Red pimple appears at site of scratch.

WHAT TO DO FOR ABDOMINAL PAIN

Don't take a laxative unless your doctor tells you to.

Do not give food or drink if you suspect appendicitis.

Do not use hot water bottle if you suspect appendicitis.

Signs of appendicitis: pain several inches below the waist, usually but not always on the right side; tenderness at a point halfway between navel and crest of hip bone; a board-like rigid abdomen. If patient has any of these signs, call the doctor immediately.

CHRONIC APPENDICITIS

Doctors now report that eliminating all sugar from the diet will stop attacks in many people. Too much sugar apparently promotes growth in the intestine of the bacteria that cause the attacks. Attacks can also be prevented sometimes by increasing the amount of roughage in the diet.

WHAT TO DO FOR ACNE

Wash your face thoroughly many times a day. Try a detergent on the acid side and with hexachlorophene, such as pHisoHex. Or try soap and lotions such as Sastid, Sulphur Soap, Acnareen, or Acne-Aid that contain sulfur, salicylic acid, resorcinol, alcohol, or acetone.

Keep your hands away from your face; don't for example lean your chin or cheek on your hand while reading or watching TV. It causes blemishes in these areas, which doctors call "TV acne."

Wash your hair often, several times a week if it is oily. Use an anti-dandruff shampoo.

Don't use hair oil or greasy lotions on hair or face. Try going without any makeup.

Change your pillow case frequently, even daily.

Test yourself on foods that seem to contribute to acne: chocolate, nuts, kelp, peanut butter, sweets, fried foods, fatty foods, spicy foods, carbonated drinks, milk and milk products. Try switching from iodized to non-iodized salt.

Use an astringent with alcohol or alum and an acid pH to cut oil and help close pores. Use clay face masks. At night: wash, use astringent, and rub a drying lotion on the face.

Steam your face frequently and use hot packs. (Soak a washcloth in very hot water and apply to face, then wash.)

Get plenty of sunshine, or try a sunlamp.

Take vitamin A, 25,000 to 50,000 units, every day. Do not take larger amounts than this because of risk of toxicity.

Check with your doctor on vitamin A acid in alcohol applied to the skin which has proved successful in recent scientific study. It is particularly good when used with tetracycline or benzoyl peroxide. The A acid goes on in the morning, the peroxide gel at night. Another doctor says the best medication is a 10 percent benzoyl peroxide lotion with 5 to 10 percent sulfur added.

Also check with him on using antibiotics daily until your acne is under control and on prescription lotions such as Neomedrol, or a mixture of erythromycin and vitamin A applied to the skin.

Use soaps with scrubbing grains and try a Buff-Puff, Buf Acne Bar, or other cleansing bars. (For free booklet on what buffing does for skin, send self-addresssed envelope to 3M Company, 135 West 50th Street, New York, N.Y. 10020.)

To remove scars: your doctor may suggest dermabrasion using a wire brush to take away top layers of scarred skin, or freezing-cold liquid nitrogen sprayed on the skin, or filling in deep scars with fibrin foam, a substance made from your own blood.

Latest news on acne: Dr. Gerd Michaelsson of Uppsala University in Sweden writes in the *Journal of the American Medical Association* that zinc sulfate tablets (three a day of the effervescent form dissolved in water and taken after meals) usually cured acne in 3 months. After 4 weeks there was a significant decrease in pimples, he said, and after 3 months acne was reduced by 85 percent.

You may be giving yourself acne. Many medications can cause acne, including bromides, cortisone, iodides, diet pills with phenobarbitol, dilantin, and some birth control pills. Working with oil and grease can do it, as can oily makeup.

WHAT TO DO FOR ANIMAL BITES

Rabies is most prevalent in dogs, cats, skunks, foxes, raccoons, and bats, but all warm-blooded animals are capable of carrying the deadly virus. The virus is transmitted by the saliva of an infected animal in the bite or entering an open wound or scratch.

Have cats and dogs vaccinated for rabies.

When tending sick farm animals or pets, take care not to be bitten.

Warn children not to handle strange-acting or sick pets or wild animals, including bats.

If bitten, immediately wash wound thoroughly and briskly with soap and water.

Identify and cage the animal if possible. Use care. Do not shoot the animal through the head.

Call a doctor immediately.

Call a veterinarian so he can examine the animal and quarantine it or send the brain to a lab for testing.

If the animal has rabies or escapes without being tested, antirabies treatment must begin immediately. A new vaccine allows treatment in 6 injections instead of the previous 14 to 21 needed, and without the bad side effects.

WHAT TO DO FOR BLISTERS

Prevent blisters by buying well-fitting shoes and breaking them in gradually.

If a sore spot develops, protect with Band-Aids.

If blister forms, do not open.

If it opens, wash and put on Band-Aid; do not use merthiolate, iodine, or alcohol on open blisters.

FOR A BLOOD BLISTER UNDER A NAIL

Take a scalpel blade or pointed knife blade and slowly and gently rotate the point on the nail over the blister, drilling a tiny hole so the blood can seep out. Do not push hard. Or unravel a paper clip, heat one end to red hot, and carefully push the heated end into the nail to release the trapped fluid.

WHAT TO DO FOR BRUISES

Apply ice bag or cold compresses for 30 minutes.

WHAT TO DO FOR BURNS

Put on ice or cold water compresses immediately and continue for at least 30 minutes. (Ice stops tissue injury, reduces pain, prevents blisters.)

If burn area is more than minor, take patient to hospital or physician at once.

Give liquids to drink (no alcohol).
Do not use ointments or greases.

CHEMICAL BURNS

Immediately flush with water, including eyes.
Seconds count.

While under shower take all clothing off.

See physician or go to hospital immediately.

IF CLOTHES CATCH FIRE

Do not run!

Roll in rug, blanket, a heavy coat to put out flames, or lie down and roll slowly on floor.

WHAT TO DO FOR CALLUSES

Put 2 cups castor oil, ½ cup paraffin wax, 1 tablespoon white soap chips or powder in top of double boiler and heat until mixed. Cool to lukewarm; add 1 teaspoon sodium thiosulfate (buy at photographic supply store). Store in plastic or glass jar. Apply to callus at bedtime; wrap with gauze to protect sheets. Wash off with hot water in morning.

WHAT TO DO FOR CONVULSIONS

Don't panic. Let the convulsion run its course. An attack usually will end by itself in a few minutes.

Don't try to restrain the person's movements. Don't try to give him liquids. Don't slap him or try to wake him up. Do not put person in bathtub or put water on him.

Lower him gently to the floor or bed, so he does not hurt himself by falling. Move away any dangerous objects he might strike during the convulsion. Put a pillow under his head so he doesn't injure his head on a hard surface.

Loosen clothing, especially collar.

Lay victim on his side with chin raised so he is less likely to draw saliva into his lungs or swallow his tongue.

If patient stays unconscious or convulsion lasts more than 15 minutes, call doctor.

After the convulsion, let the person rest or sleep. Stay with him until he has reoriented himself.

If the person is not already under treatment for epilepsy, he should see a physician for a complete workup to get proper diagnosis and treatment. Tell the doctor as much as you can of how long the seizure lasted, exactly how the person behaved during the seizure, and what events occurred before the seizure. (Many things can cause convulsions, even fever and birth control pills.)

WHAT TO DO FOR CROUP OR CHEST CONGESTION

Use a vaporizer or have patient sit near steam kettle or in bath with hot shower running.

Hot steamy wet towels held on face and throat will help also.

WHAT TO DO FOR CUTS AND SCRAPES

Wash with soap and water.

Hold sterile pad over wound until bleeding stops.

Apply Band-Aid or sterile pad with adhesive strips.

WHAT TO DO FOR DIARRHEA

Eat no food.

Take frequent sips of water, weak tea, ginger ale, clear broth, cola.

Use Kaopectate, Lomotil, paregoric, or other counteractant.

If you have severe cramps, a heating pad on the abdomen will help.

When diarrhea is under control, gradually start on bland foods such as salted crackers, dry toast, gelatins, mashed potatoes, white rice, cooked rice cereals.

Call doctor if diarrhea still continues, if it recurs frequently, or if blood is present. Diarrhea in only a day can begin to cause dehydration and upset of electrolytes. In infants and children this can be life-threatening.

WHAT TO DO FOR DIZZINESS

Lie down.

Loosen clothing and cool patient off if he is hot.

If dizziness lasts a long time, or keeps recurring, see a doctor.

ELEVEN CAUSES OF DIZZINESS YOU MIGHT NOT THINK OF:

1. Overheating
2. Anemia
3. Low blood pressure
4. Diabetes
5. Heart disease
6. Heart rhythm disturbances
7. Epilepsy
8. Stroke
9. Multiple sclerosis

10. Ear problems

11. Poor alignment of the jaw (irritating ear structures).

WHAT TO DO FOR DRY ITCHY SKIN

Do not use soap and water; instead use a water-soluble cleansing cream or lotion. Rinse well.

Use a moisturizer under makeup and at night.

Use a water mist once a week with a sauna or a steaming pot of water.

Don't take tranquilizers; they can make your skin drier.

Do not smoke cigarettes or drink alcohol (both increase dryness and wrinkles).

Stop taking so many baths and showers; make them warm, not hot.

Use a bath oil, such as Alpha-Keri, Lubath, Domol, Aveeno Oil.

Be sure to dry body thoroughly; use a body moisturizing lotion every day and after bath.

Lower the heat in your home.

Don't sit near radiators or hot air ducts.

Increase the humidity with a commercial humidifier or by putting pans of water on the stove and radiators.

Relieve itching with cool compresses, calamine lotion, or a lukewarm bath containing a cup of starch, bran, or oatmeal. If these don't work, have your doctor prescribe an ointment such as hydrocortisone plus petrolatum. If itching keeps you awake, take an antihistamine pill at bedtime.

Consider that there may be other causes to your itching and flaking: you may be allergic to a cosmetic or clothing, to a food, or to something at work. It could be scabies or lice, which used to be rare but have suddenly come back to the U.S. in epidemic proportions and can be found even in the neatest, cleanest people. It could signal a serious disorder such as diabetes, kidney disease, thyroid trouble, blood and liver diseases, and even cancer.

The Best Way to Scratch. When you scratch the center part of an itch, it can cause the release of certain chemicals that cause the itching to increase. So it's best to leave the central point alone and gently rub the surrounding area with your hands or even a brush.

WHAT TO DO FOR EAR NOISES

Ringing in the ears, buzzing, humming, or roaring can be caused by medicines such as quinine and aspirin, or by high blood pressure and rheumatic ailments. Treating these conditions may eliminate the noises.

WHAT TO DO FOR EARACHE

Place hot water bottle or heating pad to ear.

Chew gum, or yawn as strongly as possible.

Hold the nose shut and blow slightly with the mouth closed to equalize pressure.

Sometimes nose drops will help unclog ear passages.

If it occurs often, suspect an allergy.

Try steam inhalation.

Take an antihistamine to reduce swelling.

If persistent or severe, call a physician.

If an infant screams persistently for no apparent reason, consider it may have an earache.

BUG IN YOUR EAR

Hold a light up to the ear, which sometimes will attract the bug and cause him to crawl out. If this does not work, drop mineral oil into the ear canal to suffocate the insect, and have a physician remove it.

A NEW CAUSE FOR INFECTION

"Telephoner's ear" is a staph infection of the outer ear. It thrives in people who talk on the telephone for long periods of time from the telephone being held tight against the ear for long times. It is treated by compresses, antibiotics, and less telephone time.

WHAT TO DO FOR ECZEMA OR OTHER DERMATITIS

Find out what is causing it.

Protect your hands from water with cotton-lined plastic or rubber gloves while working. (Unlined ones will cause sweating and irritate the hands even more.) For non-wet work, use light cotton gloves.

Don't use excess amounts of soap and detergents when you work. Only use amounts the directions call for. Use mild soaps rather than strong ones. (Experiment with different brands, you may often have a reaction to one brand but not to another.)

Avoid wool clothing and blankets. Take special precautions to prevent contact of wool or fur around the wrists, ankles, and neck.

Don't stay in the bathtub too long. Take fewer baths. Add oil preparations to the bathwater. Sometimes all baths and soaps must be discontinued for several months and cleaning done with a lotion such as Cerephil.

Take vitamins if you think you could have a deficiency.

Keep as cool as possible; excess perspiration may cause a flare-up of the rash or irritate the skin.

Don't scratch.

Avoid pressure of clothes or jewelry over rash.

Take great care to rinse all soap from clothes.

If the eczema becomes secondarily infected, see your doctor for medication immediately.

If you have blisters, do not apply lotion or salve unless your doctor tells you to. They usually prevent blisters from healing.

Saltwater often helps. Swim frequently in the ocean or put salt into bath. (Many eczema and psoriasis sufferers show dramatic improvement after swimming in the highly salty Dead Sea.)

Useful medications available from your doctor include hydrocortisone, fluocinolone, triamcinolone, coal tars, caffeine cream, and antihistamines.

Warning: Patients with eczema should not have smallpox vaccination while they have an active rash, nor should any other members of the family living with them be vaccinated.

Caution: Some medicine, if you are sensitive to it, can make the rash even worse. If the rash becomes worse or spreads, stop treatment and contact your physician.

Caution: Coal tar may cause photosensitivity. Stay out of the sun or your skin may become discolored and rough.

WHAT TO DO FOR EYE PROBLEMS

ITCHING EYES

Lie down with cotton pads soaked in witch hazel on eyes.

Do not rub eyes.

Use eye drops recommended by your doctor.

IF YOU HAVE SOMETHING IN YOUR EYE

Do not rub eye.

Gently move lid to see if tears wash out the material, or place one lid over the other.

Use moist cotton swab to remove *gently*. Do not dig.

If object is on eyeball, blink several times so it moves to area of no danger.

If object is deep, or there is a scratch or cut, close eye and bandage lightly; see physician.

If eyeball has been scratched, it may feel as if object is still there. Rinse eye with boric acid or water and keep eye closed for short time.

BURNS

For burns caused by flames or cigarettes, the eye should be covered and a physician called immediately. For chemical burns, flood the eye with water immediately and continuously for at least 10 to 15 minutes and call your physician immediately.

FOR A BLACK EYE

Use cold compresses or ice to help reduce the swelling. If there is any change in sharpness of vision, unusual discomfort, or double images, the eye should be examined by a physician at once, since this may indicate internal damage to the eyeball.

WHAT TO DO FOR FEVER

Normal mouth temperature can range from 97° to 99° Fahrenheit. Rectal temperature runs one degree higher.

Give aspirin or aspirin substitute such as Tylenol.

Give patient a sponge bath with cool water.

Sponge off with alcohol; if necessary wrap in cold wet towels.

Put patient to bed.

Give fluids to drink.

If temperature rises to 104° in children or 105° in adults, it should be considered an emergency and brought down immediately. Call doctor without delay.

WHAT TO DO FOR HANGOVER

Drink 8 to 10 glasses of water in the first few hours in the morning or well-salted beef broth or salted tomato juice.

Take caffeine, or a caffeine-ergotamine pill (available at drugstore). Avoid aspirin and aspirin-containing products like Alka-Seltzer because alcohol makes the stomach lining more sensitive to their irritating effects.

Eat honey or fruit, or take fructose in tablet or granular form (available at drugstores or health food stores).

HOW TO PREVENT A HANGOVER

Take a vitamin B capsule before you go to bed.

Take a fructose tablet before or during drinking to decrease intoxication. Take another before going to bed and another upon awakening. (Bloody Marys or screwdrivers contain vodka, which usually causes less hangover than other alcohol forms, and they contain fructose sugar, which lessens intoxication and reduces hangover.)

WHAT TO DO FOR HICCUPS

Hold your breath several times for as long as you can. Breathe hard and fast between times of holding breath.

Swallow glass of water while holding your breath.

Breathe in and out of a paper bag.

Drink a carbonated drink.

Swallow a spoonful of sugar, dry.

If nothing works and hiccups continue for extended period, call doctor.

WHAT TO DO FOR INGROWN TOENAIL

Soak feet for 20 minutes in warm water several times a day, pushing flesh away from nail.

Use a Water-Pik on the high setting and direct the water pulses under the nail where it is growing in.

Cut a V shape out of the middle of the tip of the nail.

Use adhesive tape on the ingrown flesh, wrapping the tape around the toe to pull the flesh away from the nail and remove pressure.

WHAT TO DO FOR LICE

Lice have become epidemic. They may be caused by sexual contact or by wearing the clothes of or sleeping in the bed of an infected person.

Symptoms are: itching; a mild rash of small blue spots; sores that may lead to impetigo; tiny egg nits attached to the pubic hairs.

All persons in the household and all sexual contacts should bathe at once using a soft brush.

Apply 1 percent Kwell lotion from the neck down, concentrating on hairy areas.

Reapply lotion the following morning and evening, and on the morning of the third day (four applications in all).

Bathe again on the third evening, but apply no lotion.

Boil or launder all clothing and bedsheets.

WHAT TO DO FOR NOSEBLEED

Moisten cotton with cold water, peroxide, or nose drops and insert in nostril.

Squeeze hard against bleeding nostril for 5 minutes.

If bleeding persists, call physician.

WHAT TO DO FOR PELVIC PAIN OR URINARY RETENTION

Take a sitz bath. Sit for 5 to 30 minutes in a tub containing about 6 inches of very hot water.

WHAT TO DO FOR RAPID HEARTBEAT

Hold your breath for as long as you can.

Close your eyes and press hard on them for 20 to 30 seconds.

Drink a glass of ice-cold water.

If necessary, induce vomiting by putting a finger in the throat.

WHAT TO DO FOR SCABIES

There is a raging epidemic of scabies in the U.S. occurring in every age and socioeconomic group. The main symptom is intense itching, particularly at night. Scabies, a mite, can be spread through clothes, bed linen, or direct contact.

Get Kwell lotion from your pharmacist and apply from chin to toes for 24 hours; repeat in seven days.

Change bed linen after each treatment.

Treat other persons in the household, whether they have symptoms or not.

WHAT TO DO FOR SKIN IRRITATION

Sit in bath 10 to 30 minutes with tub two-thirds full of warm water (about 100°F), and any of the following healing baths:

Mix 1 pound of cornstarch with cold water to make paste, add hot water, then add to water in tub.

Place 2 pounds of bran in a muslin bag and soak in pot of hot water for 10 to 15 minutes, then use bag in bath to sponge the skin.

Tie 3 cups of cooked oatmeal in a cheesecloth bag and pat on skin in bath.

WHAT TO DO FOR SLIVERS AND SPLINTERS

Wash with soap and water. Remove with tweezers or forceps. Wash again.

WHAT TO DO FOR SORE THROAT

Gargle with hot salt water.

Take aspirin or aspirin substitute.

If you think a cold is coming on, take vitamin C, 1500 to 2000 mg (depending on your size) every 4 hours.

If you have fever, a rash on your body, or your throat has patches of white or yellow, call your doctor. It could be a symptom of impending serious illness.

If you have a history of rheumatic fever, always call your doctor when you have a sore throat.

Try a new technique of taking ½ teaspoon of a 0.25 percent saturated solution of dioctyl sodium sulfosuccinate in your mouth while lying on your back in bed. Let your head extend slightly over the edge of the bed while allowing the solution to reach all parts of your upper throat. Swallow several times. You need a prescription.

WHAT TO DO FOR SPRAINS AND DISLOCATIONS

A sprain is the wrenching of a joint. Signs: swelling, pain, tenderness to touch, later discoloration.

A dislocation is the slipping of a bone out of its joint. Signs: swelling, pain, tenderness, limited ability to move, may look like fracture. May actually be fractured.

SPRAIN

Elevate limb. Rest injured part.

Bandage with elastic bandage for 24 hours. (Loosen bandage if swelling gets worse.)

Use ice bag for several hours to counteract swelling and pain.

After a day or two, use hot compresses.

DISLOCATION

Keep weight off part; support it.

Apply ice packs.

Apply splint if possible.

Call doctor.

Generally one should not try to straighten out a dislocated joint or force it back into proper position. However, if there is no open wound a dislocated toe or finger can be gently pulled straight until it snaps back into place. Splint by taping to next finger or toe or to a tongue depressor or other small stick and see a doctor.

WHAT TO DO FOR STIFF NECK

Sleep flat with only a small pillow to avoid stress on neck at night.

Sleep on back or side, not with face down (which puts pressure on neck).

Apply heat with heat lamp, heating pad, hot towel, or long hot shower.

For any persistent or recurring pain, see doctor.

Pains in the arms and neck can also be caused from wearing new bifocals, if the person stretches his neck awkwardly for reading or other work at eye level. If you do a great deal of close work at eye level or above, the problem can be solved by having the reading segment of the bifocals placed at the top of the lens instead of the bottom.

WHAT TO DO FOR WARTS

Have your doctor or podiatrist remove them with an electric needle or by applying liquid nitrogen or a cauterizing chemical. Or have him trim the wart to relieve pressure, then soak your entire foot every day for 15 minutes in water heated to 120°F.

Buy a 40 percent salicylic acid plaster from your druggist, apply to wart and leave on for a week. Then scrape away the dead tissue. Reapply for several weeks until all is gone.

Some doctors recommend taking desiccated liver tablets every day (available in drugstores or health food stores).

A new vaccine technique has proved very successful in treating usually difficult-to-treat warts of the anus, according to Dr. Herand Abcarian, Chicago surgeon. Patients are treated with one or two injections of vaccine mixed with penicillin and streptomycin with excellent results.

SOME AT-HOME NURSING HINTS

HOW TO GIVE AN ALCOHOL RUB

When the body temperature is 104° or more, evaporation of alcohol cools the skin surface, reducing the fever.

Mix equal parts of rubbing alcohol and lukewarm water. Cover the patient with a sheet. Expose a leg and rub with the alcohol solution until it is dry. Cover the leg. Rub the other leg, then the arms, then the neck, covering each area when dry. Go on to the chest and abdomen and then the back. Repeat if necessary.

MAKING A BEDRIDDEN PATIENT MORE COMFORTABLE

For a back rest, use a chair turned around, a camp stool, or a board with a pillow propped in front of it.

Place a pillow under the knees.

Place a box at the foot of the bed to prop the feet against.

To take weight of bedclothes off feet, put pillow at feet and drape sheets and blankets over it.

HOW TO PREVENT BEDSORES

Nasty ulcers can occur in bedridden patients when points of their bodies are in constant contact with the bed. To prevent them, turn body at two-hour intervals to a new position. Use a water or gel mattress. (Medicare will pay for purchase or rental.) Treatment: laser beams are getting excellent results, says Dr. Eugene Seymour of Los Angeles, directing a referral center for laser treatment. Dr. James Barnes, Jr., applies sugar directly on the sore, and says it definitely improves healing.

TO PREVENT CONVALESCENT
WOBBLY KNEES

Many people after being bedridden find their legs so weak they can barely stand or walk. To avoid, do these exercises while you're still in bed:

1. Keep your heel on the bed and shrug the kneecap by trying to draw it up. Do 8 to 10 times every hour whenever you are awake.

2. Stiffen and raise your leg off the bed. Do each leg 8 to 10 times per hour.

When you are allowed to sit up, sit on the edge of the bed with your legs dangling. Then extend the leg straight out. Repeat several times a day until fatigued.

IF YOU NEED NURSING HELP

Ask your doctor or his nurse.

Call your local Visiting Nurse Association, the nursing department at your local hospital, or nurse registries in the yellow pages.

Have a cleaning woman or mother's helper take over the household chores while you do the nursing.

An *R.N.* is a registered nurse who has probably gone to college or taken a four-year nursing course in a hospital. Licensed to administer medications and treatments.

An *L.P.N.* is a licensed practical nurse who has had a shorter training period and in most states cannot administer medications unless supervised.

You can have a nurse live in full-time, come in for eight hours a day, or come in as a visiting nurse, simply stopping by to check and give any necessary medications or advice.

Check for insurance coverage on nursing care.

PRESCRIPTION EMERGENCY SERVICE

Look under Pharmacists in the yellow pages for those open all night. Or your doctor or local police station might know of a pharmacy with all night service. Some drugs can be obtained at hospitals in an emergency.

RECOMMENDED:
The Homemaker's Guide to Home Nursing
Alice M. Schmidt, R.N.
Brigham Young University Press
Provo, Utah 84602
$3.95

CHAPTER 23

How to Stay Healthy When Outdoors or Traveling

HOW TO HAVE A SUNTAN WITHOUT RISK

On the first day, expose skin to sun for no more than 15 to 20 minutes each on face and back. On the second day, increase exposure to about half an hour on each side. On the third day, you can tolerate 30 to 40 minutes.

Watch the time of day. Ultraviolet rays are most intense from 11 A.M. to 2 P.M. Go out before 8 and after 4 and you won't burn.

Remember, even when you are wearing a hat, rays reflected from sand or water can burn, and you can get a sunburn even on an overcast day.

THE SCIENTIFICALLY TESTED BEST LOTIONS TO PREVENT SUNBURN

Five percent PABA (para-aminobenzoic acid) in alcohol is most effective. Examples: PreSun, Eclipse, and Pabanol. Put it on before sunning and reapply periodically. Do not get on clothes, because sometimes the lotion will discolor fabric.

PABA esters. Chemically related, and good, but not quite as effective as regular PABA. Examples: Blockout, Pabafilm, Spectraban. The PABA esters do not discolor clothes.

Other sunscreens that got excellent ratings: lotions with benzophenones such as Uval and Solbar, ointments with zinc oxide, titanium oxide, or red petrolatum.

Be sure to read the labels on lotions. Some pro-mote tanning, some screen partially, some block completely, some counteract loss of moisture, and some are just pain-killers.

BEWARE OF PHOTOSENSITIVITY

Many cosmetics, perfumes, medicines, and even things you eat can cause your skin to be supersensitive to the sun. Sometimes you will become severely sunburned, sometimes you will get blotchy dark marks that last for months. Some of the things that can do it are:

- Lime juice
- Juice of figs, parsnip, fennel, dill, parsley, celery, and carrots
- Thiazide pills for high blood pressure
- Many oral diabetic drugs
- Some tranquilizers
- Griseofulvin (a drug used to treat fungal infections)
- Oil of bergamot (in cosmetics and perfumes)
- Saccharin (and most artificial sweeteners)
- Halogenated salicylanilides (in deodorant soaps)

OTHER TIPS

Watch high altitudes—there is less atmosphere to filter sun's rays so you may burn faster.

Never use a sun reflector.

177

PILLS TO PREVENT SUNBURN

If you are very sensitive to sun, you can obtain protection from either of these:

- PABA (para-aminobenzoic acid), available over the counter
- Solatene, a new pill containing beta-carotene, also available without prescription. (And new findings at Harvard indicate eating yellow and green vegetables which are high in beta-carotene helps build protection also.)

IF YOU DON'T HAVE AN AFTER-SUNBURN SPRAY FOR A BURN

Apply cold wet towels, cucumber slices, vinegar, or use cloth soaked in cold tea; soak in a tepid tub laced with cup of bran, oatmeal, or cornstarch, or use paste of baking soda and water, or aloe vera or vitamin E cream. Sprinkle baby powder on sheets to reduce friction. Take an aspirin to alleviate pain. Drink plenty of fluids to counteract dehydration.

NEW TREATMENT FOR SEVERE SUNBURN

A solution of indomethacin dabbed on the burned area (prescription needed).

DON'T WASH AWAY THE VITAMIN D

If you want to keep the vitamin D formed from the sun's rays and the natural oil on your skin, don't bathe or go in water before you sun or right after sunning, because it washes off the oil needed for full absorption of the vitamin into the skin.

PEELING

Help prevent it by tanning gradually with short exposures; use moisturizers heavily and frequently.

Use products from the aloe plant, or slit a leaf and apply its moisture directly.

To get rid of flaking, use a loofah sponge in the shower.

TOO MUCH HEAT

Drink huge amounts of fluid when in a hot climate.

If you exert yourself too long in extreme heat or hot sun, you can get sunstroke or heat exhaustion. *In sunstroke* the person may have hot dry skin, temperature of 100 degrees or more, may feel weak, dizzy, nauseated, and confused, or even may be unconscious. *In heat exhaustion,* the skin is pale and clammy and the person may have cramps of the legs or arms.

In either case, get the victim into a cool place, have him sit or lie down, loosen clothing. Give a cool drink (no alcohol), preferably Gatorade or water with a little salt added.

If patient still feels ill after several hours, call a doctor. If patient is unconscious and feels hot, pour cold water over him to cool body off and take him to a hospital.

NOTES ON SUNGLASSES

A quick test for sunglass quality: Stand under a light, hold the glasses so the light is reflected on the inside of the lens. Move slightly. If the image is distorted, the lens is faulty.

The mirror test: Put on your sunglasses, look at yourself in the mirror. If you can see your eyes clearly, the glasses are not dark enough.

Gray and green are best for visual acuity and color perception.

Plastic lenses filter out only ultraviolet rays; good glass lenses screen infrared rays also.

IF YOU ARE OUT IN EXTREME COLD

If you are out for a long time in extreme cold, watch for parts that look white or gray and either tingle or have no feeling. It means frostbite.

If you're outdoors, put hands under armpits or between thighs; warm ears and nose with hands. Indoors, put affected part in warm (*not hot*) water (about 102°), or cover with warm towels or blankets. Do *not* rub with snow or anything else; do *not* use strong heat such as a heat lamp or hot stove.

Give a warm drink.

Call a doctor.

After the part is warmed, encourage victim to exercise damaged part.

Also if you are exposed to severe cold for a long time, your entire body may feel cold all over; or you may show fatigue or dizziness.

Get to warm place.

Get in bathtub of warm water.

Wrap up in warm blankets.

Have warm drinks.

TO PREVENT FROSTBITE

Dress warmly enough. Dress *dryly* enough. Exercise to keep warm, especially your toes and fingers. Don't drink alcoholic beverages or smoke during or immediately before severe exposure.

IF YOU ARE EXPOSED TO POISON IVY, OAK, OR SUMAC

Shower or wash immediately being sure to soap lavishly and change clothes.

Wash contaminated clothing.

If blisters appear, don't scratch, it will spread.

Put on a soothing lotion like Ivy-Dri, calamine lotion, or cool compresses.

HOW TO KEEP BUGS AWAY

Take 100 mg of vitamin B_1 before you go out: the odor appears on your skin and bugs don't seem to like it. Eating cream of tartar tablets works too, especially to keep away chiggers.

Avoid bright patterned or dark-colored clothes and clothes with any odor. They attract bugs. Instead wear white, tan, light green. Avoid clothes that make you sweat; shower frequently.

Avoid scented hair spray, cologne, after-shave lotion.

Wear shoes, and a scarf if you have a lot of hair.

Avoid food or garbage areas or where fermented fruit lies on the ground (the alcohol from the fruit inebriates wasps and hornets, causing them to sting wildly).

In the autumn avoid areas covered with fallen leaves on humid days; bugs hover there.

If you see two wasps or bees together, be careful, you may be near a nest.

Spray picnic areas with insect repellent before spreading food. Keep food covered until served. Keep garbage wrapped.

IF STUNG

Remove stinger instantly with quick scrape of fingernail.

Leave area (bees and wasps deposit a substance that attracts others; wasps will attack again and again).

Wash with soap and water. Apply ice cube. If there is much swelling and itching, take an antihistamine pill.

Use ammonia, soda, or mud on bee or wasp stings. Or put meat tenderizer mixed with a little water on the sting site.

For chiggers: Use strong soap and leave soap paste on for two hours. Or dab on Kwell, a medicine sold for lice and scabies.

For fly and midge bites: Clean thoroughly with soap and water. If bite becomes infected, antibiotics may be necessary.

For multiple yellow jacket stings: Have physi-

cian inject stings with lidocaine (Xylocaine) or epinephrine (adrenalin).

For mosquito bites: Apply very hot water for a minute and it will magically stop the itching for up to 3 hours.

The following are scientifically effective bug repellents (no prescriptions needed).

REPELLENT	USE ON	GOOD FOR
Deet	Skin, clothes	Ticks, fleas, chiggers, mosquitoes
Indalone	Skin, clothes	Ticks
Dimethyl Carbate	Skin, clothes	Ticks, mosquitoes, chiggers
Benzyl benzoate	Clothes	Ticks, fleas, chiggers
Ethyl hexanediol	Skin, clothes	Mosquitoes, chiggers
Dimethyl phthalate	Skin, clothes	Mosquitoes, chiggers

If you have an allergic reaction to an insect (swelling of the throat, difficulty in breathing, fainting, wheezing, coughing, shortness of breath), get to a doctor or hospital emergency room *immediately*. If you know you are allergic to stings, always carry adrenalin and antihistamines with you.

ON THE COURT

EYE INJURIES

Eye doctors report more and more eye injuries from tennis balls hitting the eyes, often causing blindness. Wear a handball eye protector or sports sunglasses of impact-resistant lenses. Get lessons from a pro on proper way to play the net and protect yourself from fast balls. (Balls at net may travel 60 miles per hour.) If you do get hit in the eye, have a thorough eye examination, including careful study of the retina.

LEG CRAMPS

Get off your feet. Massage leg vigorously to get more oxygen to muscle. You may also need replacement of body salts. If it happens frequently, see your doctor.

TENNIS TOE

If the pressure from the blood under the toenail becomes painful, gently drill a hole in the nail with a knifepoint to release the pressure. Avoid narrow hard-toed and "improved" traction shoes that cause toe to slam against shoe.

TENNIS ELBOW

Major cause: an improper stroke. You either hit too far in front or too far back, the pros say, or with improperly held wrist. Or you have weak or out-of-condition forearm muscles.

Treatment: ice on elbow and aspirin to reduce immediate inflammation and pain, rest to allow healing, strengthening forearm and wrist muscles, and learning proper strokes (consult with a pro to learn what you're doing wrong).

TELEPHONE ELBOW?

You need not play tennis to get tennis elbow, says a New York specialist. You can get it from repeatedly reaching for a telephone behind your desk.

MUSCLE-STRENGTHENING EXERCISES FOR THE TENNIS PLAYER

1. Extend your arm straight forward, palm down, gripping a tennis ball. Squeeze the ball as hard as you can for a count of 5. Relax. Repeat 50 times.

2. Extend your arm forward. Make a fist. Cover your fist with other hand. Try to raise fist while holding down with other hand for a count of 5. Relax. Repeat 20 times.

ON THE FIELD

FOR FOOTBALL

Wear soccer type shoes instead of deeply cleated football shoes. The soccer shoes, with molded soles and only ⅜-inch cleats, help prevent knee and leg injuries.

THROWER'S ELBOW

Occurs in baseball pitchers and football passers, particularly in putting spin on ball.

Prevention: Always warm up before burning in your ball or throwing long passes. Strengthen arm muscles with exercise.

Thrower's exercise: Sit on a chair. Elevate your thigh by putting your foot on a stool about 4 to 6 inches high. Rest your forearm (elbow to wrist) along your thigh with your hand, palm up, extending past your kneecap. Hold a book in your hand, lift your hand by flexing your wrist, still holding your forearm down against your thigh. Count 5. Relax. Repeat 20 times. To build up strength gradually increase size of book and number of contractions. Do twice a day, both to build up strength to prevent thrower's elbow, and to treat it.

LITTLE-LEAGUE SHOULDER

Usually occurs in children, with bone damage from repeated throwing and stress. Acute pains in the shoulder when attempting to throw ball. (Can also occur in young tennis players.)

Serious damage can occur with weakness later in life. If symptoms occur, have shoulder x-rayed. If there has been damage, child must give up baseball or tennis until at least age 15.

BASEBALL FINGER

Occurs when tip of finger is hit, causing pain, swelling, and possibly tearing of ligaments.

Treatment: Put ice on finger. Tape to finger next to it to partially immobilize it. If finger is hit so last joint stays bent down (mallet finger), see doctor to have finger splinted immediately, or deformity will become permanent.

FALLING ON YOUR HAND

In any sport if you fall full force on the heel of your hand, there is danger of a fracture of the wrist bones. If there seems to be more than minor pain of the wrist by your thumb, see your doctor. It may only be a sprain, but if it is a fracture and is ignored, the wrist may be permanently disabled or require surgery.

CLINICS SPECIALIZING IN SPORT INJURIES

Institute of Sports Medicine and Athletic Trauma
　Lenox Hill Hospital
　77th Street and Park Avenue
　New York, N. Y. 10021
Orthopedic and Fracture Clinic
　750 East 11th Street
　Eugene, Ore. 97401
Temple University Sports Clinic
　Broad and Tioga Streets
　Philadelphia, Pa. 19140
Houston Orthopedic Clinic
　1315 Delauney Avenue
　Atlanta, Ga. 31901
Sports Medicine Clinic
　University of Washington School of Medicine
　Seattle, Wash. 98195

ON THE GOLF COURSE

GOLFER'S HIP

Usually caused by a faulty swing straining hip muscles, resulting in bursitis of one or both hips.

Hip strengthening exercise. Lie on your side with legs extended straight, left leg on top of right leg. Slowly raise left leg as high as you can, hold for count of 5, then slowly return. Do 20 times.

Turn and do right leg. As you gain strength, increase holding count from 5 to 10; then add weights to ankles.

ON THE SLOPES

HIGH ALTITUDE EDEMA

A big danger with skiers is high altitude pulmonary edema. It is often misdiagnosed as a cold or pneumonia, but it is much more dangerous and can kill you if not treated. It can occur as low as 8,000 feet, usually hits within a day or two after arriving at the high altitude.

Symptoms are: fatigue, weakness, headache, loss of appetite, nausea, insomnia, dizziness; often followed by shortness of breath, difficulty in breathing, mild chest pain, and a dry cough.

Treatment: bed rest and oxygen for 1 to 3 days and, if necessary, removal to a lower altitude.

SKIER'S HEEL

Straining or rupturing of the Achilles tendon from fatigue of the ankle plus under-conditioned calf muscles. Symptoms: you have extreme pain, are not able to raise your heel, and can only walk by dragging the heel behind you.

If mild: a period of rest, followed by exercise.

If serious: see orthopedic surgeon immediately for a cast or surgery to repair tendon.

Achilles exercise: Stand on the edge of a step on the balls of your feet so your heels hang well over the edge. Lower heels as far as you can, then slowly raise them to stand on your tiptoes. Hold tiptoe position for count of 5. Repeat 10 times. Work gradually up to 50.

IN AND ON THE WATER

SWIMMER'S CRAMPS

Caused by temporary insufficiency of oxygen to muscles.

Don't go swimming after you eat.

Don't panic or thrash around, which will increase cramps.

Tread water with your arms, or float; take deep breaths of air.

After cramps stop, breathe deeply for several more minutes, then call for help or go slowly to shore.

HAIR TURNING GREEN

The A.M.A. reports this startling syndrome in pool swimmers. The reason: excess copper in the water that reacts with hair. Stay out of pool till copper level is corrected; shampoo daily till removed.

MAN-OF-WAR OR JELLYFISH STING

Tentacles clinging to skin should be drenched with sand, alcohol, salt, or flour and then scraped off.

Clean area with ammonia or other alkaline substance to neutralize poison.

For rash or reddening, give antihistamines, or apply calamine lotion or corticosteroid ointment.

STING RAY WOUND

Remove sheath if visible in wound.

Rinse out puncture wound repeatedly with salt water in syringe to get rid of toxin.

Apply gauze or cotton soaked in ammonia, or if none is available, apply urine.

Immerse wound in hot water to relieve pain.

If wound is in abdomen or chest, hospitalization is necessary.

DON'T HYPERVENTILATE (OVERBREATHE) BEFORE YOU DIVE

Many deaths are being reported from loss of consciousness under water with no warning. The person passes out without even feeling the urge to come up for air. Don't try to establish records for time or distance. Always dive with a buddy.

NITROGEN EUPHORIA

Divers become tipsy and irrational at 200 feet, may take out mouthpieces or swim down instead of up without knowing it. Don't dive that deep.

THE BENDS

When a diver comes up too rapidly, air pressure can rupture the lung, an air bubble can go to the brain and cause death, or nitrogen bubbles can form in the tissue, causing the bends (decompression sickness). Any diver who has symptoms of pain or shortness of breath during or after ascending should be kept warm, given oxygen, and be taken immediately to a recompression center. (Call Coast Guard, who will transport to nearest recompression center. Do not take diver to an ordinary hospital, which usually does not have proper facilities.) Even with minor bends, have a neurological check for damage to nervous system.

To prevent the bends: learn your diving table. At 60 feet you can stay down 60 minutes; at 100 feet, only 25 minutes. Ascend slowly, no faster than 60 feet per minute.

SURFER'S EAR

Surfer's Ear is a bony growth inside the ear canal brought on by continuous exposure to cold ocean water and big waves forcing water into the ear canal over several years, says Dr. Daniel M. Seftel, in *Archives of Otolaryngology,* a publication of the American Medical Association.

If the growth becomes large enough, it can cause a plugged ear and affect hearing, says Dr. Seftel. It can be removed by surgery. Surfers may avoid the risk by wearing custom-fitted, molded ear plugs to fill the ear cavity.

SURFER'S KNEE

The knee becomes inflamed, swollen, and painful, and may develop knobs of swollen tissue. If untreated, can cause serious future knee problems.

Treatment: immediate rest from surfing; cortisone injections or draining of fluid if necessary; use knee pads in the future.

EMERGENCY LIFE-PRESERVERS

If there is no life vest or ring at hand, any of these will keep a person afloat: a board, a large beach ball, an ice chest with the lid on, a gallon or more Thermos jug.

ON THE TRAIL

RUCKSACK PALSY

If you hike with a heavy load on your back, you could get this. It used to be a common complaint of marching soldiers.

Symptoms: pain, numbness, and weakness in the shoulders and arms because of pressure of the backpack on nerves and blood vessels, according to Dr. H. David Rothner of Cleveland Clinc. He advises using a backpack with metal supports to distribute load on to hips, as well as 1-inch-thick foam rubber under shoulder straps. At the first sign of discomfort, remove and lighten pack.

HOW TO GET RID OF SKUNK SMELL

This has nothing to do with medicine, but we thought you'd like to know you can get rid of skunk stench by pouring on tomato juice.

PUFFBALL MEDICINE

If you're in the wild and have lost your first aid kit, dust powder from a crumpled giant puffball on a wound. Indians stored it for time of need.

HOW TO UNSNAG A FISH HOOK

THE USUAL WAY:

Force the hook through the skin the rest of the way.

Cut off the barb with pliers, or squeeze it down.

Pull the hook out backwards.

THE AUSTRALIAN SEAMEN'S WAY:

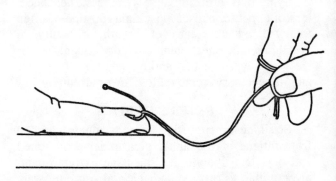

Make a string into a loop about 18 inches long. Wrap the end around your right index finger, slip the loop over the hook.

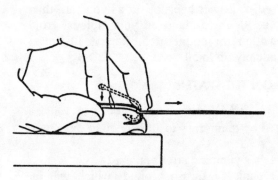

Place the victim's finger down on a flat surface. With your left hand firmly push down on the eye of the hook to disengage the barb. Put the third finger of your left hand on the loop, holding it at the point where the hook enters the skin.

Make sure the string is clear and will not tangle. Jerk the hook out with the string.

Wash the wound.

WHAT TO TAKE WITH YOU WHEN AWAY FROM YOUR DOCTOR

- A first aid booklet, or the *Whole Health Catalogue*
- Aspirin
- Stomach antacid, such as Rolaids, Tums, Maalox
- Milk of magnesia for constipation
- Antihistamine for allergies or nasal congestion (see your doctor for prescription)
- First aid spray or antiseptic
- Lotion for bug bites
- Sunburn lotion
- Tweezers
- Kaopectate (for diarrhea)
- Halizone to purify water
- Band-Aids
- Gauze bandage
- Adhesive tape
- Safety pins
- Copies of all your prescriptions
- Insect repellent
- Extra eyeglasses (and your eyeglass prescription), hearing-aid batteries, foot-care items and medicines ordinarily used
- Immersion heating coil to boil water, plus adapter for foreign sockets.

Note: If you travel out of the country, customs officers are sometimes suspicious of drugs; be sure to have all pills properly labeled.

BEFORE YOU TRAVEL, SEND FOR:

Health Information for International Travel
Center for Disease Control
U.S. Department of Health, Education and Welfare
Atlanta, Ga. 30333
Free
  Gives up-to-date information on health requirements for international travel.
Directory of English-Speaking Doctors Throughout the World
International Association for Medical Assistance to Travelers
350 Fifth Avenue
New York, N.Y. 10001
Free
  Lists physicians and hospitals in 500 cities in 116 countries.
International Medical Directory
World Medical Association
1841 Broadway
New York, N.Y. 10023
$2.00
  Guide to English-speaking physicians in 70 countries. (If you can't find a needed specialist listed for where you are going, WMA will try to locate one, free.)

Intermedic Directory
Intermedic
777 Third Avenue
New York, N.Y. 10017
  Lists doctors in 200 cities in 92 countries. Free if you become member (which also gets you somewhat lower rates than IAMAT directory).
A Foreign Language Guide to Health Care
Blue Cross Association (or local chapter)
840 North Lake Shore Drive
Chicago, Ill. 60611
Free
  Key health phrases in German, Italian, French, and Spanish to help you converse with foreign physician or hospital personnel.

THE BEST WAY TO FIND A PHYSICIAN IN ANOTHER COUNTRY

Check with your hotel, or call the American Embassy, the British Embassy, a missionary organization, an American military base, or an American or British airline or cruise ship line.

WHAT YOU NEED TO KNOW ABOUT SHOTS

Smallpox immunization, once essential, is required by the United States at present only if you are returning from Ethiopia. Governments in the Caribbean and Europe no longer insist on smallpox immunity. But all South American countries require proof of vaccination. Check with your travel agent or local passport office.

SOME QUICK HEALTH HELPS FROM THE KITCHEN WHEN YOU'RE AWAY FROM HOME

For dry skin: Put a few drops of cooking oil in the bath.

Too much sun: Put a half cup of lemon juice in the bath.

For chapped or irritated skin: Rub cucumber slice or juice onto skin.

Skin scrubber: Wet a washcloth with soap and water, sprinkle cornmeal onto the cloth, and scrub the face and neck.

Conditioner for over-sunned hair: Rub mashed avocado or mayonnaise into scalp and hair and leave on for 20 minutes before shampooing.

PREVENTING DIARRHEA

Don't drink the water in Leningrad, but it's okay in England, Scandinavia, Germany, Switzerland, Israel, Australia, New Zealand, and Canada.

Drink only boiled or bottled water, bottled beer or bottled soda. *Remember ice cubes are made from unboiled water.* Avoid raw vegetables, salads. Peel fresh fruit. Take along an immersion heater and boil water in your room.

If you get diarrhea, replenish fluids. Take Kaopectate or Lomotil or whatever your doctor advises that you take along. One doctor discovered that Pepto-Bismol works. Be careful of Entero-Viaform, said to have many side effects, and local remedies, some of which have been said to be dangerous.

PREVENTING MOTION SICKNESS

Take an anti-nausea pill such as Dramamine, Bonine, or Merezine about an hour before departure.

Get plenty of cool air.

Take vitamin B.

PREVENTING HEPATITIS

Don't swim if there is the *slightest* doubt about contaminated water. Eat shellfish only if cooked. See your doctor for a gamma globulin shot if you're going to area known to have hepatitis.

WHEN FLYING

HOW TO CURE SINUS OR EAR PAIN

Use any antihistamine pill or nasal decongestant to open blocked passages.

PROBLEM EN ROUTE?

See Travelers Aid in most transportation terminals.

HOW TO MINIMIZE JET LAG

En route wear loose fitting clothes to increase circulation; take shoes off.

Cut down on food, drink, smoking.

Drink lots of water to combat dehydration.

Don't schedule anything important on first two days: try to get plenty of relaxation.

AIR GYMNASTICS

Scrunch up your toes 10 times, then flex your ankles as though walking in plane, then contract the muscles in your legs as hard as you can and hold to the count of 5. Do 10 times each.

Take a walk in the aisle.

Roll your shoulders, making large relaxed circles forward, then backward 5 times each.

Turn your head to right, and nod 5 times. Repeat to left. Then rotate head to relax neck.

WHEN YOU GET HOME

If you develop fever or diarrhea after returning home, see your doctor and tell him where you have been; have a blood test for malaria if you may have been exposed to it.

CHAPTER 24

Do-It-Yourself Medical Tests You Can Do at Home

CHECKING FOR EARLY WARNING SIGNS

Do you really know you're healthy? Take this self-administered health quiz to check up on yourself. It is designed to detect the early warning signs that your body often gives out before serious disease strikes.

If you answer "yes" to *any* of the following questions, you should make an appointment to see your doctor as soon as possible and discuss the symptom with him. You may find a temporary condition easily treated, or you may find the appointment was life-saving.

Do you have any sores or growths on the skin, lips, mouth, or tongue that don't seem to heal? Any persistent itching that you can't explain? Any enlarged lymph glands? Moles that have changed color or size or become ulcerated or bleeding?

Do you have sweating or fever that has lasted for several weeks?

Have you developed a persistently hoarse voice? Persistent difficulty in swallowing or a constant cough? Sputum streaked with blood?

Do you have any swelling or lumps anywhere in the body?

Do you ever have shortness of breath for no apparent reason, especially doing things that never bothered you before? A squeezing or pressing feeling or a pain in your chest? Swelling of both ankles? Unexplained dizzy spells? Frequent serious nosebleeds?

Do you have pain or burning on urination? Blood in the urine? Difficulty in starting to urinate? A need to urinate much more frequently than in the past?

Do you have frequent attacks of heartburn, indigestion, or abdominal pains? Nausea or vomiting that has lasted more than a week? The recent appearance of a persistent constipation or diarrhea? Blood in the stool or a tarry black color?

Have you lost more than 10 pounds for no apparent reason? Or have you become very overweight?

Do you have severe chronic fatigue?

Do you have any swelling or persistent pain in the pelvic region? Any genital discharge that is yellow, thick, bad smelling, or that has lasted more than a few days?

Do you have problems with sexual functions that are persistent? Bleeding after intercourse?

Do you have bleeding between menstrual periods? Bleeding that has begun again after menopause? Any pains in the breast not related to menstrual periods? Any lumps in the breast? Puckering of the breast skin? Any discharge from the nipples?

Have you begun having nervous, irritable, or depressed spells? Crying jags? A feeling of a nervous breakdown coming on?

Have you developed a sudden persistent, excessive thirst? A yellow color to the skin or eyes?

Have you had any dimming or loss of vision?

Frequent earaches? Running ears? Sudden loss of hearing? Head noises? Dizziness?

Do you have headaches that are extremely severe, return again and again, or are accompanied by nausea or vomiting or blurred vision?

Do you need several drinks every day? Frequently get drunk?

Do you have convulsions? Frequently faint?

Do you have loss of sensation of any part? Loss of taste or smell? Loss of strength or function, with dropping of things or stumbling?

Have you a serious pain that won't go away? A fever that keeps coming and going? Any symptom, even minor, that persists or repeatedly returns and has no obvious cause?

TAKING AN ORAL TEMPERATURE

Wash thermometer, wipe with alcohol, and shake down.

Keep under tongue with lips closed for three minutes. (The old 1 to 2 minute time was half a degree off about a third of the time, studies show.)

TAKING A RECTAL TEMPERATURE

Adults lie on one side with knees bent.

Infants are held lying on their backs with their legs held up with one hand.

Put Vaseline or other lubricant on thermometer.

Insert gently about one inch. Do not force, let anus relax. Hold in 2 minutes.

Read temperature and write down.

Clean thermometer.

TAKING A PULSE

Place three fingers on the artery on the thumb side of the wrist. Move around till you find it. Do not use the thumb. (Or take the pulse in the neck, feeling firmly for the neck artery with your fingers on either side of the Adam's apple.)

Count pulse beats for six seconds timed by second hand on watch or clock.

Add zero for pulse per minute.

Normal pulse rates:

At birth	130–160
Infants	110–130
From 1–7 years	80–120
Older children	80–90
Women	70–80
Men	60–70

A healthy pulse has a good bounce and a regular rhythm. If your artery seems hard and brittle, your pulse is weak or irregular or you do not have a normal rate, you should see your doctor.

WHAT KIND OF SHAPE ARE YOU IN?

THREE SIMPLE TESTS FOR GENERAL FITNESS

The Hop Test

This is a test frequently used by medical examiners for life insurance companies.

1. Take your pulse while sitting at rest.
2. Hop 25 times on one foot and, immediately, 25 times on the other foot.
3. Take your pulse immediately.
4. Sit for 2 minutes and take your pulse again.

To be considered normal your pulse should be within the following ranges: before the test: 60–85 beats per minute; immediately after: an increase of 50 points. After a 2-minute rest: back to within 5 or 10 points of your resting pulse before the test.

If you have shortness of breath, chest discomfort, or dizziness while hopping, stop the test and take your pulse. If it is over 150 or if it does not return to the resting pulse value by six minutes, you should make an appointment to see your doctor.

THE STEP TEST FOR HEART-LUNG FITNESS

Warning: *Under no conditions should you take this test if you have heart or lung trouble, or are more than 20 percent overweight. If at any time during the test you have pain or discomfort, stop immediately.*

Get a stool or chair that is 15 to 18 inches off the floor. You also need a stopwatch or a watch or clock with a second hand.

First: Step up on the stool once every 10 seconds. Continue for 2 minutes. Immediately measure your pulse for 15 seconds. Multiply by 4. If your pulse is over 100, stop.

Second: Continue for 1 minute. (Stop if you feel pain.) At the end of the minute, wait 15 seconds, then count your pulse for the next 15 seconds. Wait another 15 seconds; count your pulse for 15 seconds. Again wait 15 seconds, and again count your pulse for 15 seconds. Add the three pulse scores. The lower your score, the faster your heart was able to recover, and the healthier you, your heart, and your lungs are.

IF YOUR SCORE WAS:	YOUR CONDITION IS:
61–67	Excellent
68–89	Good
90–97	Average
98–109	Below average
110 or above	Poor

DR. KENNETH COOPER'S 12-MINUTE RUN/WALK TEST

On a track or an open road, mark a starting place. Start running; when your breath gets short, walk a while, then run again. Have someone time you for 12 minutes with a watch with a second hand. Determine the distance you've traveled in your running and walking for 12 minutes. (On the road, use your car to measure the distance.)

Check your fitness against Dr. Cooper's chart.

WOMEN—UNDER AGE 30

FITNESS CATEGORY	DISTANCE COVERED
I Very Poor	.95 mile
II Poor	.95–1.14
III Fair	1.15–1.34
IV Good	1.35–1.64
V Excellent	1.65 +

WOMEN—AGE 30–39

FITNESS CATEGORY	DISTANCE COVERED
I Very Poor	.85 mile
II Poor	.85–1.04
III Fair	1.05–1.24
IV Good	1.25–1.54
V Excellent	1.55 +

WOMEN—AGE 40–49

FITNESS CATEGORY	DISTANCE COVERED
I Very Poor	.75 mile
II Poor	.75–.94
III Fair	.95–1.14
IV Good	1.15–1.44
V Excellent	1.45 +

WOMEN—AGE 50–59

FITNESS CATEGORY	DISTANCE COVERED
I Very Poor	.65 mile
II Poor	.65–.84
III Fair	.85–1.04
IV Good	1.05–1.34
V Excellent	1.35 +

WOMEN'S OPTIONAL 3-MILE WALKING TEST (NO RUNNING!)

TIME (MINUTES) REQUIRED TO WALK 3 MILES

FITNESS CATEGORY	UNDER AGE 30
I Very Poor	48:00 +
II Poor	48:00–44:01
III Fair	44:00–40:31
IV Good	40:30–36:00
V Excellent	36:00

FITNESS CATEGORY	AGE 30–39
I Very Poor	51:00 +
II Poor	51:00–46:31
III Fair	46:30–42:01
IV Good	42:00–37:30
V Excellent	37:30

FITNESS CATEGORY	AGE 40–49
I Very Poor	54:00 +
II Poor	54:00–49:01
III Fair	49:00–44:01
IV Good	44:00–39:00
V Excellent	39:00

FITNESS CATEGORY	AGE 50–59
I Very Poor	57:00 +
II Poor	57:00–52:01
III Fair	52:00–47:01
IV Good	47:00–42:00
V Excellent	42:00

FITNESS CATEGORY	AGE 60 +
I Very Poor	63:00 +
II Poor	63:00–57:01
III Fair	57:00–51:01
IV Good	51:00–45:00
V Excellent	45:00

MEN

FITNESS CATEGORY	DISTANCE COVERED
I Very Poor	less than 1.0 mile
II Poor	1.0 to 1.24 miles
III Fair	1.25 to 1.49 miles
IV Good	1.50 to 1.74 miles
V Excellent	1.75 miles or more

For men over 35 years of age, 1.40 miles in 12 minutes is consistent with the Good fitness category.

HOW TO TAKE YOUR OWN BLOOD PRESSURE AT HOME

The easiest blood pressure machines to use are ones that light up or otherwise electronically indicate your diastolic and systolic pressures. They are more expensive, but allow few mistakes and can be used alone without help. Check with your doctor for a model he recommends.

THE SPHYGMOMANOMETER– STETHOSCOPE WAY

Don't take your own pressure, because bending around can change reading. Have some other member of the family take it for you. It is best to have a nurse or doctor instruct you the first time.

Have a quiet place with a table and two chairs.

Sit down; bare patient's arm well above elbow.

Position cuff flatly and snugly on bare arm above elbow.

Raise patient's arm above shoulder and rapidly pump cuff to where pressure gauge reads 250 mm Hg.

Lower arm to table with elbow extended.

Apply stethoscope (ear tips forward), with bell flat on the soft flesh inside the crook of the elbow.

Let air out of cuff slowly so needle on pressure guage (or mercury level) falls about 2 mm Hg with each heartbeat.

Listen for blood sounds. You will hear a thudding noise in the stethoscope. The pressure when this first begins is the systolic pressure.

Continue to let the air out of the cuff. You will hear the thudding stop.

The pressure at this point is the diastolic pressure. (If the thudding does not stop, but the sound markedly changes, this can be taken as the diastolic pressure.)

SELF-EXAMINATION OF THE BREASTS

Stand as straight as you can. Place your arm above your head on the side of the body being examined to stretch the breast on that side.

Hold your opposite hand straight with fingers and feel your breast by pressing your palm against the breast.

Repeat on the other side with other arm raised. Repeat while lying down.

A tumor or cyst will feel like a peanut, pea, or lima bean.

Check not only for lumps, but also for depressions, puckering of the skin, unusual discharge, or a change in shape or size of either breast. (If you have just stopped breast-feeding, don't panic over lumps during the first month. These are glands that still have milk in them.)

You should examine your breasts every month.

If you note any abnormalities, contact your doctor immediately.

SELF-EXAMINATION OF THE TESTES

Men should examine their testes regularly to check for cancer, some doctors say. Start high in the scrotum and feel down the spermatic cord to the testis. The testis should be spongy firm and egg-shaped. Any lump or any difference in shape between the two testes should be reported to your doctor immediately.

HOW TO USE AN OTOSCOPE

You need an otoscope (ear speculum) and a little high intensity penlight to shine into the ear. Holding the ear with one hand, pull the ear out firmly to straighten out the ear canal and make it easier to see in. Insert the speculum, shine the light and peer in.

If the eardrum is normal, it will be a shiny pearly white. If there is an infection, it will be red. If it is bluish, it may be that fluid is in the middle ear. Wax will be brown or black.

(Some people's ear canals are very curved. If it is difficult to see, or if the examination is hurting the patient, stop.)

CHECKING THE EYE REFLEXES

If a patient is unconscious or has had a head injury, it is important to check the eye reflexes. Shine a flashlight on the pupils of the eyes, each eye in turn. The pupils should constrict. If they do not constrict, or one constricts and not the other, call a physician right away.

AN AT-HOME TEST YOU CAN TAKE FOR ALLERGY

Shine a flashlight into the nose and look at the lining of the nose. The normal color is pink and shiny like the lining of the mouth. If it is bright red, there is probably a bacterial infection. If it is pale, swollen, and water-logged, it means an allergy is probably at work.

A HAYFEVER ANALYSIS

If you think you are allergic to pollen, check this chart by time and place to see what pollen you are most likely allergic to. Sneezing in the spring is usually due to tree pollen; in mid-summer it is the result of the release of pollen grains of grasses; and in August and September is usually due to ragweed.

IF YOU LIVE HERE	IF YOU HAVE SYMPTOMS AT THESE TIMES	YOU PROBABLY ARE ALLERGIC TO THIS POLLEN	IF YOU LIVE HERE	IF YOU HAVE SYMPTOMS AT THESE TIMES	YOU PROBABLY ARE ALLERGIC TO THIS POLLEN
Alabama	Jan.-June	Tree	Indiana	Mar.-June	Tree
	April-Sept.	Grass		May-July	Grass
	Sept.-Oct.	Ragweed		Aug.-Oct.	Ragweed
Arizona	Feb.-April	Tree	Iowa	Mar.-May	Tree
	April-Oct.	Grass		May-Sept.	Grass
	June-Sept.	Russian thistle or salt bush		Aug.-Oct.	Ragweed
	Aug. or Sept.-Oct.	Ragweed	Kansas	Feb.-June	Tree
	May-Dec.	Amaranth		May-June	Grass
Arkansas	Feb.-May	Tree		July-Sept.	Russian thistle or amaranth
	May-Sept.	Grass			
	Aug.-Oct.	Ragweed		Aug.-Oct.	Ragweed
California	Jan. or Feb., Mar. or June	Tree	Kentucky	Mar.-June	Tree
				May-July	Grass
	Aug. or Dec.	Grass		Aug.-Oct.	Ragweed
	June or July, Oct. or Nov.	Ragweed, sage, or Russian thistle	Louisiana	Jan.-April	Tree
				April-Dec.	Grass
	May-Aug.	Dock or plantain		Aug.-Oct.	Ragweed
Colorado	Mar.-April	Tree	Maine	April-June	Tree
	June-July	Grass		May-July	Grass
	Aug.-Sept.	Ragweed or sage		Aug.-Sept.	Ragweed
	July-Sept.	Russian thistle or kochia	Maryland	Mar.-May	Tree
				May-July	Grass
Connecticut	Mar.-May	Tree		Aug.-Sept.	Ragweed
	May-July	Grass	Massachusetts	April-May	Tree
	Aug.-Oct.	Ragweed		May-July	Grass
Delaware	Mar.-May	Tree		Aug.-Sept.	Ragweed
	May-July	Grass	Michigan	Mar.-June	Tree
	Aug.-Oct.	Ragweed		May-July	Grass
District of Columbia	Feb.-May	Tree		Aug.-Sept.	Ragweed
	May-July	Grass	Minnesota	April-May	Tree
	Aug.-Oct.	Ragweed		May-July	Grass
Florida	Feb.-April or May	Tree		June-Oct.	Chenepod or amaranth
	Spring-fall, or year-round	Grass		Aug.-Sept.	Ragweed
	May-Sept. or Aug.-Nov.	Ragweed	Mississippi	Feb.-April	Tree
				May-Aug.	Grass
Georgia	Jan.-May	Tree		Aug.-Sept.	Ragweed
	May-Sept.	Grass	Missouri	Mar.-May	Tree
	Aug.-Oct.	Ragweed		May-July	Grass
Idaho	Mar.-May	Tree		Aug.-Sept.	Ragweed
	May-Aug.	Grass	Montana	April-May	Tree
	July-Sept.	Russian thistle or salt bush		May-Sept.	Grass
				July-Sept.	Russian thistle
	Aug.-Sept.	Ragweed or sage		Aug.-Oct.	Ragweed or sage
Illinois	Mar.-May	Tree	Nebraska	Mar.-May	Tree
	May-July	Grass		May-July	Grass
	Aug.-Oct.	Ragweed		July-Sept.	Russian thistle
				Aug.-Sept.	Ragweed or hemp

IF YOU LIVE HERE	IF YOU HAVE SYMPTOMS AT THESE TIMES	YOU PROBABLY ARE ALLERGIC TO THIS POLLEN	IF YOU LIVE HERE	IF YOU HAVE SYMPTOMS AT THESE TIMES	YOU PROBABLY ARE ALLERGIC TO THIS POLLEN
Nevada	April-May	Tree	South Carolina	Feb.-May	Tree
	June-July	Grass		May-July	Grass
	July-Sept.	Russian thistle		Aug.-Oct.	Ragweed
	Aug.-Oct.	Sage	South Dakota	Mar.-April	Tree
	Sept.-Oct.	Ragweed		May-July	Grass
New Hampshire	April-May	Tree		June-Sept.	Russian thistle
	May-July	Grass		July-Sept.	Ragweed
	Aug.-Sept.	Ragweed		Aug.-Sept.	Sage
New Jersey	Mar.-May	Tree	Tennessee	Feb.-May	Tree
	May-July	Grass		May-Sept.	Grass
	Aug.-Sept.	Ragweed		Aug.-Oct.	Ragweed
New Mexico	Feb.-April	Tree		Sept.-Oct.	Sage or tree
	May-Oct.	Grass	Texas	Jan.-April; Aug.-Sept.	Tree
	July-Sept.	Amaranth or salt bush		April-Sept.	Grass
	Sept.-Oct.	Ragweed or sage		Sept.-Oct.	Ragweed
New York	Mar.-May	Tree	Utah	April-May	Tree
	May-July	Grass		May-July	Grass
	Aug.-Sept.	Ragweed		July-Sept.	Russian thistle
North Carolina	Feb.-May	Tree		Aug.-Sept.	Ragweed
	May-July	Grass		Aug.-Oct.	Sage
	Aug.-Sept.	Ragweed	Vermont	April-May	Tree
North Dakota	April-May	Tree		May-July	Grass
	June-July	Grass		Aug.-Sept.	Ragweed
	July-Sept.	Russian thistle or ragweed	Virginia	Feb.-June	Tree
				May-July	Grass
	Aug.-Sept.	Sage		Aug.-Sept.	Ragweed
Ohio	Mar.-June	Tree	Washington	Feb. or Mar.-Apr.	Tree
	June-July	Grass		Apr.-July or Oct.	Grass
	Aug.-Sept.	Ragweed		May-Oct.	Dock or plantain
Oklahoma	Feb.-June	Tree		Aug.-Sept.	Sage or ragweed
	May-Sept.	Grass		July-Sept.	Russian thistle or salt bush
	July-Oct.	Amaranth			
	Aug.-Oct.	Ragweed	West Virginia	Mar.-June	Tree
Oregon	Feb.-April	Tree		May-July	Grass
	April-June or Aug.	Grass		Aug.-Sept.	Ragweed
	May-Sept.	Dock or plantain	Wisconsin	Apr.-May	Tree
	July-Sept.	Russian thistle or salt bush		June-July	Grass
				Aug.-Sept.	Ragweed
	Aug.-Sept.	Ragweed	Wyoming	Mar.-April	Tree
Pennsylvania	Mar.-May	Tree		June-July	Grass
	May-July	Grass		Aug.-Oct.	Sage
	Aug.-Oct.	Ragweed		July-Sept.	Russian thistle or ragweed
Rhode Island	Mar.-May	Tree			
	May-July	Grass			
	Aug.-Sept.	Ragweed			

A SIMPLE SENSITIVITY TEST FOR A COSMETIC

If you are going to use a cosmetic product regularly, here's how to test to see if you are allergic to it. Take a small amount of the product, rub it into your forearm, and leave it for 24 hours. Wait a week and do it again. Wait another week and do it again. If there's no reaction any of the times, the product will probably not cause you to react. If you do have hives, redness, or rawness, don't use it.

HOW TO TELL IF YOUR SKIN IS DRY OR OILY

Dry skin is flaky in cold weather, sometimes feels very tight and drawn.

With oily skin you shine instead of glowing, are prone to blemishes and enlarged pores.

The Tissue Test: At night wash your face and rinse, put on no creams. In the morning blot your forehead, cheeks, nose, chin, and upper lip with tissue, holding it up to the light each time to check for traces of oil. If there is no oil, your skin is dry.

If there is lots of oil, your skin is oily. If there are traces of oil only in the forehead, nose, and chin zone, you have a normal combination skin.

EXAMINE YOUR HANDS FOR CLUES TO YOUR HEALTH

CLUE	WHAT IT MAY MEAN
Clubbing (enlargement) of fingertips and pale blue-gray fingernails	Congenital heart defect, lung disease such as emphysema, or cancer
Yellow palms	High levels of fats in the blood
Reddening of the palms	Pregnancy, cirrhosis of the liver
Moist, thin-skinned, warm hand and weak grip	Rheumatoid arthritis
Icy cold fingers	Constricted blood vessels, sometimes from smoking cigarettes
Pale nails instead of pink	Poor circulation
White spots on nails	Zinc deficiency
Horizontal white bands on nails	Arsenic or other metal poisoning; poor circulation; arthritis
Brittle nails	Vitamin deficiency or lack of moisture
Weak nails	Iodine, calcium or vitamin A needed
Separation of nails	Upset in thyroid metabolism; allergy to nail polish
Excessive hangnails	Low protein, vitamin C, or folic acid.

HOW TO TELL IF YOU HAVE FLAT FEET (FALLEN ARCHES)

Dip your feet in water and stand on a newspaper so you can see the outline of how your foot touches the ground.

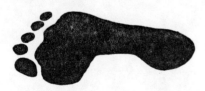

A normal foot

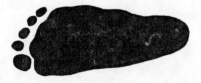

Fallen arch

MUSCLE IMBALANCE

If you have pains in the legs, knees, hip, back, or neck, they could be caused by the muscles being shorter or tighter on one side of the body, throwing your body a tiny bit off balance. Here are two simple tests so you can check your family.

SOME TESTS FOR MUSCLE IMBALANCE

1. Analyze footprints in the sand or by wetting the feet and walking on newspapers.

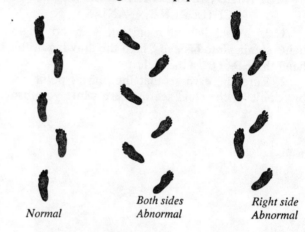

Normal   *Both sides Abnormal*   *Right side Abnormal*

2. Have the person stand up straight. Is one hip higher than the other?

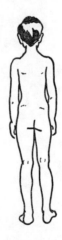

3. Is there difficulty in bending over and touching the toes?
4. Does it hurt to sit up straight on the floor with legs fully extended?

If these tests indicate you might have muscle imbalance, see an orthopedic surgeon. He may be able to cure your chronic pain with simple exercise or even a heel pad in one shoe.

Drawings courtesy of Dr. Arthur Michele, *Orthotherapy* (M. Evans Publishing Co. New York, N.Y.).

A HOME SCREENING EYE TEST FOR CHILDREN

When one eye is much stronger than the other so that vision becomes blurred and double, a condition called amblyopia ex anopsia occurs. The child shuts out the image from the weaker eye. The unused eye becomes weaker and weaker and finally almost blind.

You can check your child's eyes with this test.

MODIFIED SJOGREN HAND CARD FOR CHILDREN 3, 4, AND 5

1. In a well-lighted room but with no bright lights shining into his eyes, hold the drawing of the hand three feet from the child.

2. Turn the card so that the fingers point up, but don't let the child see the card while you turn it. Ask him to point his hand in the same direction as the hand on the card or to tell you if the fingers point to the sky, floor, wall, or window.

3. Repeat with the fingers pointing down, to the left and to the right. Then repeat any two positions.

4. Have someone cover one of the child's eyes with a small paper cup or tablespoon. Tell the child to keep both eyes open.

5. Repeat the six card positions, using a different order, so they won't be memorized.

6. Repeat with other eye covered.

7. *Screening.* Then move back to twelve feet and repeat the series. (If the child cannot answer correctly to at least four of the six positions, he may have an early case of amblyopia ex anopsia. See your doctor.

A DO-IT-YOURSELF URINE TEST

Take three glasses. When you urinate, catch the first part of the urine in the first glass, the middle part of the urination in the second glass, and the end in the third glass. Try to divide the urine equally among the three glasses.

Hold the urine up to the light. If all three are clear, with no clumps or shreds, you can be fairly certain there is no infection. If the first and third are cloudy, the second clear, doctors say you most likely have an inflammation of the urethra if a female, or of the prostate if a male. If all three glasses are cloudy, it is probably an infection of the upper urinary tract.

Note: A new test for urinary tract infection that can be done at home is Microstix. You dip a small plastic strip in the urine. If it turns pink in 30 seconds, it means a probable urinary tract infection, and you should see your doctor for treatment. Available from your pharmacist or Ames Division, Miles Laboratories, Elkhart, Indiana 46514.

A TEST FOR HYPOGLYCEMIA—THE DO-IT-YOURSELF GLUCOSE TOLERANCE TEST

Eat normally for three days, with plenty of carbohydrates. On the third day eat nothing after supper.

In the morning drink an entire bottle of glucola (you can get it from the drugstore). Do not eat or drink anything else (except lots of water) for six hours.

During the six hours, write down exactly how you feel at least every hour and note any symptoms you have such as fatigue, headache, trouble concentrating, a cold clammy feeling. If any of these symptoms occur, it strongly suggests you have hypoglycemia.

At the same time you can test your urine for sugar. Collect a urine sample every hour or two and test it with urine glucose testing sticks or strips (such as Tes-Tape) available at your drugstore. Keep drinking lots of water.

If there is sugar in your urine, the sticks or tape will turn green or blue.

If you have sugar in your urine or had symptoms during the glucose tolerance test, you should see your physician and have a regular six-hour laboratory glucose tolerance test.

HOW TO TEST YOUR URINE FOR VITAMIN C LEVEL

If you take more vitamin C than you need, it is excreted in your urine. Here's how to test.

Buy a 5 percent solution of aqueous silver nitrate from a drugstore. Put 10 drops in a clean cup. Add 10 drops of your urine (collected in a container).

Wait 2 minutes. The solution turns white to gray to charcoal in color. The darker it is, the more vitamin C you are spilling. If you excrete little or no vitamin C, it means your system is using all it can get and you can increase your dose. If it is dark charcoal, you can decrease the amount you are taking.

HOW TO USE KETOSTIX

Many people lose weight by going on a diet low enough in carbohydrates to cause their body to burn up fat and produce ketones. They test for the ketones being produced by using Ketostix (available in any drugstore without prescription).

To use a Ketostix, hold the strip where the urine will wet it, or collect a sample of urine in a cup and put the tip of the stick in it. The stick will turn lavender to purple if your body is producing ketones. The deeper the purple, the more ketones are present.

DIRECTORY

A GUIDE OF WHERE TO GO
FOR INFORMATION AND HELP
ON SPECIFIC
MEDICAL PROBLEMS.

There are hundreds of services available in this country free or almost free that the public, and often even the medical profession, is not completely aware of. A voluntary health organization exists for almost every disease there is, providing some free services as well as counseling and tons of literature. Many also give financial help to patients. Medical schools, hospitals, and government agencies are available to help you. You can write for booklets, write or call about specific problems, and often can use their diagnostic, counseling, or treatment facilities.

Planned Parenthood chapters, for example, provide contraceptive information and products, Pap tests, VD tests and treatment, pregnancy tests, abortion counseling, and information on sterilization and adoption. Ob-gyn advice is given at neighborhood women's health centers. Free Pap smears and breast checkups are available at many hospitals and through American Cancer Society neighborhood screening units.

Free and low-cost mental health facilities are offered by several mental health associations.

Community health fairs, mobile units, and hospital programs often offer free testing, free inoculations, and literature on lead poisoning, diabetes, sickle cell, high blood pressure, and glaucoma.

Most city health departments have free services for alcoholism, birth control, cancer detection, dentistry for children, diabetes, immunizations, infant care, mental health, narcotics addiction, smoking, nutrition, pregnancy testing, prenatal care, sickle cell anemia, tuberculosis, venereal disease.

Most public health services have free blood tests for syphilis and other diseases, free or inexpensive x-rays.

Some 200 inner-city neighborhood clinics have counseling services, referral services, and they help with problems such as drug abuse, illegitimate pregnancies, and venereal disease on a confidential walk-in basis.

We have listed the addresses of the national offices of organizations in this directory. But most national agencies have local chapters, so check your telephone directory to see if there is a chapter in your city where you can visit personally to discuss your problem. If you cannot find a local chapter in your area, write to the national headquarters and ask them for help.

To find government services, you usually must look under the name of the city or state. For example, if you live in Chicago, you would look under several listings: *Chicago, City of; Cook, County of; Illinois, State of;* and *United States.* Under these you will then find *Department of Health, U.S.*

Public Health Service, Social Services, Department of Welfare, Diabetes Detection Center, and many more.

Other local sources to check into for services and information are hospitals, medical schools, dental schools, and clinics near your neighborhood.

If you are writing for a booklet or advice from any of the organizations listed, you will get faster service if you enclose a stamped, self-addressed business-sized envelope.

ABORTION

Abortion Rights Association of New York
    250 West 57th Street
    New York, N.Y. 10019
National Abortion Council (formerly Association for the study
      of Abortion)
    120 West 57 Street
    New York, N.Y. 10019
National Abortion Rights Action League
    706 Seventh Street, S.E.
    Washington, D.C. 20003
National Clergy Consultation Service
    55 Washington Square South
    New York, N.Y. 10012
    Phone 212-254-6230
        Gives free abortion information, counseling, and referral by clergymen of all faiths.
National Association for Repeal of Abortion Laws
    250 West 57th Street
    New York, N.Y. 10019
Task Force on Reproduction and Its Control
    National Organization for Women
    1957 East 73rd Street
    Chicago, Ill. 60649
Zero Population Growth
    353 West 57th Street
    New York, N.Y. 10019
Women's Health and Abortion Project
    36 West 22nd Street
    New York, N.Y. 10010
Women's National Abortion Action Coalition
    156 Fifth Avenue
    New York, N.Y. 10010
        Each of these has programs of education in family planning, including counseling and referral for abortion and sterilization; and they have information on political programs to repeal restrictive abortion and contraception laws.

ACCIDENT PREVENTION

American Automobile Association
    1712 G Street, N.W.
    Washington, D.C. 20006
Council on Family Health
    201 East 42nd Street
    New York, N.Y. 10017
        Programs on home safety and first aid.

National Insitute for Occupational Safety & Health
    U.S. Department of Health, Education and Welfare
    5600 Fishers Lane
    Rockville, Md. 20852
        Information on occupational problems. Testing of occupational safety and health equipment.
National Safety Council
    425 North Michigan Avenue
    Chicago, Ill. 60649
        International clearinghouse of information about causes of accidents and accident prevention. Advises companies, traffic authorities, industrial management, transportation officials, school administrators, and farm organizations; works with organized labor, churches, clubs, colleges, and traffic authorities as well as with industry.

ADOPTION

Birthright
    2800 Otis Street, N.E.
    Washington, D.C. 20018
        Provides information and referral on adoption agencies, medical care, and financial assistance to women with unwanted pregnancies.
Child Welfare League of America
    67 Irving Place
    New York, N.Y. 10003
        Information on adoption and well-being of children.
International Social Service
    345 East 46th Street
    New York, N.Y. 10017
        Helps families to adopt children from abroad.

AGING

Administration on Aging
    U.S. Department of Health, Education and Welfare
    Washington, D.C. 20201
        Information on aging, retirement, senior citizens' centers, job opportunities, and housing. Lists senior citizens' social centers in country.
National Geriatrics Society
    165 North Pearl Street
    Albany, N.Y. 12207
U.S. Dept. of Housing and Urban Development
    Publications Division
    Washington, D.C. 20410
        Guide to elderly housing and related facilities.
American Association of Homes for the Aging
    315 Park Avenue South
    New York, N.Y. 10010
American Association of Retired Persons
    1090 K Street, N.W.
    Washington, D.C. 20049
        Information on aging and retirement. Travel, pharmacy, nursing-home services, and health, life, and auto insurance programs are available.
American Geriatrics Society
    10 Columbus Circle
    New York, N.Y. 10019

Gerontological Society
    110 South Central Avenue
    Clayton, Mo. 63105
Institute of Lifetime Learning
    Dupont Circle Building
    1346 Connecticut Avenue, N.W.
    Washington, D.C. 20036
        Continuing education program with classes at cen-
        ters throughout the country.
Manpower Administration
    U.S. Department of Labor
    Washington, D.C. 20210
        Coordinates programs of occupational training for
        unemployed and under-employed persons.
Mature Temps
    521 Fifth Avenue
    New York, N.Y. 10017
        National temporary-help service for people over 55.
National Council of Senior Citizens
    1627 K Street, N.W.
    Washington, D.C. 20006
        Sponsors Medicare supplemental insurance and
        drug-discount programs for members. Low-cost
        travel benefits.
National Council on the Aging
    1828 L Street, N.W.
    Washington, D.C. 20036
        Extensive library of literature on aging. A national
        directory of housing for older people. $5.50
        Also see *Nursing Homes*

ALCOHOLISM

Al-Anon
    P.O. Box 182
    Madison Square Station
    New York, N.Y. 10010
        Information for relatives and friends of alcoholics.
Alcholics Anonymous
    P.O. Box 459
    Grand Central Station
    New York, N.Y. 10017
        Meetings, group help, and literature for men and
        women with alcoholism.
National Committee on Alcoholism
    2 East 103rd Street
    New York, N.Y. 10029
National Council on Alcoholism
    2 Park Avenue
    New York, N.Y. 10016
Alcohol and Drug Problems Association
    1130 17th Street, N.W.
    Washington, D.C. 20036
National Institute on Alcohol Abuse and Alcoholism
    National Institutes of Health
    P.O. Box 2345
    Rockville, Md. 20852
        Programs to prevent and treat alcohol abuse. Public
        information, education, consultation, and referral
        services. Advice to labor and management on estab-
        lishing employee alcoholism programs.

ALLERGIES

Allergy Foundation of America
    801 Second Avenue
    New York, N.Y. 10017
American Academy of Allergy
    756 North Milwaukee Street
    Milwaukee, Wis. 53202
Children's Asthma Research Institute and Hospital
    3401 West 19th Avenue
    Denver, Colo. 80204
        Free treatment and care to children.
National Institute of Allergy and Infectious Diseases
    Office of Information
    Bethesda, Md. 20014
        Conducts and coordinates research on diseases
        caused by infectious organisms and allergies.

ARTHRITIS

The Arthritis Foundation
    3400 Peachtree Street, N.E.
    Atlanta, Ga. 30326
        Clinic, home-care programs, and centers for care
        and rehabilitation to arthritis patients. Many chap-
        ters also have facilities for occupational therapy. In-
        formation on rheumatic conditions.
National Institute of Arthritis and Metabolic Diseases
    Office of Information
    Bethesda, Md. 20014
        Information on causes, prevention, and treatment of
        various arthritic, rheumatic, collagen, and metabolic
        diseases.

ASTHMA

    See *Respiratory Disease; Allergies*

BIRTH CONTROL

    See *Family Planning*

BIRTH DEFECTS

National Foundation—March of Dimes
    Public Education Department
    Box 2000
    White Plains, N.Y. 10602
        Patient service centers for diagnosis, treatment, and
        prevention of birth defects. Free prenatal clinics.

BLINDNESS

American Foundation for the Blind
    15 West 16th Street
    New York, N.Y. 10011
        Information, counsel, and services to blind persons.
        Books, magazines, monographs, and leaflets in con-
        ventional print and large type, on recordings and in

braille. Special appliances for use by blind people. Also has *Directory of Agencies Serving Blind Persons in the United States* with more than 500 listings. $4.00

The Library of Congress
Division for the Blind and Physically Handicapped
1291 Taylor Street, N.W.
Washington, D.C. 20542
Library services for the blind and physically handicapped.

Braille Institute of America
741 North Vermont Avenue
Los Angeles, Calif. 90029
Information, casework, books in braille for the blind at cost; lending library service.

Eye Bank for Sight Restoration
210 East 64th Street
New York, N.Y. 10021
Arranges for donation of eyes for corneal transplants.

Fight for Sight
41 West 57th Street
New York, N.Y. 10019

American Printing House for the Blind
1839 Frankfort Avenue
Louisville, Ky. 40206
Braille publications, large-type textbooks, cassettes.

The Associated Blind
135 West 23rd Street
New York, N.Y. 10010

Kinlock National Mission for the Blind
407 Lenox Avenue
New York, N.Y. 10037
Helps the black blind.

Jewish Braille Institute
110 East 30th Street
New York, N.Y. 10016
Sends braille and talking books free anywhere in the world in Hebrew and Yiddish. Free review with magazine articles translated into braille.

Jewish Guild for the Blind
1880 Broadway
New York, N.Y. 10023
Open to all for assistance.

National Aid for Visually Handicapped
3201 Balboa Street
San Francisco, Calif. 94121
Large print materials for children and adults with defective eyesight.

National Council to Combat Blindness
41 West 57th Street
New York, N.Y. 10019

National Industries for the Blind
1120 Avenue of the Americas
New York, N.Y. 10036
Rehabilitation of the blind.

National Society for the Prevention of Blindess
79 Madison Avenue
New York, N.Y. 10016
Information on glaucoma, cataract, eye health and safety.

Research to Prevent Blindness
598 Madison Avenue
New York, N.Y. 10022

New Eyes for the Needy
549 Millburn Avenue
Short Hills, N.J. 07078
Provides eyeglasses for those unable to pay.

The Seeing Eye
Morristown, N.J. 07960
Trains Seeing-Eye dogs. Trains blind persons in proper care and handling of the dogs.

Guiding Eyes for the Blind
106 East 41st Street
New York, N.Y. 10017

Recording for the Blind
215 East 58th Street
New York, N.Y. 10022

Louis Braille Foundation for Blind Musicians
112 East 19th Street
New York, N.Y. 10003
Scholarships and braille music scores for blind musicians.

National Association for Visually Handicapped
305 East 24th Street
New York, N.Y. 10010
Produces and distributes large-print books. Clearinghouse of information about services available for the partially seeing. Free loan library of large-type books.

National Eye Institute
National Institutes of Health
Bethesda, Md. 20014

National Retinitis Pigmentosa Foundation
Rolling Park Building
8331 Mindale Circle
Baltimore, Md. 21207

BLOOD

American Association of Blood Banks
30 North Michigan Avenue
Chicago, Ill. 60602

American Red Cross
150 Amsterdam Avenue
New York, N.Y. 10023
Provides blood and blood derivatives to individuals and groups who donate, and also sells it.

Children's Blood Foundation
342 Madison Avenue
New York, N.Y. 10017
Children with blood diseases are treated and given blood transfusions free.

National Rare Blood Club
164 Fifth Avenue
New York, N.Y. 10010
Rare blood free to patients or hospitals.
See also *Sickle Cell Disease*

CANCER

American Cancer Society
777 Third Avenue
New York, N.Y. 10017
Information and service to cancer patients.

Cancer Care
National Cancer Foundation
1 Park Avenue
New York, N.Y. 10016

Cancer Care (*cont.*)
>   Professional counseling for cancer patients and their families who live within 50 miles of New York City. Financial assistance for self-supporting families of low and middle income.

Children's Cancer Fund of America
>   15 East 67th Street
>   New York, N.Y. 10021

National Cancer Institute
>   Information Office
>   Bethesda, Md. 20014
>   Information on causes, prevention, and treatment of cancer.

United Ostomy Association
>   1111 Wilshire Boulevard
>   Los Angeles, Calif. 90017
>   Information and counseling for patients who have had colostomy surgery.

The Candlelighters
>   133 C Street, S.E.
>   Washington, D.C. 20003
>   Self-help program for parents of young cancer victims. Newsletter.

International Association of Laryngectomy
>   777 Third Avenue
>   New York, N.Y. 10017
>   Information and counseling for patients who have had their larynx removed. Help in learning to speak again.

Reach for Recovery
>   777 Third Avenue
>   New York, N.Y. 10017
>   Also check with your local chapter of the American Cancer Society for counseling if you have had a mastectomy, including personal visits by other mastectomy patients with aids on coping.

Hospice
>   765 Prospect Street
>   New Haven, Conn. 06511
>   The hospice specializes in caring for terminally ill patients, and aims to make their final days as comfortable and humanistic as possible.

Make Today Count
>   218 South Sixth Street
>   Burlington, Iowa 52601
>   Provides group sessions for the terminally ill, led by the terminally ill, and tries to help with both emotional and practical problems. Newsletters. $10

Society for the Rehabilitation of the Facially Disfigured
>   550 Fifth Avenue
>   New York, N.Y. 10017
>   Treatment and counseling.
>   Also see *Leukemia*

CEREBRAL PALSY

American Academy for Cerebral Palsy
>   1520 Louisiana Avenue
>   New Orleans, La. 70015

United Cerebral Palsy Association
>   66 East 34th Street
>   New York, N.Y. 10016
>   Local centers for treatment and study of persons with cerebral palsy. Vocational training and sheltered workshops.

CHILDREN

American Academy of Pediatrics
>   1801 Hinman Avenue
>   Evanston, Ill. 60204

American Association for Maternal and Child Health
>   116 South Michigan Avenue
>   Chicago, Ill. 60603

American School Health Association
>   515 East Main Street
>   Kent, Ohio 44240

Child Study Association of America
>   9 East 89th Street
>   New York, N.Y. 10028
>   Mental health education through parent counseling, discussion groups, and training of professionals.

Commission for Community Control of Day Care
>   458 Columbus Avenue
>   New York, N.Y. 10024

Day Care and Child Development Council of America
>   1426 H Street, N.W.
>   Washington, D.C. 20005

Office of Child Development
>   Department of Health, Education and Welfare
>   P.O. Box 1182
>   Washington, D.C. 20013

National Institute of Child Health and Human Development
>   National Institutes of Health
>   Bethesda, Md. 20014

Association for Children with Learning Disabilities
>   5225 Grace Street
>   Pittsburgh, Pa. 15236

Parents Anonymous
>   250 West 57th Street
>   New York, N.Y. 10019
>   A self-help group of parents who counsel parents who feel they are abusing or neglecting their children.

National Association of Children's Hospitals and Related Institutions
>   1308 Delaware Avenue
>   Wilmington, Del. 19805

National Foundation for Sudden Infant Death
>   1501 Broadway
>   New York, N.Y. 10036

National Sudden Infant Death Syndrome Foundation
>   310 South Michigan Avenue
>   Chicago, Ill. 60604
>   Information and assistance to families who've suffered infant loss.
>   You can also obtain guidance and counseling on programs for youth, advice on juvenile deliquency and other problems of child care at the local offices of your City Youth Board, Police Athletic League, State Division for Youth, Community Council, Children's Aid Society, Bureau of Child Welfare, and religious agencies.

CLEFT PALATE

American Cleft Palate Association
>   Parker Hall
>   University of Missouri
>   Columbia, Mo. 65202

American Dental Association
211 E. Chicago Avenue
Chicago, Ill. 60611
Also contact your nearest dental school.

COUNSELING
Family Service Association of America
44 East 23rd Street
New York, N.Y. 10010
Confidential counseling for family, marriage, and personal problems.
American Association of Marriage Counselors
270 Park Avenue
New York, N.Y. 10017
National Council on Family Relations
5737 Drexel Avenue
Chicago, Ill.
Also see *Mental Health*

CYSTIC FIBROSIS
National Cystic Fibrosis Research Foundation
3379 Peachtree Street, N.E.
Atlanta, Ga. 30326
Information, equipment, and financial aid. Directory of diagnosis and treatment clinics.

DENTAL
American Dental Association
Bureau of Health Education
211 East Chicago Avenue
Chicago, Ill. 60611
Information on dental health.
American Society of Oral Surgeons
211 East Chicago Avenue
Chicago, Ill. 60611
National Institute of Dental Research
Office of Information
Bethesda, Md. 20014
Information on causes, prevention, and treatment of oral conditions.

DIABETES
American Diabetes Association
18 East 48th Street
New York, N.Y. 10017
Juvenile Diabetes Foundation
23 East 26th Street
New York, N.Y. 10010

DIGESTIVE DISEASES
National Foundation for Ileitis and Colitis
295 Madison Avenue
New York, N.Y. 10017
National Institute of Arthritis, Metabolism and Digestive
Diseases
National Institutes of Health
Bethesda, Md. 20014

DRUG ADDICTION
Addicts Anonymous
Box 2000
Lexington, Ky. 40501

American Social Health Association
1740 Broadway
New York, N.Y. 10019
Comprehensive material on drug abuse.
National Clearinghouse for Drug Abuse Information
National Institute of Mental Health
5600 Fishers Lane
Rockville, Md. 20852
Programs and information against drug abuse. Has a 24-hour hot line on drug abuse information: (301) 496-7171.
Synanon House
1910 Ocean Front
Santa Monica, Calif. 90405
Community houses. Clinics for confidential help.

EPILEPSY
National Epilepsy League
6 North Michigan Avenue
Chicago, Ill. 60602
American Epilepsy Society
50 North Medical Drive
Salt Lake City, Utah 84101
Epilepsy Foundation of America
1828 L Street, N.W.
Washington, D.C. 20006
All have information on epilepsy and services including medical, social, psychological, and vocational. Some have drugs at discount.

EYE CARE
American Association of Ophthalmology
1100 17th Street, N.W.
Washington, D.C. 20036
American Optometric Association
P.O. Box 13157
St. Louis, Mo. 63119
Better Vision Institute
230 Park Avenue
New York, N.Y. 10017
National Eye Institute
9000 Rockville Pike
Bethesda, Md. 20014
Contact Lens Association of Ophthalmology
40 West 77th Street
New York, N.Y. 10024
Illuminating Engineering Society of North America
345 East 47th Street
New York, N.Y. 10017
Contact Lens Manufacturers Association
435 North Michigan Avenue
Chicago, Ill. 60611
Contact Lens Society of America
167 West Main Street
Lexington, Ky. 40507
Also see *Blindness*

FAMILY PLANNING
American Fertility Society
944 South 18th Street
Birmingham, Ala. 35205

IDANT Corporation
    645 Madison Avenue
    New York, N.Y. 10022
        Commercial sperm-banking facility, artificial insemi-
        nation available.
Association for Voluntary Sterilization
    14 West 40th Street
    New York, N.Y. 10018
        Information on voluntary sterilization. Referral ser-
        vice to physician in your area who performs opera-
        tion.
Planned Parenthood—World Population
    515 Madison Avenue
    New York, N.Y. 10022
        Family planning centers for free and low-cost ser-
        vice. Counseling for abortion, sterilization, and con-
        traception.

FINANCIAL AID

To apply for public assistance, you must appear in person at the
Welfare Department center nearest your home. The criteria for
receiving public assistance is not enough money to meet the
needs of a family, as calculated on a public assistance budget,
which is very low. Categories of welfare are:

        Home Relief, for a person who does not earn enough
        money to maintain his family or himself and is un-
        able to secure additional support.
        Old Age Assistance, for persons over 65 unable to
        support themselves.
        Aid to the Disabled, for persons permanently or to-
        tally disabled and unable to support themselves.
        Assistance to the Blind, for blind persons who have
        no means of support.
        Veteran Assistance, for aid to veterans falling under
        any of the above categories.
        Aid to Dependent Children, for children under 16,
        18, or 21 if in school, whose parents cannot support
        them. Aid is also given to the mother.

FOOT CARE

American Podiatry Association
    20 Chevy Chase Circle, N.W.
    Washington, D.C. 20015
        Foot-health screening examinations in schools and
        community health programs. Free literature.

GASTROINTESTINAL PROBLEMS

American College of Gastroenterology
    33 West 60th Street
    New York, N.Y. 10023
American Gastroenterological Association
    11 East 100th Street
    New York, N.Y. 10029

GENETIC COUNSELING

National Genetics Foundation
    250 West 57th Street
    New York, N.Y. 10019
        Genetic counseling and treatment centers to help
        people who have, or suspect they have, hereditary
        diseases. Diagnosis and treatment in family plan-
        ning.

National Foundation—March of Dimes
    P.O. Box 2000
    White Plains, N.Y. 10602
        Genetic counseling and diagnosis. Complete interna-
        tional list of genetic counseling services by area.

HANDICAPPED

See *Rehabilitation*

HEARING

American Speech and Hearing Association
    9030 Old Georgetown Road
    Washington, D.C. 20014
        Information on speech and hearing. Free list of clini-
        cal services in speech pathology and audiology.
National Association of the Deaf
    314 Thayer Avenue
    Silver Spring, Md. 20910
        Information on employability and status of the deaf.
Alexander Graham Bell Association for the Deaf
    1537 35th Street, N.W.
    Washington, D.C. 20007
        Information, aid, and education for the deaf.
National Association of Hearing and Speech Agencies
    919 18th Street, N.W.
    Washington, D.C. 20006
        Helps local communities and agencies to establish,
        maintain, and improve hearing, speech, and lan-
        guage services. Information on deafness.
National Hearing Aid Society
    24261 Grand River Avenue
    Detroit, Mich. 48219
        Information on and standards for hearing aids.
The Volta Bureau
    3417 Volta Place, N.W.
    Washington, D.C. 20007
        Offers a free bibliography on deafness and hearing
        aids.
The Deafness Research Foundation
    366 Madison Avenue
    New York, N.Y. 10017

HEART AND CIRCULATORY DISEASES

American College of Cardiology
    9650 Rockville Pike
    Bethesda, Md. 20014
American Heart Association
    7320 Greenville Avenue
    Dallas, Tex. 75231
        Professional and public information and community
        service on heart disease and high blood pressure.
        Publishes newsletter and booklets.
Associated Cardiac League Inc.
    1 Union Square
    New York, N.Y. 10003
        Referral through clinics and doctors only. Camps for
        children aged 8 to 15.
Deborah Hospital
    Browns Mills, N.J. 08015
        Hospital for the correction of operable heart defects
        and lung diseases. Admission through sponsorship
        by chapters.

National Heart and Lung Institute
Office of Information
Bethesda, Md. 20014
Information on cause, prevention, diagnosis, and treatment of circulatory diseases, including high blood pressure, hardening of the arteries, and heart attacks.

National Institute of Neurological Diseases and Stroke
National Institutes of Health
Bethesda, Md. 20014
Information on strokes.

National Hemophilia Foundation
25 West 39th Street
New York, N.Y. 10018
Referrals to blood banks and clinics. Vocational rehabilitation, educational and social service programs. Volunteers assist with home transfusions, transport patients to clinics and hospitals.

HIGH BLOOD PRESSURE

National High Blood Pressure Information Program
120/80
Bethesda, Md. 20014
Also see *Heart and Circulatory Diseases*

HOMEMAKER SERVICES

National Committee on Homemaker Service
12 South Lake Avenue
Albany, N.Y. 12203
Homemaker service programs and advisers to programs.

National Council for Homemaker—Home Health Aide Services
1740 Broadway
New York, N.Y. 10019
Gives care and help to people in their homes.

HUNTINGTON'S DISEASE

Committee to Combat Huntington's Disease
299 Clinton Street
Brooklyn, N.Y. 11201
Information and counseling for patients with Huntington's disease.

KIDNEY DISEASE

American Urological Association
1120 North Charles Street
Baltimore, Md. 21201

National Association of Patients on Hemodialysis and Transplantation
505 Northern Boulevard
Great Neck, N.Y. 11022

Kidney Disease Control Program
5600 Fishers Lane
Rockville, Md. 20852
Has list of kidney disease services and programs in the U.S.

National Kidney Foundation
116 East 27th Street
New York, N.Y. 10016
Programs of community services, information on kidneys and kidney disease, and National Organ Donor project. Funds for chronic kidney dialysis treatments and kidney transplants.

LEPROSY

Leonard Wood Memorial for the Eradication of Leprosy
79 Madison Avenue
New York, N.Y. 10016

U.S. Public Health Service Center
Carvill, La. 70721
Free treatment and care for leprosy patients.

LEUKEMIA

Leukemia Society
211 East 43rd Street
New York, N.Y. 10017
Aid to patients with leukemia.

LUPUS ERYTHEMATOSIS

Lupus Erythematosis Foundation
44 East 23rd Street
New York, N.Y. 10010

MATERNITY

See *Pregnancy*

MEDICAID

Medical Services Administration
Social and Rehabilitation Service
U.S. Department of Health, Education and Welfare
Washington, D.C. 20201
Information on federal and state medical assistance programs.

MEDICINES

Food and Drug Administration
Consumer Enquiry
5600 Fishers Lane
Rockville, Md. 20852
Information on drug side effects and medicines.

Pharmaceutical Manufacturers Association
1155 15th Street, N.W.
Washington, D.C. 20005
Information on prescription medicines.

Proprietary Association
1700 Pennsylvania Avenue, N.W.
Washington, D.C. 20006
Information on non-prescription medicines.

MENTAL HEALTH

American Psychiatric Association
1700 18th Street, N.W.
Washington, D.C. 20009

American Psychological Association
1200 17th Street, N.W.
Washington, D.C. 20036

American Schizophrenia Association
56 West 45th Street
New York, N.Y. 10036

National Association for Mental Health
1800 North Kent Street
Rosslyn, Va. 22209

American Group Psychotherapy Association
1865 Broadway
New York, N.Y. 10023

National Institute of Mental Health
>   Bethesda, Md. 20014
>   > Information on mental illness. Support for patients in hospitals and newly returned home.

National Association of Private Psychiatric Hospitals
>   353 Broad Avenue
>   Leonia, N.J. 07605
>   > Their Mental Health Directory lists hundreds of agencies by state that provide mental health prevention, treatment, and rehabilitation services and their fees.

Mental Health Film Board
>   8 East 93rd Street
>   New York, N.Y. 10028
>   > Write for their current film catalogue.

Neurotics Anonymous International
>   1341 G Street, N.W.
>   Washington, D.C. 20005

Recovery
>   116 South Michigan Avenue
>   Chicago, Ill. 60614
>   > Peer help for those with emotional problems and also those hospitalized for same.

Schizophrenics Anonymous
>   Box 1134
>   Linden Hills Station
>   Flushing, N.Y. 11354
>   > Helps members recovering from their illness.

MENTAL RETARDATION

National Association for Retarded Children
>   420 Lexington Avenue
>   New York, N.Y. 10017

Exceptional Children's Foundation
>   2225 West Admas Boulevard
>   Los Angeles, Calif. 90018
>   > Complete range of services for mentally retarded of all ages.

National Association for Retarded Citizens
>   P.O. Box 6109
>   Arlington, Va. 76011
>   > Helps families cope with problems.

Joseph P. Kennedy Jr. Foundation
>   1701 K Street, N.W.
>   Washington, D.C. 20006

Retarded Infants Services
>   386 Park Avenue South
>   New York, N.Y. 10016

Council for Exceptional Children
>   1920 Association Drive
>   Reston, Va. 22091
>   > Educational program for mentally retarded pupils as well as teacher training, instructional materials.

MULTIPLE SCLEROSIS

National Multiple Sclerosis Society
>   257 Park Avenue South
>   New York, N.Y. 10010
>   > Services to patients in chapter clinics. Many publications.

MUSCULAR DYSTROPHY

Muscular Dystrophy Associations of America
>   1790 Broadway
>   New York, N.Y. 10019
>   > Community services to patients and families. Diagnostic workups, wheelchairs, physical therapy.

MYASTHENIA GRAVIS

Myasthenia Gravis Foundation
>   230 Park Avenue
>   New York, N.Y. 10017
>   > Information about the cause, cure, and prevention of myasthenia gravis and services for people with the disease.

National Foundation of Neuromuscular Diseases
>   250 West 57th Street
>   New York, N.Y. 10019

NARCOTICS

> See *Drug Addiction*

NURSES

National League for Nursing
>   10 Columbus Circle
>   New York, N.Y. 10019
>   > Information on nursing and visiting nurse service.

NURSING HOMES

American Health Care Association
>   1025 Connecticut Avenue, N.W.
>   Washington, D.C. 20036
>   > Information on proprietary and non-proprietary nursing homes.

American Association of Homes for the Aging
>   529 Fourteenth Street, N.W.
>   Washington, D.C. 20004

NUTRITION

American Dietetic Association
>   620 North Michigan Avenue
>   Chicago, Ill. 60611

Food and Drug Administration
>   Office of Consumer Affairs
>   5600 Fishers Lane
>   Rockville, Md. 20852
>   > Information on standards on the composition, quality, nutrition, and safety of foods.

Nutrition Foundation
>   99 Park Avenue
>   New York, N.Y. 10016
>   > Nutrition education.

U.S. Department of Agriculture
>   Office of Information
>   Washington, D.C. 20250

Information on nutrition, food grading, and food economics. Booklets about buying meat, fruit, poultry, egg, and other foods.

Vitamin Information Bureau
575 Lexington Avenue
New York, N.Y. 10022
Provides information on vitamins and minerals.

OSTEOPATHIC MEDICINE

American Osteopathic Association
212 East Ohio Street
Chicago, Ill. 60611

PARKINSON'S DISEASE

American Parkinson Disease Association
147 East 50th Street
New York, N.Y. 10022
National Parkinson Disease Insitute
1501 N.W. 9th Avenue
Miami, Fla. 33136
Parkinson's Disease Foundation
640 West 168th Street
New York, N.Y. 10032

PHYSICAL FITNESS

President's Council on Physical Fitness and Sports
7th and D Streets, S.W.
Washington, D.C. 20202
Promotes home and school exercise programs.

PLASTIC SURGERY

American Society of Plastic & Reconstructive Surgeons
18 Laughlin Lane
Philadelphia, Pa. 19118
American Academy of Facial Plastic Reconstructive Surgery
1111 Tulane Avenue
New Orleans, La. 70112

POISON CONTROL

American Association of Poison Control Centers
44th and Dewey Avenues
Omaha, Neb. 68105
Bureau of Product Safety
Medical Review and Poison Control Branch
200 C Street, S.W.
Washington, D.C. 20204
National clearinghouse of information for poison control centers. First-aid information on poisoning.

POLIOMYELITIS

Georgia Warm Springs Foundation
120 Broadway
New York, N.Y. 10005
Aids sufferers from after-effects of polio.
The National Foundation—March of Dimes
P.O. Box 2000
White Plains, N.Y. 10602
(Formerly the National Foundation for Infantile Paralysis.) Provides information and aids patients.

POLLUTION

Environmental Protection Agency
Office of Public Affairs
Washington, D.C. 20460
Information on what you can do about clean air, water, and living environment.
Izaak Walton League of America
1326 Waukegan Road
Glenview, Ill. 60025
Information on conservation of natural resources and protection of environmental quality.

PREGNANCY

American College of Obstetricians and Gynecologists
79 West Monroe Street
Chicago, Ill. 60603
American Association for Maternal and Child Health
116 South Michigan Avenue
Chicago, Ill. 60603
La Leche League International
9616 Minneapolis Avenue
Franklin Park, Ill. 60131
Information on breast feeding.
Maternal and Child Health Service
5600 Fishers Lane
Rockville, Md. 20852
Provides health services to expectant mothers and children.
Maternity Center Association
48 East 92nd Street
New York, N.Y. 10028
Educational programs for expectant parents and professionals on parental care. Trains nurse-midwives.
American Society for Psycho-Prophylaxis in Obstetrics
1523 L Street, N.W.
Washington, D.C. 20005
Information on the Lamaze method of education for "natural" childbirth.

PSORIASIS

National Psoriasis Foundation
6415 S.W. Canyon Street
Portland, Ore. 47221

REHABILITATION

American Academy of Physical Medicine and Rehabilitation
30 North Michigan Avenue
Chicago, Ill. 60602
American Occupational Therapy Association
251 Park Avenue South
New York, N. Y. 10010
American Physical Therapy Association
1740 Broadway
New York, N. Y. 10019
American Rehabilitation Committee
28 East 21st Street
New York, N. Y. 10010
Maintains a rehabilitation center for the disabled.
National Information Center for the Handicapped
Box 1492
Washington, D.C. 20013

Association for the Aid of Crippled Children
345 East 46th Street
New York, N. Y. 10017
Association for the Aid of Crippled Children and Adults
239 Park Avenue South
New York, N. Y. 10010
Children's Bureau
Office of Child Development
330 Independent Ave., S.W.
Washington, D.C. 20201
Will tell you where there is a clinic in your area that offers services for handicapped children.
Department of Defense
Washington, D.C. 20301
Employs disabled civilians and rehabilitates disabled servicemen and women.
Paralyzed Veterans of America
7315 Wisconsin Avenue
Washington, D.C. 20014
Many publications including Wheelchair House Plans (50¢) and guidebooks for handicapped travelers.
Disabled American Veterans
1425 East McMillan Street
Cincinnati, Ohio 45206
Aids disabled veterans with hospitals, insurance, and employment.
Goodwill Industries of America
1913 N Street, N.W.
Washington, D.C. 20006
Provides employment opportunities for the handicapped and disabled.
Institute for the Achievement of Human Potential
8801 Stenton Avenue
Philadelphia, Pa. 19119
Treatment for severely handicapped and brain-injured children.
Institute for the Crippled and Disabled
400 First Avenue
New York, N. Y. 10010
Vocational advice for rehabilitation.
President's Committee on Employment of the Handicapped
Washington, D.C. 20210
Promotional opportunities for training and employment for handicapped.
International Society for Rehabilitation of the Disabled
219 East 44th Street
New York, N. Y. 10017
Sister Kenny Rehabilitation Institute
1800 Chicago Avenue
Minneapolis, Minn. 55404
National Amputation Foundation
12–45 150th Street
Whitestone, N. Y. 11357
Members visit patients who have undergone amputation. A limb shop fits limbs. Help is given amputees seeking employment, free admission to shows and sports events.
National Association of the Physically Handicapped
76 Elm Street
London, Ohio 43140

National Center for Law and the Handicapped
1235 North Eddy Street
South Bend, Ind. 46617
Legal assistance on rights of handicapped persons.
National Association of Sheltered Workshops and Homebound Programs
1522 K Street
Washington, D.C. 20005
National Easter Seal Society for Crippled Children and Adults
2023 West Ogden Avenue
Chicago, Ill. 60612
Vocational and educational services. Sheltered workshops, treatment centers, mobile therapy units, camps. "New York City Guide for the Handicapped" lists where to find wheelchair ramps and other special facilities free.
National Rehabilitation Association
1029 Vermont Avenue, N.W.
Washington, D.C. 20005
Rehabilitation services for the mentally and physically handicapped.
Institute of Physical Medicine and Rehabilitation
400 East 34th Street
New York, N. Y. 10016
Homemakers program for disabled.
Office of Vocational Rehabilitation
Washington, D.C. 20201
Information on federal-state programs for rehabilitating handicapped persons.
Shriner's Hospital for Crippled Children
323 North Michigan Avenue
Chicago, Ill. 60601
Shut-in Society, Inc.
11 West 42nd Street
New York, N. Y. 10036
Provides correspondence and other services for the handicapped.
U.S. Department of Health, Education and Welfare
Social and Rehabilitation Service
330 C Street, S.W.
Washington, D.C. 20201
Coordinates government services to the handicapped.
Veterans Administration
Washington, D.C. 20420
Rehabilitates disabled veterans.
National Park Guide for the Handicapped is available (95¢) from Superintendent of Documents, Government Printing Office, Washington, D.C. 20402.

RESPIRATORY DISEASE

Children's Asthma Research Institute and Hospital
Denver, Colo. 80204
Treatment of asthma. Children remain in residence 18 to 24 months.
National Heart and Lung Institute
Office of Information
Bethesda, Md. 20014
Information on diseases of the lungs, heart, and circulation.

National Jewish Hospital and Research Center
    Denver, Colo. 80204
        Research center for chronic respiratory diseases.
        Some free care for emphysema, asthma, and other
        allergic disorders, and tuberculosis.
American Lung Association
    1740 Broadway
    New York, N. Y. 10019
        Information on prevention and control of tuberculo-
        sis and other respiratory diseases, prevention of air
        pollution, elimination of smoking. Testing programs
        in many chapters.

SCHIZOPHRENIA

   See *Mental Health*

SEX

American College of Obstetricians and Gynecologists
    1 East Wacker Drive
    Chicago, Ill. 60601
National Woman's Health Coalition
    1120 Lexington Avenue
    New York, N. Y. 10021
        Educational information on women's health, consul-
        tant services for other groups that want to set up
        low-cost women's health centers, free pregnancy di-
        agnosis.
Healthright, Women's Health Forum
    175 Fifth Avenue
    New York, N. Y. 10010
American Social Health Association
    1740 Broadway
    New York, N. Y. 10019
        Family life education material for schools and for
        training teachers.
SIECUS (Sex Information and Education Council of the U.S.)
    1855 Broadway
    New York, N. Y. 10023
        Works with physicians, educators, clergymen, and
        social scientists to develop programs in sex educa-
        tion for all ages.

SICKLE CELL DISEASE

Association for Sickle Cell Anemia
    520 Fifth Avenue
    New York, N. Y. 10036
Black Athletes Foundation for Sickle Cell Disease
    1312 Grant Boulevard
    Pittsburgh, Pa. 15219
Foundation for Research and Education for Sickle Cell Disease
    423 West 120th Street
    New York, N. Y. 10027
Midwest Association for Sickle Cell Anemia
    841 East 63rd Street
    Chicago, Ill. 60637
Mid-South Association for Sickle Cell Disease
    2316 Alameda
    Memphis, Tenn. 38108
National Sickle Cell Disease Research Foundation
    520 Fifth Avenue
    New York, N. Y. 10036

Sickle Cell Anemia Research and Education
    P. O. Box 40118
    1930 Sutter Street
    San Francisco, Calif. 94140
Volunteers in Aid of Sickle Cell Anemia, Inc.
    P. O. Box 1839
    Philadelphia, Pa. 19105
The Sickle Cell Guild of America
    P. O. Box 47947
    Los Angeles, Calif. 90047
United Sickle Cell Anemia Association
    P. O. Box 17254
    Philadelphia, Pa. 19105

SKIN CARE

American Academy of Dermatology
    2250 N.W. Flanders Street
    Portland, Ore. 97210

SMOKING

National Clearinghouse for Smoking and Health
    5600 Fishers Lane
    Rockville, Md. 20852
        Information on the hazards of smoking and how to
        become a non-smoker.
National Interagency Council on Smoking and Health
    419 Park Avenue
    New York, N. Y. 10016
        Coordinates smoking education programs for organi-
        zations concerned with smoking and health pro-
        grams. Publishes *Smoking and Health Newsletter*.

SOCIAL SECURITY

Social Security Administration
    Baltimore, Md. 21235
        Information about Social Security, disability insur-
        ance benefits, old age and survivors insurance.

SPEECH

American Speech and Hearing Association
    9030 Old Georgetown Road
    Washington, D.C. 20014
        Free guide to clinical services in speech pathology
        and audiology.
Audiology and Speech Correction Center
    Walter Reed Army Hospital
    Washington, D.C. 20012
National Association of Hearing and Speech Agencies
    919 18th Street, N.W.
    Washington, D.C. 20006
        Helps establish community speech and language ser-
        vices. Publishes "Hearing and Speech News."
National Hospital for Speech Disorders
    61 Irving Place
    New York, N. Y. 10003
Speech Rehabilitation Institute
    61 Irving Place
    New York, N. Y. 10003
        Offers diagnostic and therapeutic services to speech-
        handicapped clients of every age and economic
        level. Write for: "If Your Child Stutters." Free.

STERILIZATION

Association for Voluntary Sterilization
  14 West 44th Street
  New York, N. Y. 10036
      Facts on sterilization procedures for men and
      women. Lists of physicians in your area who will
      perform vasectomy or tubal ligation.
Planned Parenthood—World Population
  515 Madison Avenue
  New York, N. Y. 10022
      Gives information on where to get help. Several vas-
      ectomy clinics in major cities.

STROKE

Stroke Club of America
  Box 15186
  860 North Highway
  Austin, Tex. 78761
      Also see *Heart and Circulatory Diseases*

SUICIDE

Center for Studies of Suicide Prevention
National Institute of Mental Health
  5600 Fishers Lane
  Rockville, Md. 20652
      Sponsors educational efforts in suicide prevention.
National Save-A-Life League
  20 West 43rd Street
  New York, N. Y. 10036
      Provides 24-hour telephone service for crisis coun-
      seling and potential suicides.
      Also see *Mental Health*

TAY-SACHS DISEASE

Tay-Sachs and Allied Disease Association
  200 Park Avenue South
  New York, N. Y. 10003

TUBERCULOSIS

  See *Respiratory Disease*

UNMARRIED MOTHERS

Children's Bureau
Department of Health, Education and Welfare
  Washington, D.C. 20201
Florence Crittenton Homes Association
  608 South Dearborn Street
  Chicago, Ill. 60605
      Services for unwed mothers.
Maternity Service for Unmarried Mothers
  225 Park Avenue South
  New York, N. Y. 10003
National Association on Service to Unmarried Parents
  171 West 12th Street
  New York, N. Y. 10011
National Council on Illegitimacy
  44 East 23rd Street
  New York, N. Y. 10010
      Pre- and postnatal health care for mother and child,
      advises local communities on program development,

and serves as a clearinghouse for information for
news media, researchers, program planners, and leg-
islators. Publishes a directory of maternity homes
and residential facilities for unmarried mothers.

VENEREAL DISEASE

American Public Health Association
  1015 18th Street, N.W.
  Washington, D.C. 20036
American Social Health Association
  1790 Broadway
  New York, N. Y. 10019
      Supplies many publications free or at low cost on
      venereal disease.
Center for Disease Control
  Office of Information
  Atlanta, Ga. 30333
      Information on major communicable diseases, in-
      cluding VD.
      Also check your local department of health for con-
      fidential free diagnostic and treatment services.

VETERAN'S HEALTH CARE

Veterans Administration
  810 Vermont Avenue, N.W.
  Washington, D.C. 20420
      Benefits for medical treatment to all eligible veterans
      and certain dependents.

ZOONOSES

Health Services Administration
  5600 Fishers Lane
  Rockville, Md. 20852
      Information and programs for prevention and con-
      trol of diseases communicated by animals.

MISCELLANEOUS

American Medical Association
  535 North Dearborn Street
  Chicago, Ill. 60610
      Films, booklets, and other educational information
      on everything from acne, alcoholism, arthritis, and
      athlete's foot to ulcer, venereal disease, warts, and
      what to do after the baby comes.
American National Red Cross
  Washington, D.C. 20005
      Disaster aid. Local chapters provide services such
      as driving patients to and from treatments.
Benevolent and Protective Order of Elks
  425 West Diversey Parkway
  Chicago, Ill. 60614
      Mobile vans to bring therapy to the home for cere-
      bral palsy patients. Aid to the visually handicapped.
      X-ray mobile units to detect chest disease.
Lions International
  209 North Michigan Avenue
  Chicago, Ill. 60601
      Aid to disaster victims. Sponsor glaucoma clinics.
      Purchase eye-testing equipment, Braillewriters, and
      tape recorders for schools and individuals, and oper-
      ate summer camps for blind children.

National Institutes of Health Clinical Center
  Bethesda, Md. 20014

> A free medical research center for certain chronic conditions. A physician must recommend the patient and supply medical information. Among conditions treated: asthma, juvenile rheumatoid arthritis, sarcoidosis, diabetes mellitus and insipidus, systemic lupus erythematosus, intestinal malabsorption syndrome, severe obesity, thyroid diseases, anemia, calcium disorders, Hodgkin's disease, malignant melanoma, urinary tract tumors, speech disabilities, abnormal patterns of growth, maxillo-facial defects, coronary artery disease, congenital and acquired heart disease, cardiac failure, essential hypertension, schizophrenia, manic-depression, sleep disturbance, muscular dystrophy, cataract, epilepsy, and Parkinsonism.

Salvation Army
  120 West 14th Street
  New York, N. Y. 10011

> Residential centers for homeless men in many cities, programs for the destitute and alcoholics, maternity homes and hospitals for unmarried mothers, camping for children, senior citizens, and physically handicapped persons, emergency disaster service, homes for the aged, Senior Citizens' Clubs, Red Shield Clubs and USO units for servicemen and women, halfway houses for drug addicts, aids to prisoners and parolees and their families, family service bureaus with caseworkers to aid troubled families and individuals and community centers to inner-city areas.

Superintendent of Documents
  Government Printing Office
  Washington, D.C. 20402

> Clearinghouse for U.S. Government publications on many subjects.

Volunteers of America
  340 West 85th Street
  New York, N. Y. 10024

> Maternity homes for unmarried mothers, aid to the handicapped, clubs and homes for the aged, and services for the destitute.

RELIGIOUS ORGANIZATIONS WITH NATIONAL HEALTH AND SOCIAL SERVICES

American Baptist Homes & Hospitals Association
  Valley Forge, Pa. 19481

Catholic Charities
  122 East 22nd Street
  New York, N. Y. 10010

Council of Jewish Federations and Welfare Funds
  315 Park Avenue South
  New York, N. Y. 10010

National Jewish Welfare Board
  145 East 32nd Street
  New York, N. Y. 10022

Federation of Protestant Welfare Agencies
  281 Park Avenue South
  New York, N. Y. 10010

The Lutheran Church—Special Ministries
  315 Park Avenue South
  New York, N. Y. 10010

National Association of Methodist Hospitals & Homes
  1200 Davis Street
  Evanston, Ill. 60201

U.S. Catholic Conference—Bureau of Health and Hospitals
  1312 Massachusetts Avenue, N.W.
  Washington, D.C. 20005

HEALTH RECORDS

Keep Records. Get a health record book, or file folder, or use the back of this book to keep key medical facts about each member of your family. At each visit to your doctor write down your blood pressure, cholesterol level, any abnormal findings, and keep track of immunizations, diseases, operations, and other key facts. Take this record with you when you go to a new doctor. It will save time and money by telling him results of past tests and details of your medical history.

OPERATIONS, ACCIDENTS, HOSPITALIZATIONS

NAME	AGE	PROCEDURE DONE	ANY COMPLICATIONS

FAMILY HEALTH RECORD

Write dates of immunizations, allergies and sensitivities, blood types, and blood pressure readings for each person. Leave space for several entries for each person.

NAME	Whooping Cough	Diphtheria	Tetanus	Smallpox	Polio	Blood Type	Blood Pressure	Allergies— Sensitivities	Other Shots

Any abnormal laboratory results that bear watching (include dates):

FAMILY MEDICAL HISTORY

Check off the diseases that you know any member of your family has had. Show the list to any doctor you go to for the first time.

	Cancer	Diabetes	Heart Disease	Stroke	High Blood Pressure	Kidney Disease	Allergy	Drug Use or Alcoholism	Emotional Problems	Tuberculosis	Rheumatic Fever	Measles	Strep Throat	Hepatitis	Mumps	If deceased – age and cause of death
GRANDPARENTS																
PARENTS																
HUSBAND																
WIFE																
CHILDREN																

INDEX

MEDICAL IDENTIFICATION CARD

If you have any chronic condition, have a copy of this identification card made and place it in your wallet where it can be seen in any emergency.

MEDICAL IDENTIFICATION CARD

I am taking the following medications:

Drug	Dosage	For
_____	_____	_____
_____	_____	_____
_____	_____	_____

I have the following allergies or other problems:

_____

_____

Doctor _____   My name _____

Telephone _____   Address _____

                                       Telephone _____

MEDICAL IDENTIFICATION BRACELETS

If you are diabetic, are a bleeder, are epileptic, or have any other special problems, you should wear an identification tag. You can order them from:

Medic Alert Foundation
Turlock, Calif. 95380